Atlas of Oral Diseases

Isaäc van der Waal

Atlas of Oral Diseases

A Guide for Daily Practice

Springer

Isaäc van der Waal
Dept. of Oral and Maxillofacial Surgery/
Oral Pathology of the VU University
Medical Center/ACTA
Amsterdam
The Netherlands

ISBN 978-3-662-51726-0 ISBN 978-3-662-48122-6 (eBook)
DOI 10.1007/978-3-662-48122-6

Springer Heidelberg New York Dordrecht London

The Work was first published in 2015 by Bohn Stafleu van Loghum with the following title: Mond - en kaakziekten - Een atlas voor de dagelijkse praktijk.

Printed on acid-free paper

Springer-Verlag GmbH Berlin Heidelberg is part of Springer Science+Business Media (www.springer.com)

Preface

This Atlas is intended for use by all dental and medical professionals who are involved in the diagnosis and treatment of lesions and disorders of the oral mucosa and the jaw bones. The choice has been made to prepare a concise, science-based but practice-oriented, text. This approach has always been well received during numerous continuing education courses presented worldwide for dentists, dental hygienists, physicians, and specialists, such as oral and maxillofacial surgeons, dermatologists, otolaryngologists, and pathologists.

The introductory chapter will deal with the intraoral examination, the referral procedure, and the biopsy. It is perhaps tempting for the reader to skip such introductory chapter, but I wholeheartedly recommend to read it.

A general chapter on diseases of the oral mucosa will be followed by four additional chapters of diseases that occur mainly or exclusively on the lips, the tongue, the gingiva and alveolar mucosa, and the palate, respectively. The final chapter on diseases of the jaw bones discusses the various osseous diseases, as well as odontogenic cysts and tumors and generalized diseases that may affect the jaw bones.

A sincere word of thanks is due to the publisher Springer Verlag for the way in which it committed to produce an Atlas as fine as this one.

Amsterdam, The Netherlands　　　　Isaäc van der Waal

Acknowledgment of the Figures

The majority of the pictures used in this Atlas are taken at the Department of Oral and Maxillofacial Surgery/Oral Pathology of the VU University Medical center/ACTA, Amsterdam, the Netherlands. In this respect I am grateful to our photographers, in particular Mr. J.T. van Velhuisen and Mr. T. Dijkstra. In addition, a number of pictures have been kindly provided by various colleagues as listed below.

Fig. 1.4 R.B. Greebe, Netherlands
Fig. 1.6 T. Daniels, U.S.A.
Fig. 2.29 W.H. Groenenberg, Netherlands
Fig. 2.62 C. de Baat, Netherlands
Fig. 2.109. J.P. van Hooff, Netherlands
Fig. 2.152. P.A. Reichart, Germany
Fig. 3.1 V. Ramirez-Amador, Mexico
Fig. 3.12 J.P.W. DonGriot, Netherlands
Fig. 3.21 M.J.P.F. Ritt, Netherlands
Fig. 4.6 C.R. Leemans, Netherlands
Figs. 5.7 and 5.14 J. Hes, Netherlands
Fig. 5.15 N.P.J.B. Sieverink, Netherlands
Fig. 5.31 J.P.A. van den Bergh, Netherlands
Fig. 5.43 J.G.A.M. de Visscher, Netherlands
Fig. 5.44 J.J. Pindborg, Denmark
Fig. 6.4 E. Cataldo, U.S.A.
Fig. 6.37 R.B. Greebe, Netherlands
Fig. 7.1 E.W. van Roessel, Netherlands
Fig. 7.11 J.J. Pindborg (Denmark) and M. Shear (South Africa)
Fig. 7.22 J.A. Baart, Netherlands
Fig. 7.23 D.B. Tuinzing, Netherlands
Fig. 7.33 C.A. Bertheux, Netherlands
Fig. 7.65 J.P.A. van den Bergh, Netherlands
Fig. 7.99 J.G.A.M. de Visscher, Netherlands
Fig. 7.113 I. Cruz, Netherlands
Fig. 7.115 J.M. Kwakman, Netherlands

Contents

1 Examination of the Oral Cavity, Referral to a Specialist, and the Biopsy Procedure

1.1 Examination of the Oral Cavity

1.1.1 Inspection

Examination of the oral cavity requires a proper source of illumination. The patient should be situated in a comfortable way, and there should be an adequate headrest device. Partial or full dentures should be taken out in order to allow proper inspection of the borders of the tongue and the floor of mouth in particular.

To be able to properly inspect the buccal mucosa, the use of two dental mirrors or cheek retractors is advised (Fig. 1.1). A piece of gauze enables to carefully grasp the tip of the tongue and to properly inspect the dorsal surface and the borders of the tongue as well as the floor of the mouth (Fig. 1.2).

In evaluating a mucosal lesion, one should not only observe the extent and the texture of the lesion but also its color. There may be some advantage in using special light devices (e.g., a fluorescent light source) or special dyes, e.g., toluidine blue, for the detection of early cancerous lesions.

In case of a lesion of the mucosal lining of the jaws, a radiograph may be required in order to assess possible changes in the underlying bone.

It is beyond the present treatise to discuss how to examine the neck. It is, of course, well recognized that a swelling in the neck, particularly a cervical lymph node metastasis, may lead to the detection of an oral or oropharyngeal squamous cell carcinoma.

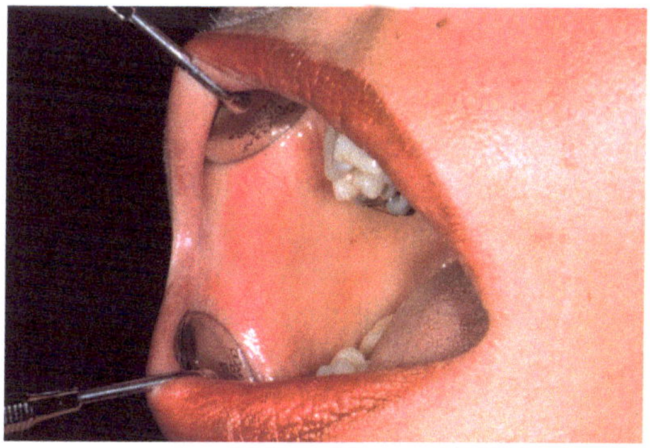

Fig. 1.1 Inspection of the buccal mucosa using two dental mirrors

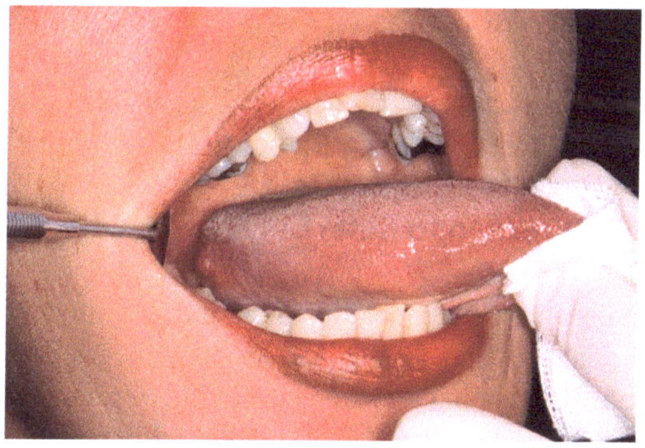

Fig. 1.2 Inspection of the borders of the tongue with the use of a piece of gauze

I. van der Waal, *Atlas of Oral Diseases: A Guide for Daily Practice*,
DOI 10.1007/978-3-662-48122-6_1

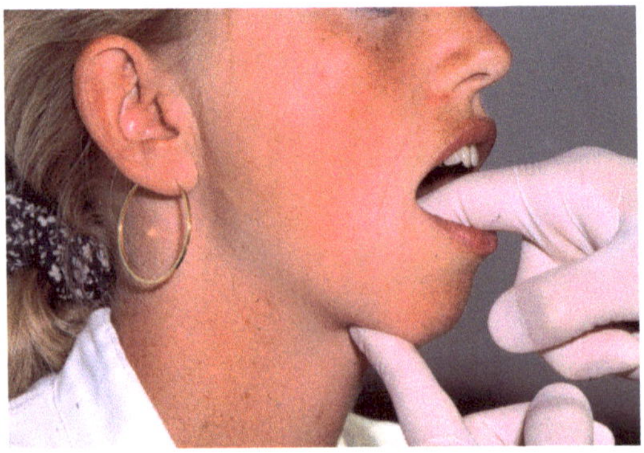

Fig. 1.3 Bimanual palpation of the floor of the mouth

1.1.2 Palpation

Manual palpation with gloved hands is an important part of the inspection of a mucosal lesion since it gives information about the consistency of the lesion, including the possible presence of induration. Such induration may indicate the presence of a malignancy.

Inspection of a lesion of the lips, the buccal mucosa, and particularly of the floor of the mouth may require bimanual palpation (Fig. 1.3).

1.1.3 Exfoliative Cytology

The diagnostic value of exfoliative cytology in oral mucosal lesions is rather limited. Particularly in case of a suspected malignancy, a confirmatory biopsy remains required to establish a more reliable diagnosis.

1.2 Referral to a Specialist

1.2.1 When to Refer?

In general, each patient in whom the practitioner is unable to diagnose an oral lesion, either in the soft tissues or in the jaw bones, should be referred to a specialist, irrespective of the suspicion of malignancy.

Occasionally, a patient insists on being referred to a specialist ("a higher echelon"), while there is actually no need for it. In such instance, there is not much use in trying to prevent such referral.

1.2.2 To Whom to Refer?

The referral should be directed to a colleague with recognized knowledge and experience in that particular field, irrespective of the specialty of that colleague. For instance, in some parts of the world, an oral medicine specialist or a maxillofacial surgeon may be the appropriate colleague to refer to, while in other parts of the world, the dermatologist or the otolaryngologist may be the proper colleague for a given problem. In general, family doctors have had limited training in the diagnostic and therapeutic aspects of oral lesions and, therefore, are usually not the appropriate colleagues to whom to refer a patient with an oral problem.

1.2.3 What Information Should Be Given to the Patient?

The patient should be properly informed about the reason of the referral and, preferably, should be informed about the content of the referral letter.

In general, it seems better not to express one's concern about a possible malignancy, if applicable, since this may erroneously cause anxiety. The same applies to a suspicion of venereal diseases or an underlying systemic disease, e.g., an HIV infection.

Avoid explaining to the patient what the specialist is going to do (e.g., "a biopsy will be performed"), since the taking of a biopsy or ordering blood examination may not be indicated at all. Avoid to create high expectations from the referral, since this may frustrate not only the consulted specialist but, above all, the patient if the specialist is unable to solve the problem.

1.2.4 Content of the Referral Letter

Properly specify your question to the specialist, including the exact location of the lesion(s).

The referral letter should preferably be worded in a neutral way without speculation about the possible (malignant or infectious) nature of a lesion. For instance, in case of suspicion of cancer of the border of the tongue, one may use the sentence: "I kindly ask your help for the diagnosis and possible treatment of an ulcer of the right border of the tongue, being present for at least several weeks"; the same applies to the possibility of an infectious lesion, e.g., a syphilitic lesion or a possible manifestation of an underlying HIV infection.

Provide the specialist with proper documentation, e.g., good-quality clinical and radiographic pictures, if available, thereby avoiding unnecessary radiation exposure.

1.2.5 Timely Referral

In case of the possible presence of a malignancy, the referral should preferably be arranged within a week, not so much because of medical reasons, but to avoid feelings of frustration from the patient's side in case of a proven malignancy ("Why did you not arrange an earlier appointment with the specialist? Now the cancer has been growing and spreading in the meantime").

1.2.6 Feedback from the Specialist

The specialist to whom the patient has been referred to should arrange timely written feedback to the referring doctor. One may consider to send a copy of such letter to the patient, written in a way that is understandable for the patient.

1.3 The Biopsy

1.3.1 When to Take a Biopsy?

In many oral mucosal lesions, no biopsy is required for a proper diagnosis. Nevertheless, a biopsy may be performed in such instances because of a request by the patient or because of medicolegal reasons.

Preferably, a biopsy should be taken in order to confirm the preliminary diagnosis rather than to detect the diagnosis. The preliminary diagnosis more or less dictates the type of biopsy one is going to perform and the type of medium in which the specimen should be transported.

1.3.2 Who Should Take the Biopsy?

In general, the taking of a biopsy does not require advanced surgical skills and could be performed by every health care worker, provided he or she has been properly trained to do so. Furthermore, the clinician should be familiar with the logistic aspects with regard to the handling of the specimen and the sending of the specimen to the pathologist.

In case of a suspected vesiculobullous disease, one may need an additional biopsy taken from perilesional tissue in order to enable immunofluorescent examination; besides, in such instance, a special transport medium is required in order to avoid destruction of proteins by the regular formalin fixative.

In case of a suspected malignancy, the biopsy should preferably be performed by the specialist who will perform the final treatment.

1.3.3 The Importance of Proper Anesthesia

If not properly anesthesized, the resulting biopsy may be of insufficient quality to allow reliable histopathologic examination.

The use of local infiltration anesthesia into a lesion is to be avoided when a malignancy is suspected because of the risk of spreading tumor cells by the needle. In the latter instance, topical application of an anesthetic solution or spray put on a gauze and firmly held in situ for a few minutes usually allows to perform a biopsy more or less painless. In some locations, e.g., the lower lip, the mental nerve can be anesthesized.

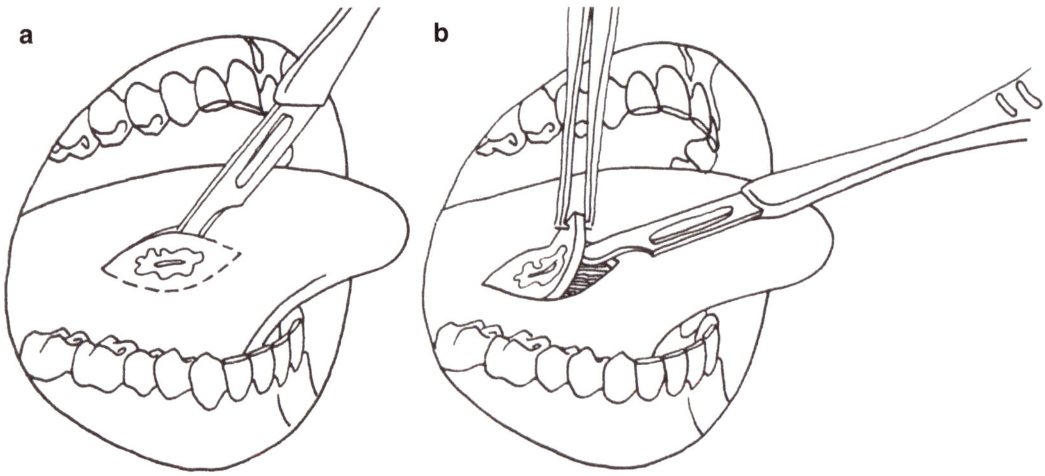

Fig. 1.4 (**a**) Schematic drawing of an excisional biopsy of a supposedly benign mucosal lesion. (**b**) The biopsy specimen is carefully excised

1.3.4 The Importance of Proper Tissue Handling

When taking a biopsy, the tissue should be handled as gently as possible. This is particularly relevant in case of a vesiculobullous lesion in which the fragile epithelium can be easily damaged. Delicate tissue handling is also important in case of lymphoreticular disease. In the latter case, the lymphoid tissue can be severely crushed by the instruments, not allowing reliable histopathologic examination anymore.

1.3.5 Excisional Versus Incisional Biopsy

In the absence of suspected malignancy, small lesions (up to 1–2 cm) of the mucosal surface may be biopsied in toto (excisional biopsy) using local anesthetics (Fig. 1.4a, b).

In case of a larger lesion of the mucosal surface, particularly when a malignancy is suspected, an excisional biopsy is rarely justified. The main objection is that in case of a cancer, the obtained surgical margins of the excisional biopsy are usually not sufficient from an oncologic point of view.

In case of an incisional biopsy of a suspicious lesion, the biopsy should be taken at the clinically most suspicious site, being, e.g., an area of induration or an abnormal texture or color. Areas of necrosis are to be avoided since such areas may not be suitable for proper histopathologic examination.

1.3.6 Dimensions of the Biopsy Specimen; Multiple Biopsies

The specimen should be of proper dimensions, being some 0.3 cm in length, having a width of some 0.2 cm and a depth of approximately 0.2 cm.

In extensive mucosal lesions, one may consider to take multiple biopsies.

The biopsy should be taken perpendicularly to the mucosal surface in order to prevent tangential cutting.

1.3.7 Which Instruments to Use for a Biopsy?

One may use a cold knife or a punch instrument with a diameter of 0.3 cm (Fig. 1.5a–d).

Thermal instruments are less suitable for a biopsy procedure since these may damage the specimen, making it less suitable for proper histopathologic examination. If needed, the biopsy wound can be sutured.

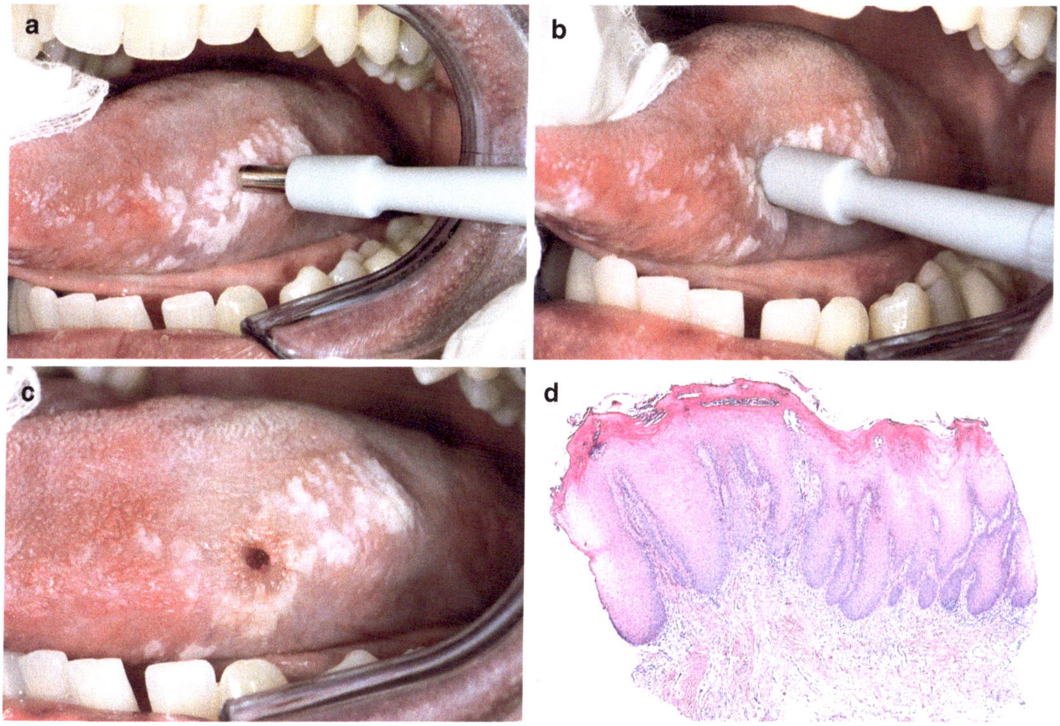

Fig. 1.5 (**a**) Punch instrument with a diameter of 0.3 cm for performing a biopsy. (**b**) The instrument can carefully be screwed into the lesion at a proper depth. (**c**) The wound of the punch biopsy usually does not require suturing. (**d**) Low-power view of a punch biopsy from a different patient

1.3.8 Perilesional Biopsy in Case of a Clinical Diagnosis of Vesiculobullous Disease

In case of a vesiculobullous disease, a biopsy is required in order to obtain a more accurate diagnosis, e.g., pemphigus vulgaris versus mucous membrane pemphigoid, by the use of immunofluorescent examination. It is advisable to discuss the biopsy procedure beforehand with the pathologist, particularly with regard to the type of medium that should be used.

Preferably, the biopsy should be taken at the junction of the lesion and the adjacent, peripheral, clinically normal looking mucosa. With an adequate size of the biopsy, the specimen can be carefully divided in a part that can be put in formalin for routine histopathologic examination and a part that can be offered to the pathologist immediately, unfixed, or put in saline as a transport medium allowing immunofluorescent examination. An alternative option is to take two biopsies – of which one should be taken perilesionally at a distance of not more than 0.5 cm–1 cm – to allow proper immunofluorescent examination.

Immunofluorescent examination can only be performed if an epithelial lining is present.

1.3.9 Labial Biopsy in the Diagnostic Work-Up of the Diagnosis of Sjögren's Syndrome

In the diagnostic work-up of a patient who may suffer from Sjögren's syndrome, either a parotid or a labial salivary gland biopsy may be required. Most clinicians prefer to do a labial biopsy rather than a parotid one.

The labial biopsy should contain some 4–5 salivary gland lobules. The technique on how to perform the biopsy is well illustrated in Fig. 1.6. The biopsy specimen can be put in a regular fixative medium.

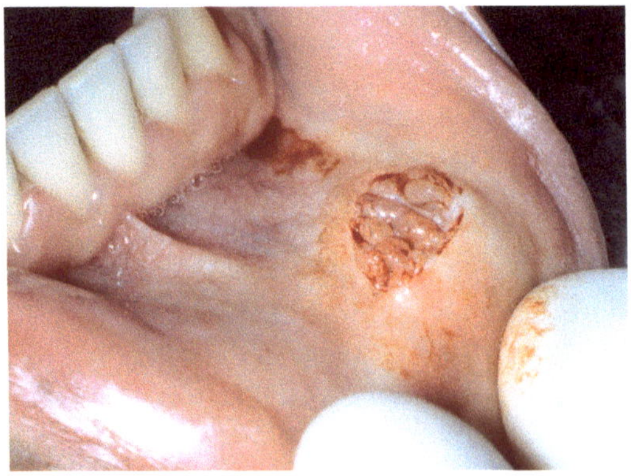

Fig. 1.6 Labial biopsy in the diagnostic work-up for the possible presence of Sjögren's syndrome

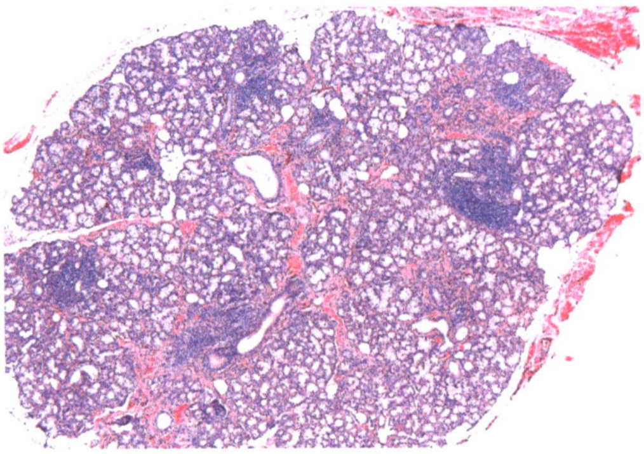

Fig. 1.7 Low-power view of a labial salivary gland biopsy

The pathologist will calculate a focus score. A focus is defined as a cluster of 50 lymphocytes per 4 mm^2 salivary gland tissue (Fig. 1.7). The presence of more than 1 focus is supportive of the diagnosis of Sjögren's syndrome.

1.3.10 Biopsy of a Bony Lesion

In case of a biopsy of a small bony lesion (up to a few centimeters), enucleation is usually easy to perform unless one is dealing with a sclerotic lesion. In the latter instance, one may need to use a bur or a hollow trephan to obtain a biopsy; proper cooling is essential in order to maintain the integrity of the tissue.

The specimen can be placed in a regular fixative. The pathologist should be informed about the bony nature of the specimen, since decalcification is required before being able to cut the tissue for histopathologic examination.

Diseases of the Oral Mucosa and Soft Tissues: General Aspects

2

2.1 Introduction

In this chapter, diseases arising from the oral mucosa and soft tissues, such as connective tissue, fat tissue, blood vessels, nerves, and also minor salivary glands, will be discussed. The choice has been made to follow an alphabetical order. Some lesions are grouped together, e.g., fibroma and fibroma-like lesions. A number of the presently discussed lesions and disorders will also be briefly covered in the chapters of the various oral subsites.

2.2 Angioedema

Definition
Sudden vasodilatation caused by histamines and histamine-like substances, followed by plasmatic transudate.

Etiology
C1-esterase inhibitor deficiency in the serum (hereditary type). Allergic reaction, e.g., to drugs such as antibiotics or angiotensin converting enzyme inhibitors (acquired type).

Clinical Aspects
Mainly involvement of the face, lips, eyes, and tongue (Fig. 2.1); occasionally also involvement of the hand and feet. Glottic edema can lead to a life-threatening situation.

Treatment
In case of glottis involvement, it is important to secure a free airway; occasionally, a tracheostomy may be required. In the hereditary type administration of C1-esterase inhibitor concentrate is indicated. In the acquired type, antihistamines may be administered.

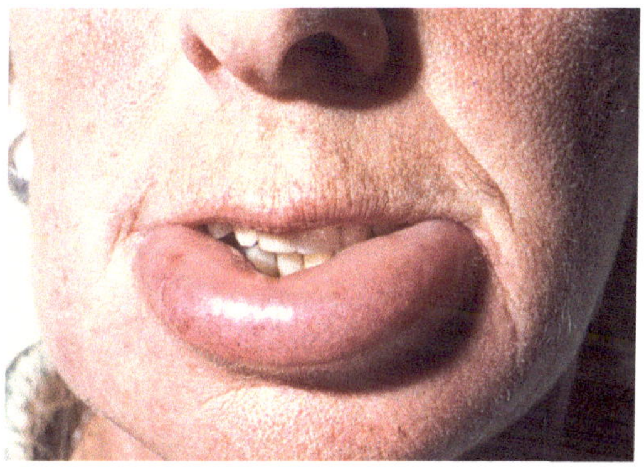

Fig. 2.1 Suddenly arising swelling of the lower lip due to angioedema

I. van der Waal, *Atlas of Oral Diseases: A Guide for Daily Practice*,
DOI 10.1007/978-3-662-48122-6_2

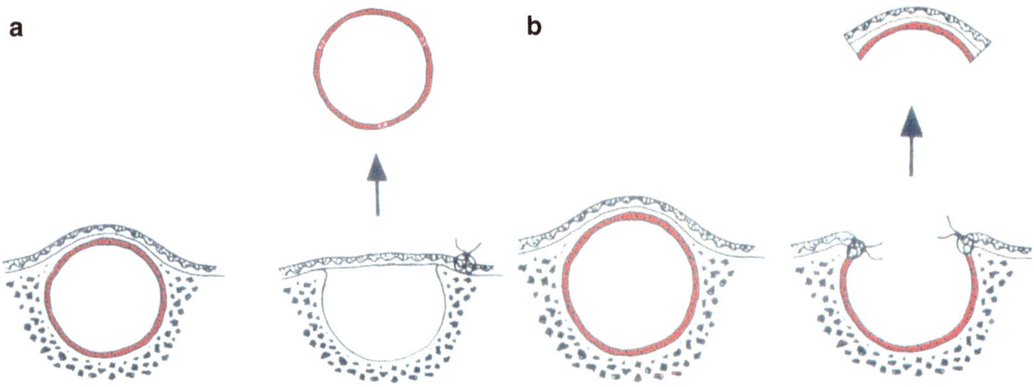

Fig. 2.2 (**a**) Schematic drawing of enucleation of a cyst followed by primary closure. (**b**) Schematic drawing of marsupialization of a cyst

2.3 Cysts in the Soft Tissues

Cysts, in general, may be treated by enucleation or by marsupialization (Fig. 2.2a, b). Enucleation aims at removal of the entire cyst, followed by primary closure. In marsupialization just the roof of the cyst is removed, thereby connecting the epithelial cyst lining with the mucosal epithelium.

Enucleation is usually performed in small cysts in which complete removal does not interfere with vital structures, e.g., nerves or large blood vessels. Marsupialization is performed in large cysts in which enucleation would carry a risk to damage nerves, e.g., the mandibular nerve, or teeth. The challenge in marsupialization is to prevent the mucosal margins to close again during the postoperative period since that event would result in a "new" cyst. For this purpose, a temporary gauze or an acrylic device can be inserted temporarily into the cavity.

2.3.1 (Epi)dermoid Cyst

Definition
Developmental cyst arising from gastrointestinal epithelium.

Epidemiology
Rather rare cyst.

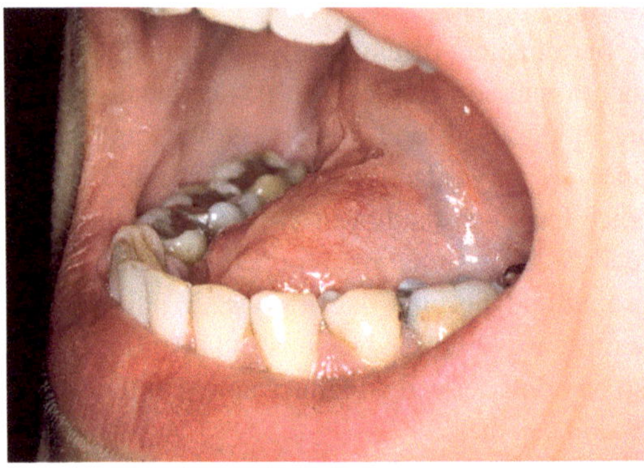

Fig. 2.3 Dermoid cyst of the floor of the mouth

Clinical Aspects
May become manifest already during infancy or childhood. The most common location is the midline of the floor of the mouth (Fig. 2.3).

Histopathology
Histopathologic examination will show a cyst lined by stratified squamous epithelium (epidermoid cyst); in the presence of adnexal structures (e.g., sebaceous glands or hair follicles), one is dealing with a dermoid cyst (Fig. 2.4b, c).

Treatment
Enucleation; recurrences are rare.

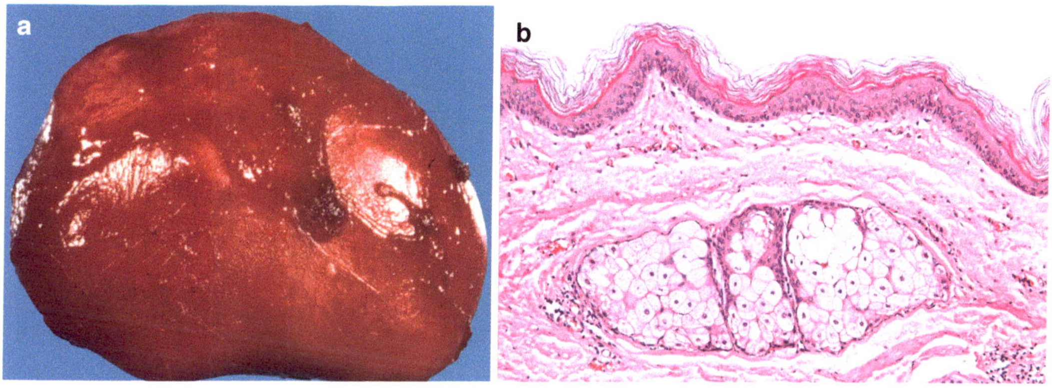

Fig. 2.4 (a) Gross specimen of well-encapsulated dermoid cyst. (b) Wall of a dermoid cyst containing sebaceous glands

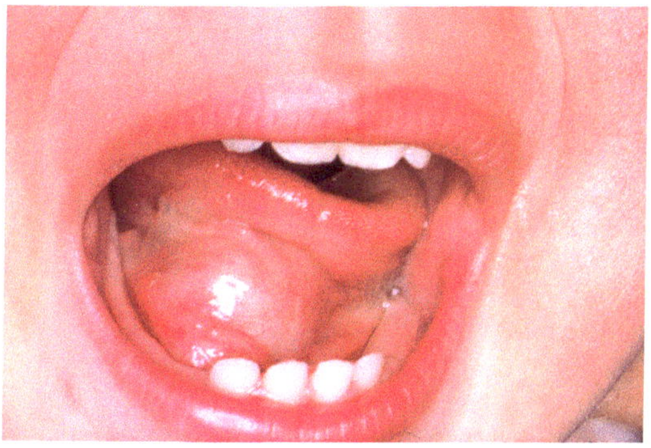

Fig. 2.5 Heterotopic gastrointestinal cyst in a young child

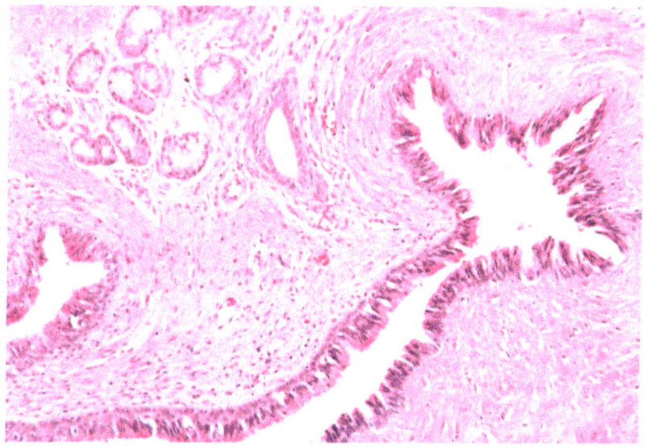

Fig. 2.6 Low-power view of a heterotopic gastrointestinal cyst

2.3.2 Heterotopic Gastrointestinal Cyst

Definition
Developmental cyst characterized by presence of a gastrointestinal epithelial lining of the cyst wall.

Epidemiology
Rare cyst with less than 100 cases published in the literature.

Clinical Aspects
Usually already present at birth or shortly thereafter. Presents itself as a cystic swelling in the anterior part of the floor of the mouth (Fig. 2.5).

Histopathology
The cyst wall is lined by gastrointestinal epithelium (Fig. 2.6). Sometimes it is difficult to really demonstrate the gastrointestinal origin of the epithelial lining.

Treatment
Enucleation; recurrences are rare.

2.3.3 Lymphoepithelial Cyst ("Oral Tonsil")

Definition
Developmental cystic lesion, sometimes forming a crypt like in the tonsils, arising from epithelium

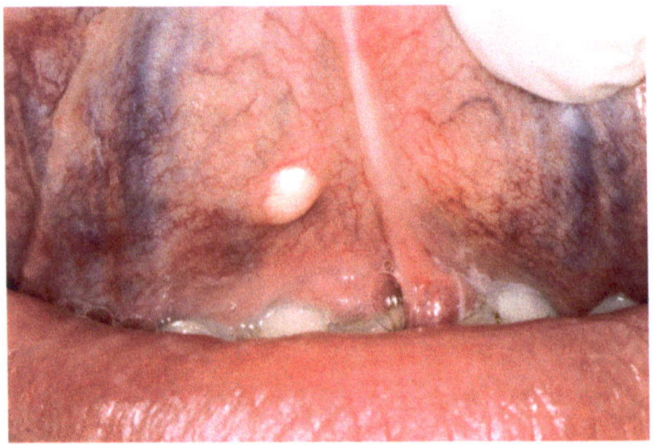

Fig. 2.7 Lymphoepithelial cyst ("oral tonsil") at the ventral aspect of the tongue

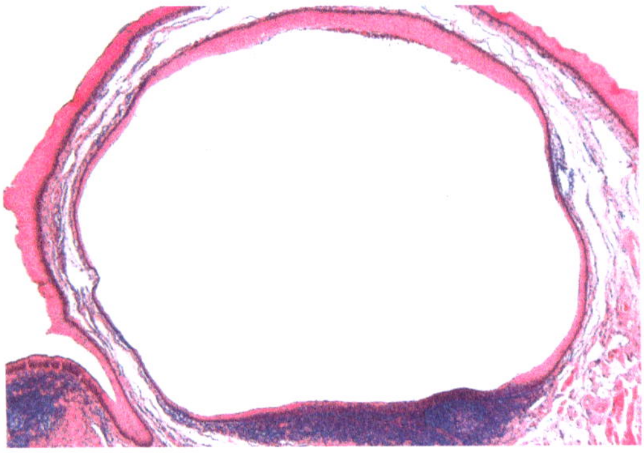

Fig. 2.8 Low-power view of a lymphoepithelial cyst

that has been entrapped in lymphoid tissue; is also referred to as "oral tonsil."

Epidemiology
Rather rare cyst; may occur at all ages.

Clinical Aspects
Yellowish, circumscribed swelling, asymptomatic otherwise (Fig. 2.7). Usually solitary or multiple presentation. The floor of the mouth and ventral aspect of the tongue are the most common locations. The differential diagnosis includes mainly ranula and lipoma.

Histopathology
The cyst is lined by stratified squamous epithelium and surrounded by lymphoid tissue (Fig. 2.8).

Treatment
In general removal is recommended, mainly for histopathologic verification. Recurrences have not been reported.

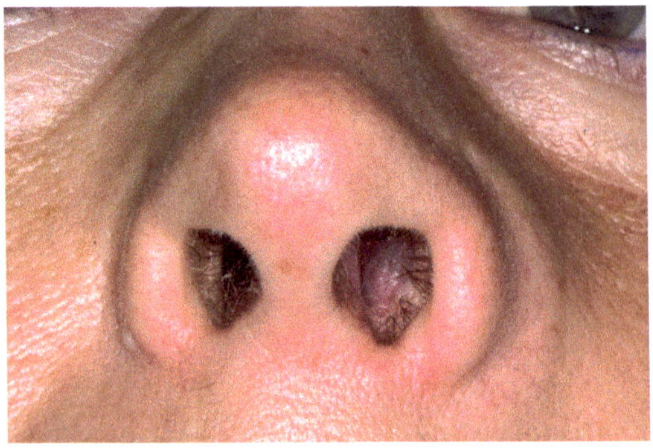

Fig. 2.9 Nasolabial cyst; notice swelling of left nasolabial fold and the bluish swelling in the left nostril

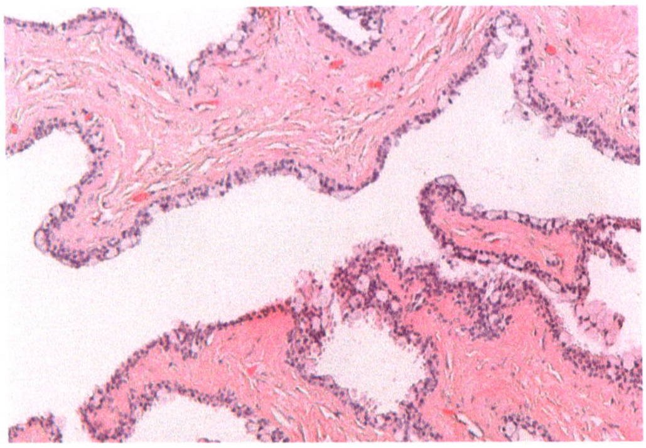

Fig. 2.10 Rather typical histology of nasolabial cyst

2.3.4 Nasolabial Cyst

Definition
Developmental cyst arising from epithelium enclosed in the lower part of the nasolacrimal duct.

Epidemiology
Rare cyst; mainly diagnosed during adulthood.

Clinical Aspects
Paramedian swelling in the upper mucobuccal fold and, extraorally, of the nasolabial fold (Fig. 2.9). Radiographically, some erosion of the underlying maxillary bone may be observed.

Histopathology
The cyst is lined by cylindrical epithelium (Fig. 2.10). Occasionally, the lining consists of squamous epithelium.

Treatment
Enucleation through an intraoral approach; recurrences are rare.

2.3.5 Mucous Retention Phenomenon or Mucous Cyst (Mucocele, Ranula)

Definition
Retention of mucous material in the excretory duct of minor salivary gland or the sublingual gland in case of involvement of the floor of the mouth; occasionally, extravasation in the surrounding connective tissue.

Etiology
Most likely caused by traumatic obstruction of the orificium of the duct.

Epidemiology
Rather common cyst; may occur at all ages.

Clinical aspects
Bluish, non-painful, recurrent cystic swelling. Occurs mainly in the lower lip (mucocele) and in the floor of the mouth (ranula) (Fig. 2.11a, b). Rarely occurs at the ventral aspect of the tip of the tongue (see also Chap. 4) or the palate.

A special variant of the ranula is the "plunging" ranula, in which the cyst herniates through the mylohyoid muscle, presenting itself as a submental or submandibular swelling. The differential diagnosis of a mucous cyst includes a cystic salivary gland neoplasm, (arterio)venous malformation, and phlebectasia, particularly when located on the lower lip.

Histopathology
Histopathologically, a lumen is seen filled with mucous and cell debris. The lumen may be lined by ductal epithelium ("retention type"); in case of absence of an epithelial lining, one is dealing with the "extravasation type."

Treatment
A mucocele of the lower lip can usually easily be removed in toto; recurrences are rare. In case of a mucocele at the ventral aspect of the tip of the tongue, the removal of the associated, surrounding minor salivary glands is indicated in order to prevent recurrences.

A ranula is usually primarily treated by marsupialization. In case of recurrence, the removal of the underlying sublingual gland may be required. In case of a "plunging ranula" intraoral removal of the associated sublingual gland usually suffices.

2.3.6 Thyroglossal Duct Cyst

The thyroglossal duct cyst is discussed in the chapter of diseases of the tongue see (Chap. 4).

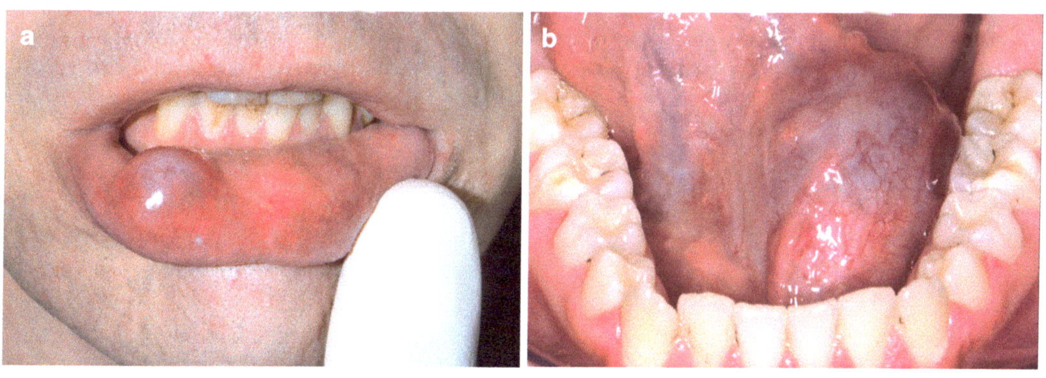

Fig. 2.11 (**a**) Typical presentation of a mucocele. (**b**) Typical presentation of a ranula in the floor of the mouth

2.4 Erythroplakia

Definition
Flat erythematous lesion of the oral mucosa that cannot be recognized as any other known erythematous lesion. In fact, it is a definition by exclusion, similarly as applies for the definition of leukoplakia.

Erythroplakia is a premalignant or potentially malignant condition that carries a much higher risk of malignant transformation than leukoplakia. No exact annual malignant transformation figures are available from the literature.

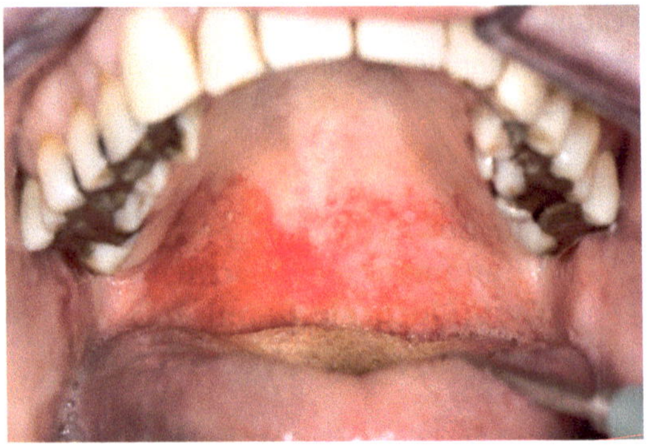

Fig. 2.12 Erythroplakia of the palate

Etiology
Almost exclusively seen in heavy smokers and drinkers.

Epidemiology
Rather rare condition; the estimated prevalence is less than 0.01 %. Rarely occurs below the age of 40 years.

Clinical Aspects
Usually smooth, but sometimes granular, reddish aspect of the mucosa (Fig. 2.12). Often causes symptoms, such as burning or itching. May occur at all sites of the oral cavity.

Clinical Differential Diagnosis
Erythematous candidiasis (usually bilateral and symmetrical), particularly on the dorsal surface of the tongue and on the hard palate.

Erythematous lichen planus (almost always bilateral and symmetrical distribution).

A patient with erythroplakia should always be referred to a specialist for further evaluation.

Histopathology
Histopathologic examination will usually show severe dysplasia, carcinoma in situ, or even squamous cell carcinoma (Fig. 2.13).

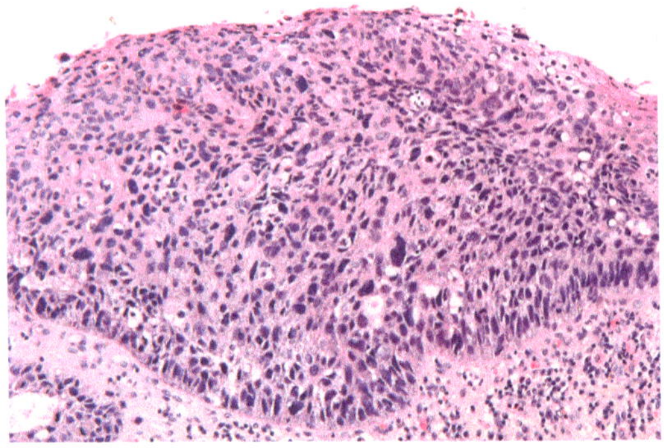

Fig. 2.13 Severe dysplasia or carcinoma in situ

Treatment
Treatment usually consists of surgical removal. CO_2-laser vaporation may be considered but has the disadvantage of not providing a surgical specimen for additional histopathologic examination. Photodynamic therapy may be considered in widespread erythroplakia but carries the same disadvantage as being mentioned for laser vaporation.

Long-term (lifelong?) follow-up after treatment is recommended with intervals of not more than 4–6 months.

2.5 Fibroma and Fibroma-Like Lesions

2.5.1 Fibroma

Definition
A fibroma of the oral mucosa represents a hyperplastic lesion rather than a neoplastic one; sometimes the term "fibroepithelial polyp" is used.

The rare "solitary fibrous tumor" of the oral mucosa will not be discussed here; this tumor does not have a characteristic clinical presentation, and the diagnosis is solely based on histologic criteria, resembling the somewhat questionable entity of hemangiopericytoma.

Etiology

Chronic, mechanical irritation caused by habitual biting on the mucosa, by a broken-down dental restoration, or by an ill-fitting partial or full denture. The etiology of "symmetrical fibromas" of the palate or the lingual aspect of the mandible near the trigonum region is unknown.

Clinical Aspects

Often pedunculated, usually solitary lesion, occurring particularly at sites of mechanical irritation such as the buccal mucosa, the tip of the tongue, and along the borders of a denture. In the latter event, the term "denture hyperplasia" or "epulis fissuratum" is used (Figs. 2.14 and 2.15a, b). The consistency of a fibroma may vary from soft to firm elastic. Fibromas are asymptomatic otherwise.

Symmetrical fibromas may occur on the hard palate and on the lingual aspect of the trigonum region of the mandible (Fig. 2.16).

Clinical Differential Diagnosis

The differential diagnosis includes lipoma, pyogenic granuloma, and other neoplasms either benign or malignant such as a non-Hodgkin lymphoma or a metastasis. A unilateral fibroma-like lesion on the palate may also be caused by a salivary gland neoplasm.

Multiple fibroma-like swellings may be part of the multiple hamartoma syndrome (Cowden syndrome; a rare hereditary syndrome in which the patient is prone to develop a variety of benign or malignant tumors; see also Chap. 4).

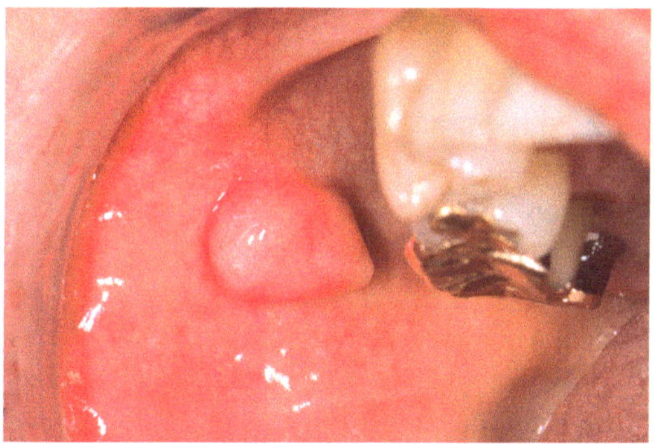

Fig. 2.14 Pedunculated fibroma of the buccal mucosa

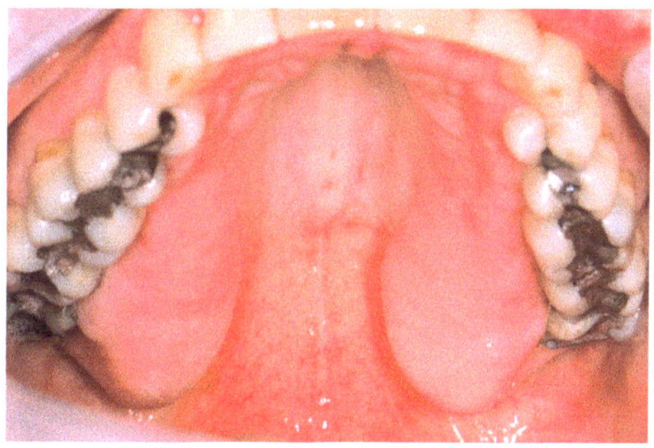

Fig. 2.16 Symmetrical fibromas of the palate; unknown etiology

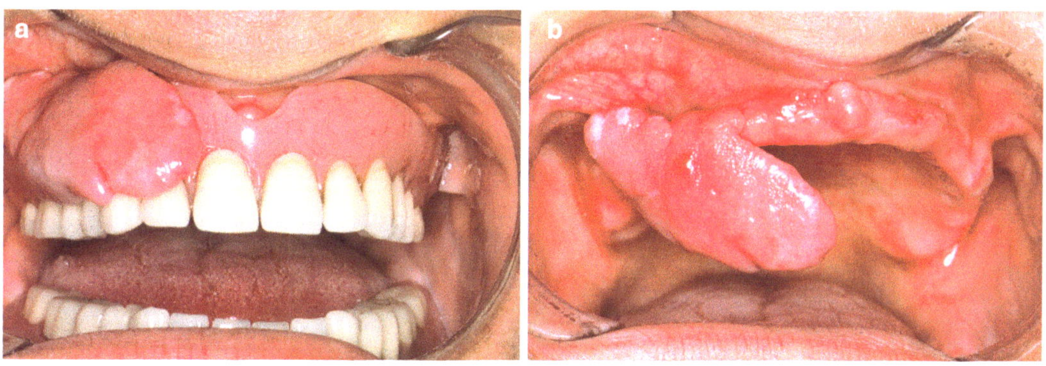

Fig. 2.15 (**a**) Fibrous hyperplasia along the border of an ill-fitting denture (Epulis fissuratum). (**b**) Clinical aspect after removal of the denture

In tuberous sclerosis, a (sometimes hereditary) syndrome in which a variety of abnormalities may occur, oral involvement consists a.o. of fibrous hyperplasia of the oral mucosa and the gingiva (Figs. 2.17 and 2.18), enamel pitting, and radiolucencies in the jaws based on fibrous connective tissue that may cause eruption disturbancies.

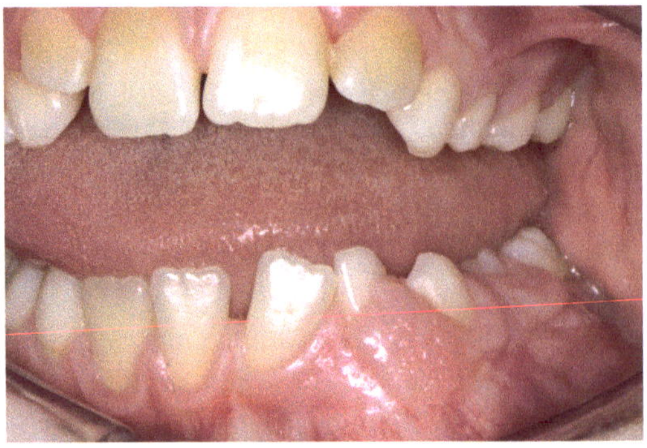

Fig. 2.17 Fibrous hyperplasia in left part of the mandible in a patient suffering from tuberous sclerosis

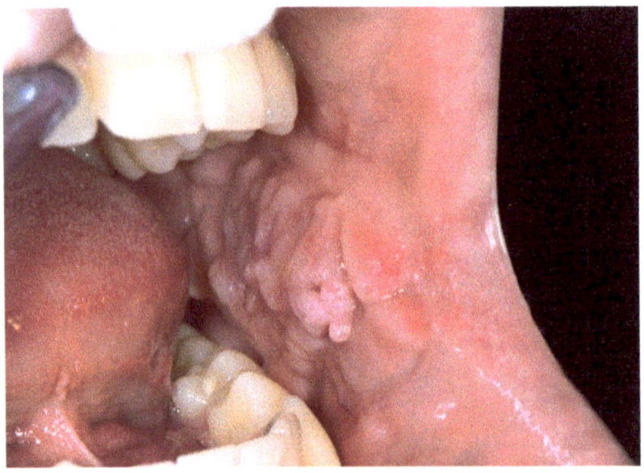

Fig. 2.18 Fibrous hyperplasia of buccal mucosa in a patient suffering from tuberous sclerosis

In Crohn's disease, fibroma-like swellings of the buccal mucosa may occur. These swellings may have a cobble stone appearance (Fig. 2.19a, b).

Histopathology

On histopathologic examination of a fibroma fibrous tissue is seen with or without the presence of an inflammatory infiltrate. Occasionally, stellate-like, large fibroblasts are observed, referred to as "giant cell fibroma"; this histopathologic subtype does not have any clinical relevance (Fig. 2.20a, b).

Treatment

Elimination of the etiologic factor, if identified, is sometimes effective. If not, excision and histopathologic verification may be considered. Recurrences are rare.

2.5.2 Lipoma

Definition

Benign neoplasm of fat cells.

Clinical Aspects

Fibroma-like appearance, sometimes showing a somewhat yellowish color, having a soft consistency (Fig. 2.21), being otherwise asymptomatic. Bilateral, symmetrical occurrence is extremely rare.

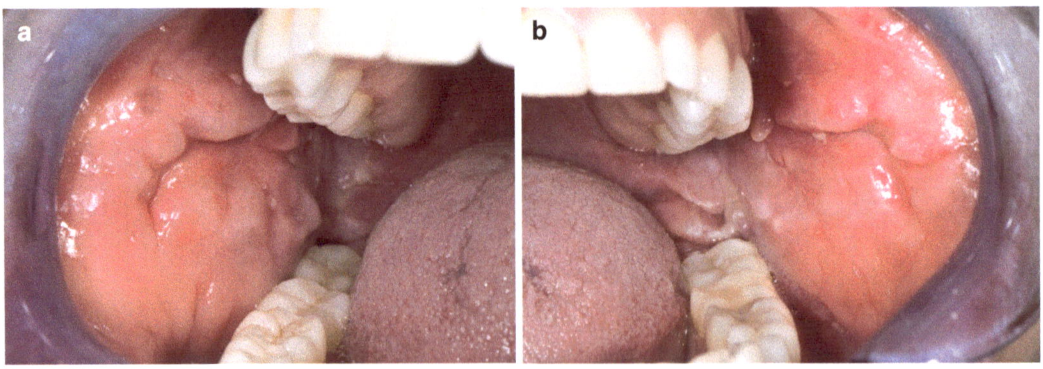

Fig. 2.19 (**a**) Fibrous swellings in a patient suffering from Crohn's disease. (**b**) Notice the cobble stone appearance of the buccal mucosa

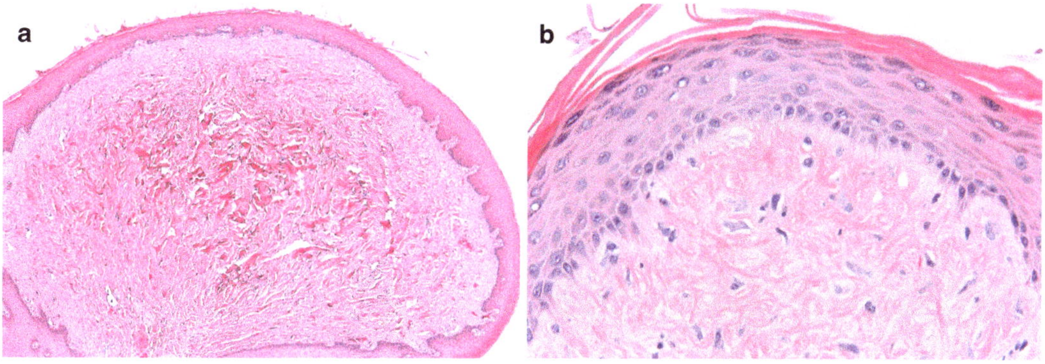

Fig. 2.20 (**a**) Low-power view of a fibroma. (**b**) Stellate-like, large fibroblasts in giant cell fibroma

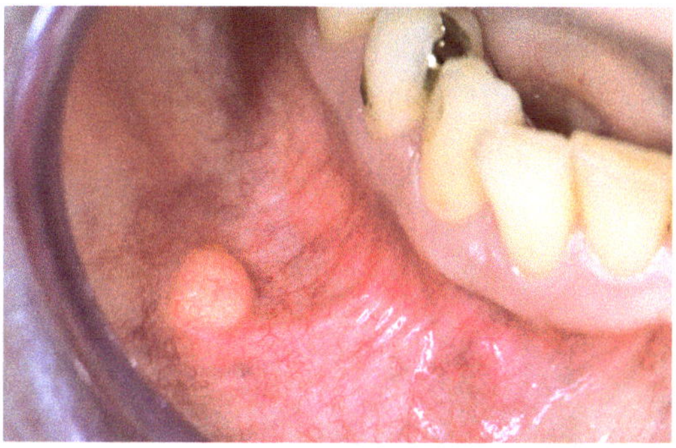

Fig. 2.21 Lipoma in the mucobuccal fold of the mandible

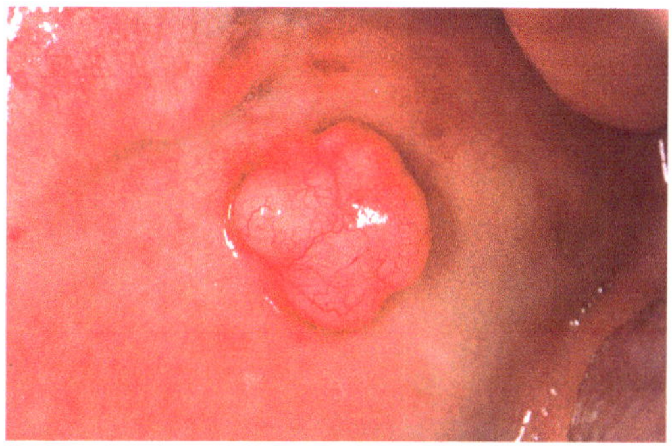

Fig. 2.23 Fibroma-like swelling of focal mucinosis

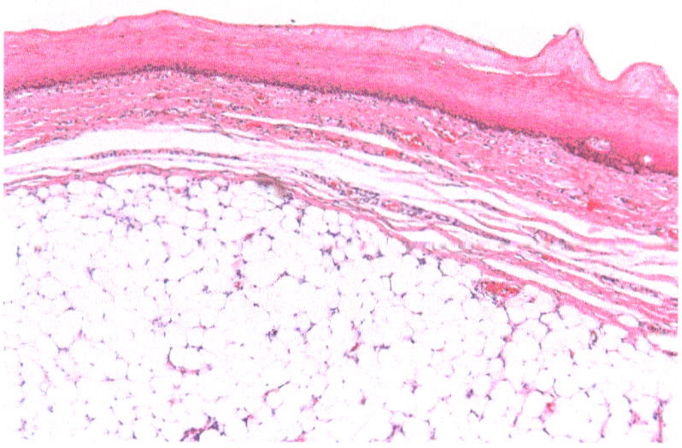

Fig. 2.22 Low-power view of a lipoma

Histopathology

Histopathologically, mature, well-encapsulated fat cells are seen (Fig. 2.22). There are a few histologic subtypes such as fibrolipoma and angiolipoma; these subtypes are not of clinical significance. The malignant variant of a lipoma, referred to as liposarcoma, rarely occurs in the mouth.

Treatment

Surgical removal. Lipomas rarely, if ever, recur.

2.5.3 Mucinosis, Focal

Definition

Rare, somewhat questionable entity of unknown etiology, possibly representing the counterpart of cutaneous focal mucinosis; may be just a fibroma with myxoid changes of the connective tissue.

Clinical Aspects

Pedunculated, fibroma-like swelling that may occur on the gingiva, palate, and buccal mucosa, being asymptomatic otherwise (Fig. 2.23).

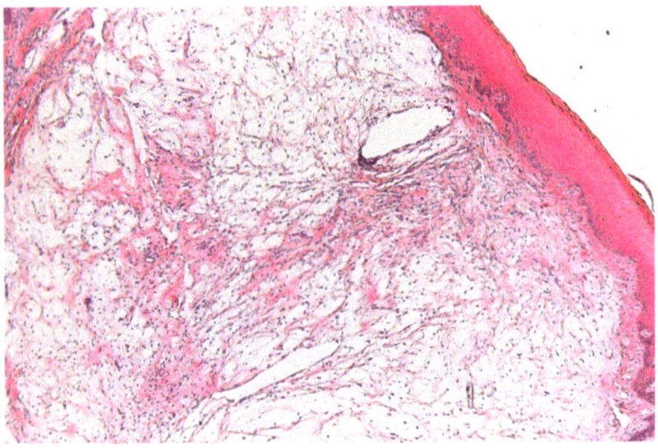

Fig. 2.24 Low-power view of focal mucinosis

Histopathology
Histopathologically, a somewhat circumscribed myxoid fibromatous lesion can be observed without the presence of an inflammatory infiltrate (Fig. 2.24).

Treatment
Surgical removal.

2.5.4 Neurofibroma

Definition
Benign neoplasm derived from perineural fibroblasts and Schwann cells; can be part of hereditary neurofibromatosis type I.

Epidemiology
Rather uncommon tumor of the oral soft tissues.

Clinical Aspects
Solitary or multiple firm-elastic swelling of the oral mucosa, usually asymptomatic otherwise. The tongue and the buccal mucosa are the sites of predilection. Occasionally, the palate is involved (Fig. 2.25).

Histopathology
Histopathologically, the lesion is usually well circumscribed. Proliferation of spindle cells in a collagen-rich matrix can be observed (Fig. 2.26).

Treatment
A solitary neurofibroma can be removed by surgical excision. In patients suffering from neurofibromatosis type I, malignant transformation may occur. Because of the often widespread occurrence throughout the body, prophylactic removal of these neurofibromas is not feasible. Instead, regular, lifelong follow-up is recommended.

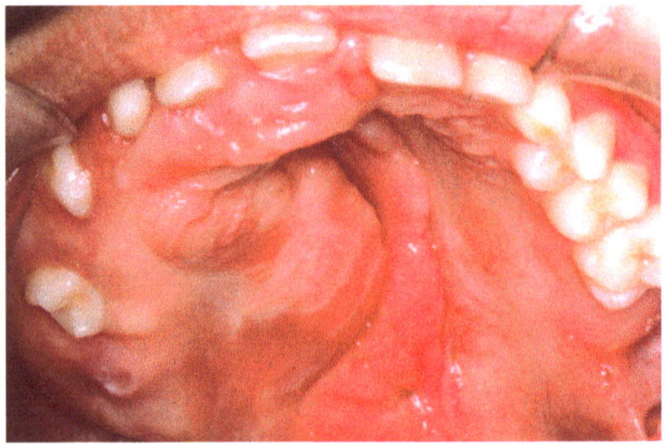

Fig. 2.25 Neurofibroma of the palate in patient suffering from neurofibromatosis

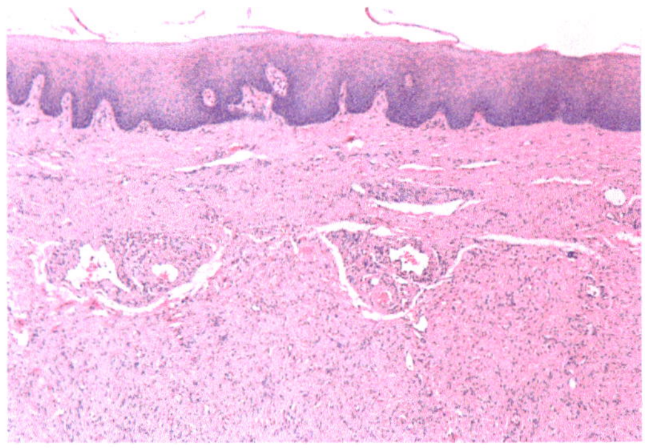

Fig. 2.26 Low-power view of neurofibroma

2.5.5 Neurilemmoma (Schwannoma)

Definition
Benign neoplasm derived from Schwann cells.

Epidemiology
Rare intraoral neoplasm.

Clinical Aspects
Circumscribed firm-elastic swelling, usually asymptomatic otherwise (Fig. 2.27).

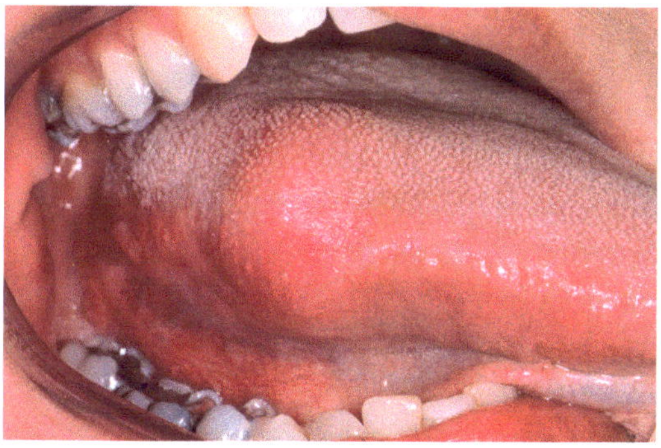

Fig. 2.27 Neurilemmoma at the border of the tongue

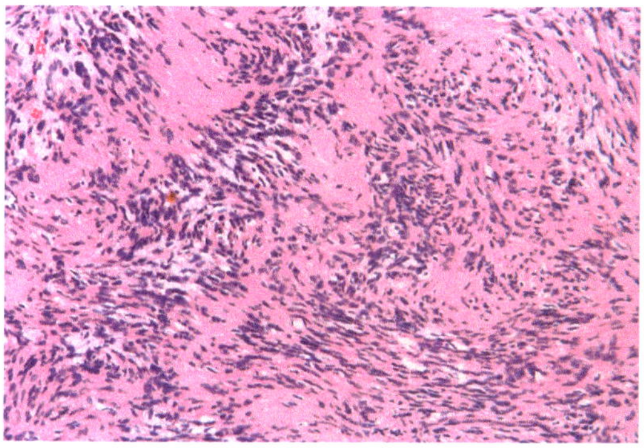

Fig. 2.28 Neurilemmoma; the pinkish material represents the Verocay bodies

Histopathology

Histopathologically characterized by two cell types, being " Antoni-A cells" (with elongated nuclei and arranged in a palisade pattern around acellular collagen-like structures, so-called Verocay bodies) and Antoni-B cells (Fig. 2.28).

Treatment

Surgical removal.

2.5.6 Neuroma

Definition

Proliferation of neural structures caused by trauma ("traumatic neuroma"). Multiple mucosal neuromas are indicative of the hereditary multiple endocrine neoplasia (MEN) type 2B syndrome, also referred to as Sipple syndrome (Fig. 2.29).

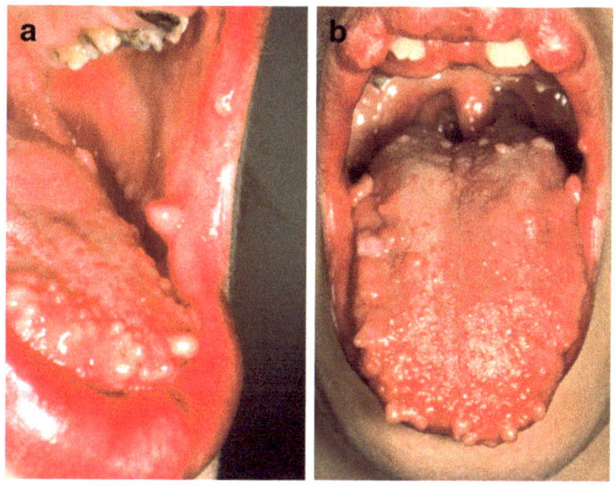

Fig. 2.29 Multiple neuromas in MEN type 2B (**a** and **b**)

Clinical Aspects

Circumscribed solitary or multiple swellings of the lower lip or the tongue, sometimes painful. In case of multiple neuromas, the lips, tongue buccal mucosa, gingiva, and palate may be involved.

Histopathology

The histopathology is characterized by a haphazard proliferation of nerve bundles. In MEN type 2B syndrome, distinct hyperplasia of nerve bundles can be seen.

Treatment

A traumatic neuroma can be excised, together with a part of the associated nerve bundle.

In MEN type 2B, the emphasis is on early detection of the possible development of thyroid cancer.

2.5.7 Pyogenic Granuloma ("Lobular Capillary Hemangioma")

Definition

Excessive tissue reaction to nonspecific local irritation. In the past believed to be caused by pus-producing microorganisms, hence the adjective "pyogenic." Is by some regarded as a vascular lesion ("lobular capillary hemangioma").

Clinical Aspects

Soft, pedunculated, and usually partly ulcerative swelling, usually asymptomatic otherwise

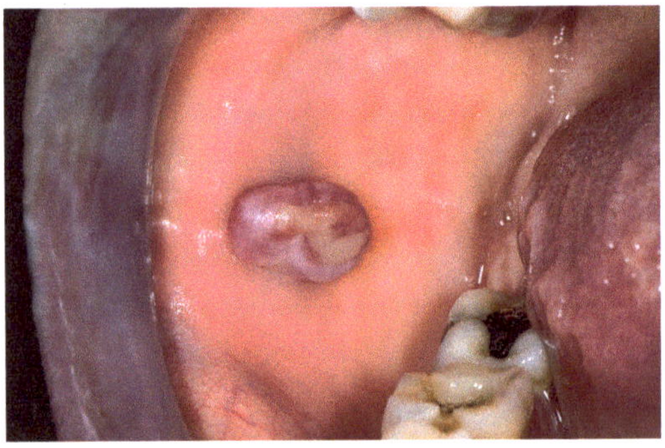

Fig. 2.30 Pyogenic granuloma of the buccal mucosa

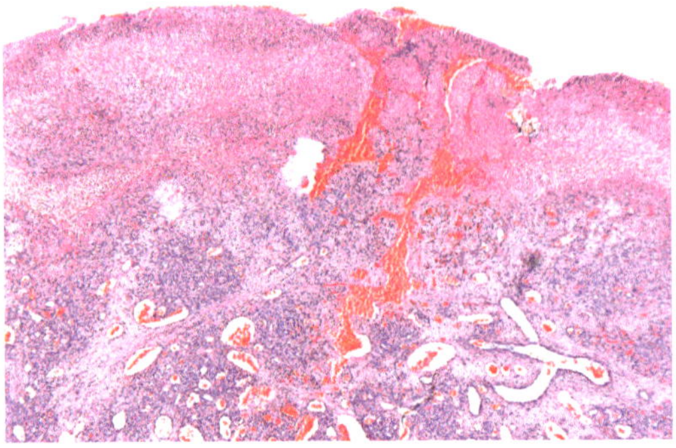

Fig. 2.31 Low-power view of pyogenic granuloma

(Fig. 2.30). May occur at any site in the oral cavity, except for the floor of the mouth.

Histopathology

Vascular spaces surrounded by clusters of endothelial cells ("lobular capillary hemangioma"); there may be secondary signs of inflammation (Fig. 2.31).

Treatment

Conservative surgical excision; recurrences are rare.

2.5.8 Mucosal Nodules in Sarcoidosis

Definition

Generalized granulomatous disease.

Etiology

Unknown.

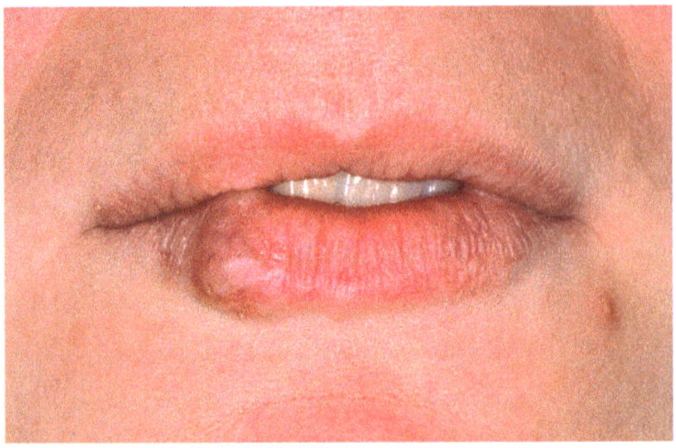

Fig. 2.32 Nodular swelling caused by sarcoidosis

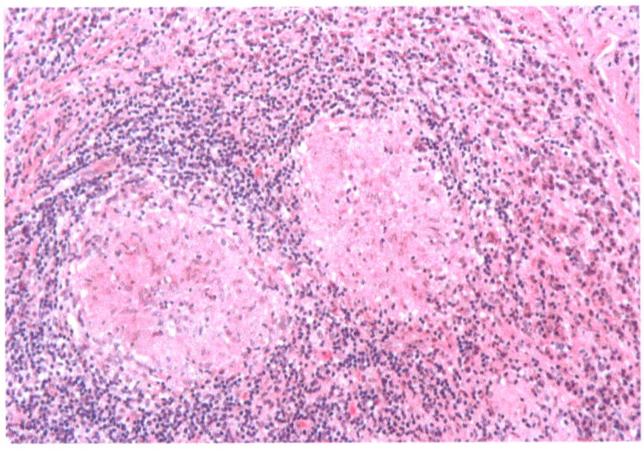

Fig. 2.33 Sarcoid granulomas, suggestive but not diagnostic of sarcoidosis

Epidemiology

Rather uncommon disease; may become manifest during adolescence.

Clinical Aspects

In 90 % of patients suffering from sarcoidosis, the lungs are involved. Oral involvement is rare and consists of solitary or multiple nodules of the oral mucosa (Fig. 2.32).

Histopathology

Histopathologically, noncaseating granulomas are observed ("sarcoid granulomas"); these do not allow to make a firm diagnosis of sarcoidosis and require additional medical examination (Fig. 2.33).

Treatment

Treatment is only indicated in active disease and usually consists of systemic administration of corticosteroids.

2.5.9 Nodular Presentation of Sialoadenitis of Minor Salivary Glands

Definition
Inflammation of minor salivary glands. Subacute necrotizing sialadenitis (SANS) of the palate is a separate entity that will be discussed in Chap. 6.

Epidemiology
Usually in adults and elderly patients.

Etiology
Probably the result of an ascending infection from the oral flora through the excretory ducts of the minor salivary glands ("retrograde" infection).

Clinical Aspects
Occurs mainly in the upper and lower lip (cheilitis glandularis; see also Chap. 3) and the buccal mucosa. Presents as recurrent, solitary, or multiple firm-elastic swellings of the mucosa (Fig. 2.34). Sometimes painful and occasionally resulting on abscess formation. On careful massage of the nodule(s), some mucopurulent discharge may be observed.

In case of a solitary swelling of the oral mucosa, the possibility of a salivary gland neoplasm should be considered as well as the rare event of a sialolith. The final diagnosis can only be established by histopathologic examination.

Nodular lesions of the lips and the cheek may also be the result of a foreign body reaction to fillers.

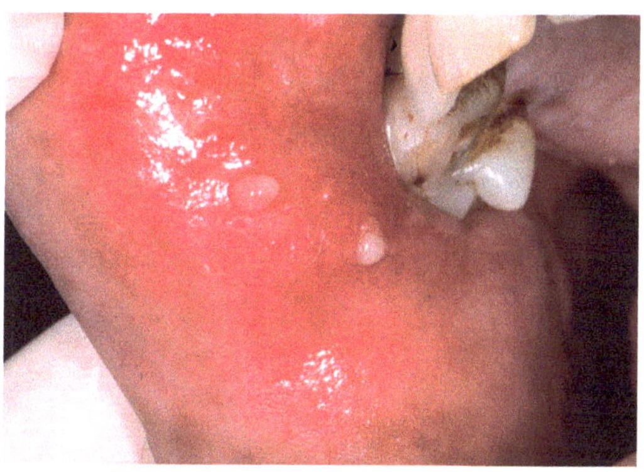

Fig. 2.34 Sialoadenitis of minor salivary glands; notice the mucous discharge

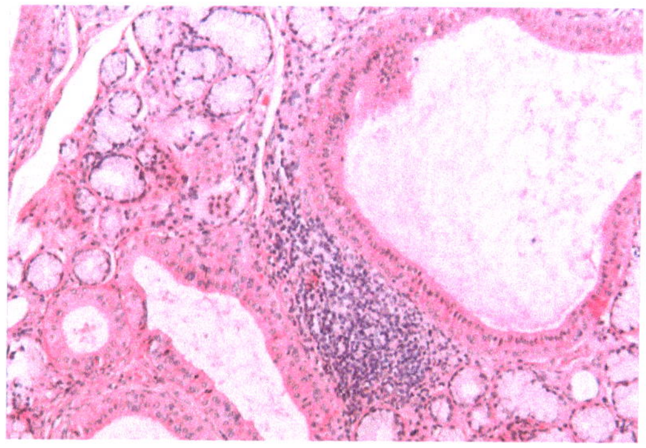

Fig. 2.35 Dilated excretory ducts surrounded by an inflammatory infiltrate in sialoadenitis

Histopathology
Histopathologic examination shows a nonspecific inflammatory reaction in the salivary gland tissue (Fig. 2.35).

Treatment
In case of a solitary lesion, a biopsy is usually sufficient; in case of multiple lesions, the treatment policy is mainly guided by the presence of symptoms.

2.5.10 Fibroma-like Lesions or Nodules Caused by Salivary Gland Tumors of the Intraoral Glands

Definition
Tumor usually arising from the parenchymal epithelial salivary gland tissue and rarely from the stromal part of the salivary glands.

Etiology
Unknown; in an occasional patient, there is a history of previous irradiation in the head and neck region that may have caused the tumor.

Epidemiology
The incidence of salivary gland tumors, including the ones that occur in the major salivary glands, is approximately 3 per 100,000 population per year, for benign and malignant tumors together. May occur at all ages, although occurrence in children is rather rare.

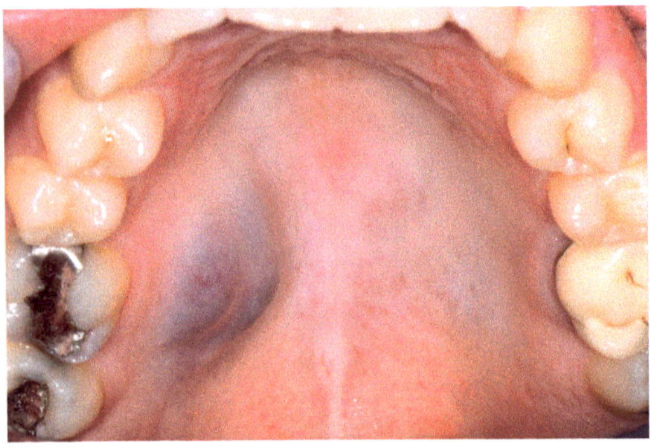

Fig. 2.36 Salivary gland tumor; the biopsy showed a mucoepidermoid carcinoma

Clinical Aspects

Usually a slowly growing, firm-elastic fibroma-like swelling, sometimes of cystic consistency, of the oral mucosa, being asymptomatic otherwise. Sites of preference are the palate, particularly at the junction of the hard and soft palate (see also Chap. 6), the upper lip and, rarely, the buccal mucosa and the floor of the mouth (see also Chap. 3) (Fig. 2.36).

The percentage of occurrence in all salivary glands is as follows:

Parotid gl. : submandibular gl. : sublingual gl.: intraoral (accessory gl.) = 100: 10: 1: 10. In the parotid gland, the majority of the neoplasms is benign, while in the intraoral glands some 50 % are malignant.

Based on the clinical signs and symptoms, no reliable distinction can be made between a benign or a malignant salivary gland tumor, and in all instances, a biopsy is required, preferably taken in the center of the swelling and deep enough to obtain representative tissue.

Histopathology

Histopathologically, there is a wide range of benign and malignant salivary gland tumors (Table 2.1). It may be difficult for the pathologist to provide a firm histopathologic subtype of a salivary gland tumor based on a biopsy.

The adenoid cystic carcinoma is a rare intraoral salivary gland tumor known for its perineural spread (Fig. 2.37) and rather poor prognosis.

Table 2.1 Classification of salivary gland tumors

Benign
Pleomorphic adenoma
Basal cell adenoma
Warthin tumor
Canalicular adenoma
Ductal papilloma
And several other, rare subtypes
Malignant
Acinic cell carcinoma
Mucoepidermoid carcinoma
Adenoid cystic carcinoma
Salivary duct carcinoma
Adenocarcinoma, not otherwise specified
Carcinoma ex pleomorphic adenoma
And several other, rare subtypes

WHO (2005); slightly modified

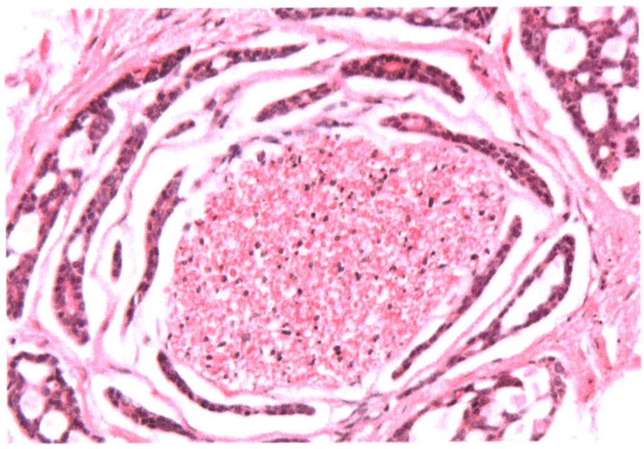

Fig. 2.37 Perineural spread of adenoid cystic carcinoma

Treatment

Surgical removal; postoperative irradiation on indication. Malignant salivary gland tumors may metastasize to the cervical lymph nodes. The adenoid cystic carcinoma often produces distant metastases, skipping the regional lymph nodes in the neck.

2.5.11 Fibroma-Like Swelling Caused by a Sialolith

Definition

A sialolith (calculus formation) in the duct of a minor or major salivary gland; occasionally in the gland itself, e.g., in the submandibular or the parotid gland.

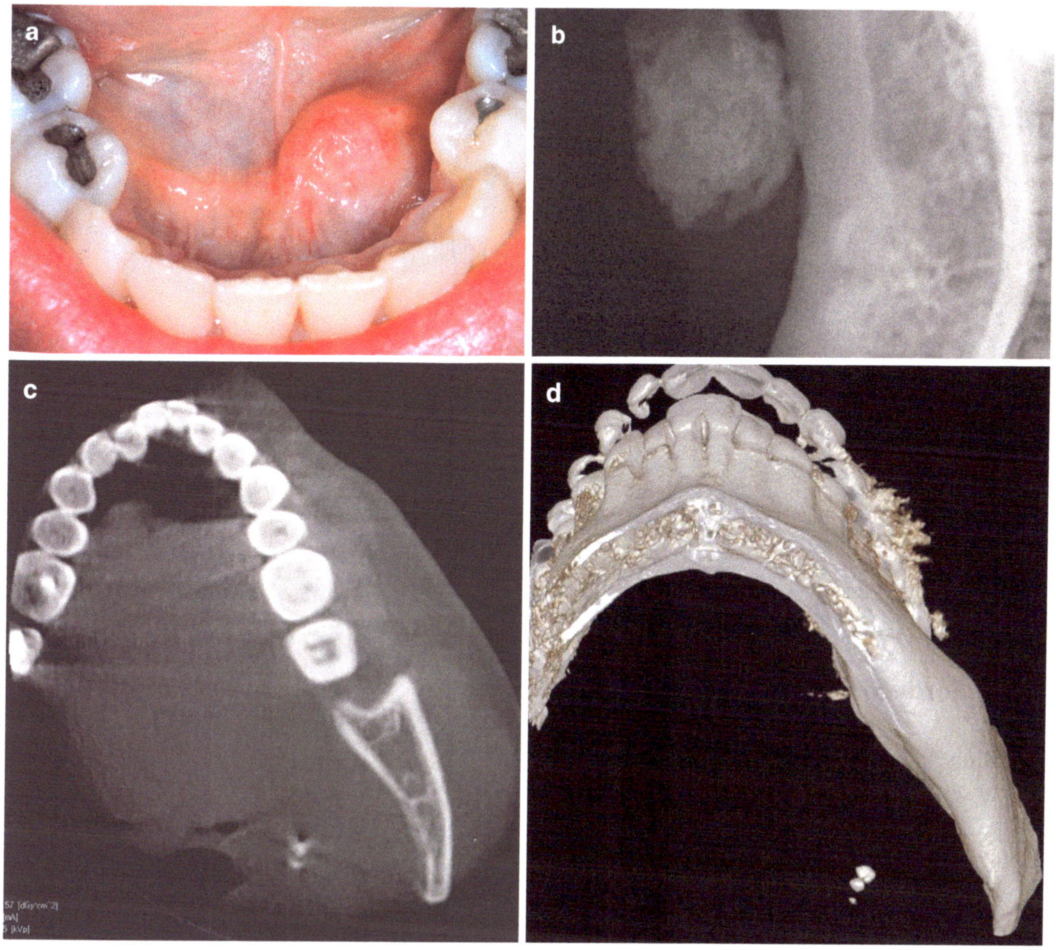

Fig. 2.38 (**a**) Swelling in the floor of the mouth caused by an underlying sialolith. (**b**) Occlusal radiograph shows a sialolith. (**c**) CT scan of another patient shows a small sialolith. (**d**) 3D image of **c**.

Etiology

Deposition of debris possibly caused by infection and followed by calcification. There is no association between calculus formation in the salivary glands and other organs, e.g., kidney and gall bladder.

Epidemiology

Rather rare event; usually at middle age but may occur in children as well.

Clinical Aspects

Sialoliths mainly occur in the submandibular glands or their excretory ducts and are usually associated with symptoms of a painful, recurrent submandibular swelling, particularly during meals. Occasionally presents as a swelling in the floor of the mouth (Fig. 2.38a). The diagnosis is confirmed by the findings on an occlusal radiograph (Fig. 2.38b) or a (cone beam) CT (Fig. 2.38c, d).

Occurrence of a sialolith in a minor salivary gland is quite rare; the usual presentation is a small nodule in the upper lip.

Treatment

Treatment consists usually of surgical removal. In most cases of involvement of the submandibular ductal system, there is no need to also remove the associated submandibular gland. Some clinicians prefer to apply lithotripsy. Removal of a sialolith in the parotid gland is more cumbersome;

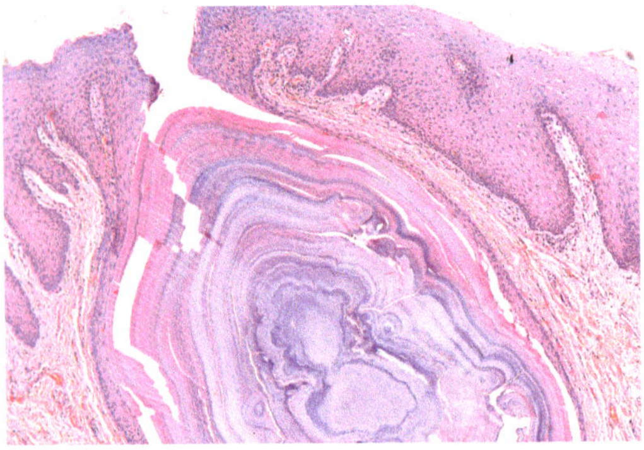

Fig. 2.39 Sialolith removed from the upper lip

sometimes sialoendoscopic removal is possible. An intraoral sialolith can be simply enucleated (Fig. 2.39).

2.6 Fordyce's Spots

Definition
Ectopic sebaceous glands in the oral mucosa.

Etiology
Developmental anomaly.

Epidemiology
Is present in various amounts in almost all people. Fordyce's spots become manifest during adulthood.

Clinical Aspects
Usually multiple pinpoint-sized yellowish granules; may occur everywhere in the oral cavity but sites of preference are the buccal mucosa and the upper lip (Fig. 2.40). Fordyce's spots do not cause any symptoms. In rare cases, Fordyce's spots become hyperplastic or even cystic. There is rarely a need for histopathologic confirmation.

Histopathology
Normal sebaceous glands without hair follicles (Fig. 2.41).

Treatment
No treatment required.

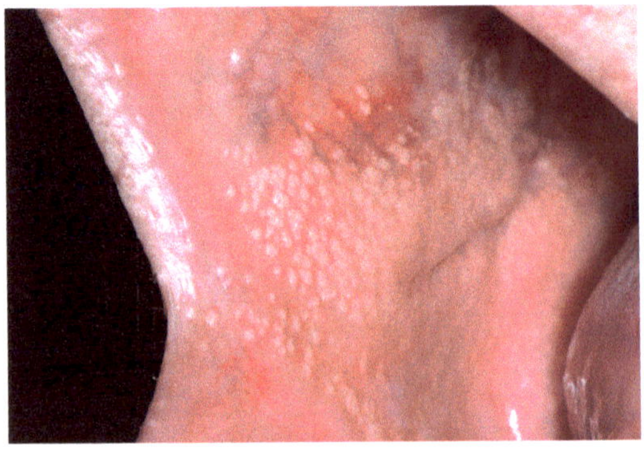

Fig. 2.40 Fordyce's spots in the buccal mucosa

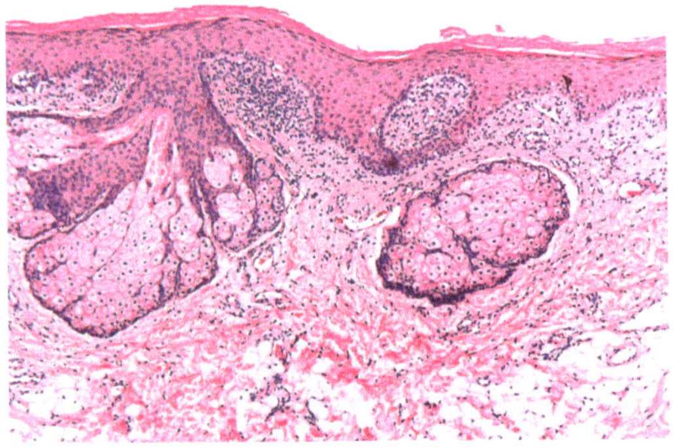

Fig. 2.41 Low-power view of Fordyce's spots

2.7 Fungal Diseases

2.7.1 Actinomycosis

Definition
Acute or chronic infection of the cervicofacial region caused by actinomycetes. Actinomycetes are actually no fungi but normal, saprophytic bacteria of the oral flora. There are several subclasses of actinomycetes such as *A. israelii* and *A. viscosus*.

Etiology
Trauma, e.g., a tooth extraction, may be the "port d'entrée" of the infection, resulting in abscess formation that ultimately may cause a cutaneous fistula. In most cases, there is an interval of some months between the extraction and the clinical presentation of the disease.

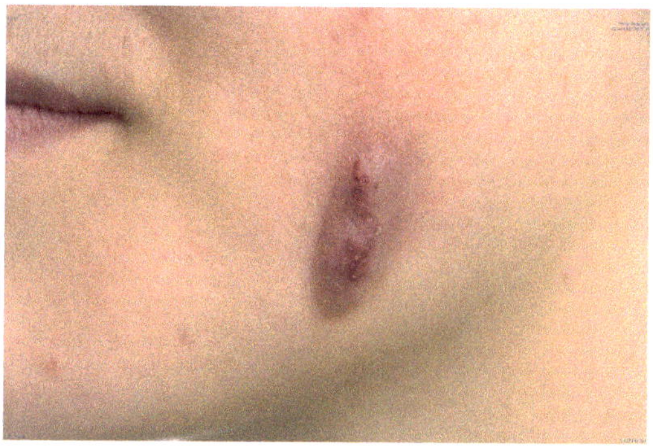

Fig. 2.42 Cervicofacial actinomycosis 2 months after a tooth extraction

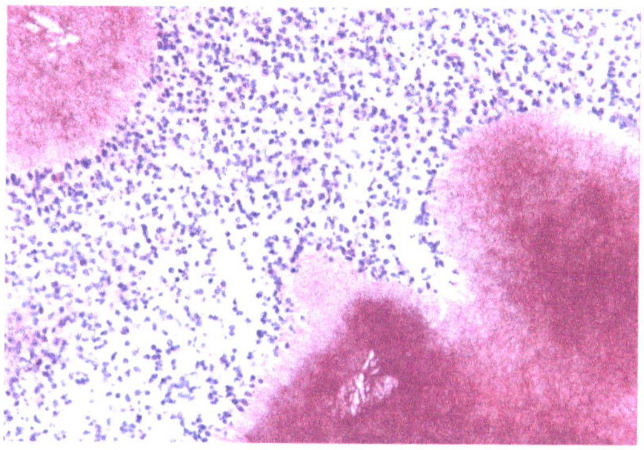

Fig. 2.43 Actinomyces colonies (PAS stain)

Epidemiology
Rather rare disease in the head and neck region.

Clinical Aspects
Usually presenting as a firm infiltrate or abscess, showing a bluish-reddish discoloration of the overlying skin (Fig. 2.42).

Laboratory Examination
Culturing of pus or infected tissue does not always demonstrate the presence of actinomycetes; in a number of such cases, histopathologic examination is helpful (Fig. 2.43).

Treatment
Surgical drainage and debridement followed by a 6–12-week course of penicillin.

2.7.2 Candidiasis

Definition
Fungal infection caused by one of the *Candida* species, most often being *C. albicans*.

Etiology
C. albicans occurs in the oropharyngeal cavity in approximately 40 % of the population without causing signs or symptoms. Local and systemic factors may lead to a disease state, referred to as candidiasis. Local predisposing factors may be poor oral hygiene, dry mouth, topical use of corticosteroids, e.g., in the form of inhalers, smoking, and irradiation of the head and neck.

Systemic predisposing factors consist of immunodeficiencies (e.g., HIV infection), diabetes mellitus, malnutrition, hematologic disorders such as leukemia, and prolonged use of antibiotics.

Clinical Aspects
There are several clinical manifestations; these may occur simultaneously in an individual patient. There is almost always a bilateral, more or less symmetrical pattern.

The *pseudomembranous type* ("thrush") is characterized by white plaques that can be easily wiped off from the mucosal surface (Fig. 2.44); this type mainly occurs on the buccal mucosa and the tongue. Symptoms may consist of a burning sensation and an abnormal taste.

The *erythematous type* is characterized by sometimes painful, fiery red changes of the mucosa, particularly occurring on the palate and the dorsum of the tongue (Fig. 2.45). Median rhomboid glossitis is regarded as a variant of erythematous candidiasis (see Chap. 4), being sometimes associated with erythematous candidiasis of the palate ("kissing lesion"); *C. albicans* may also play a role in angular cheilitis ("perlèches"); furthermore, denture stomatitis may be a variant of erythematous candidiasis, although the etiologic role of *C. albicans* in this condition is less convincing than has been thought in the past. In the absence of a bilateral distribution, the clinician should consider a diagnosis of erythroplakia, being a rare but serious premalignant disorder.

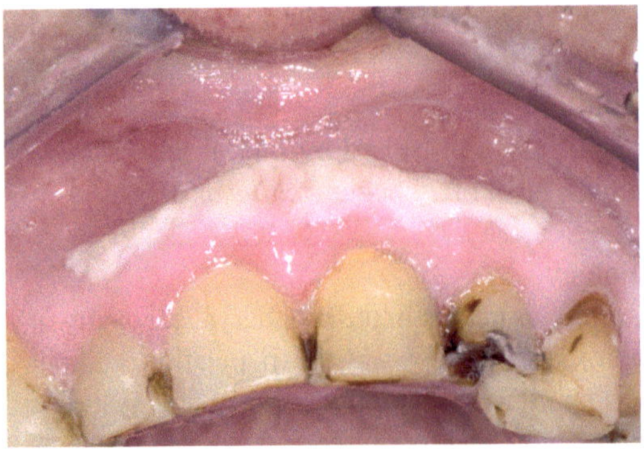

Fig. 2.44 Pseudomembranous candidiasis; notice the bilateral distribution

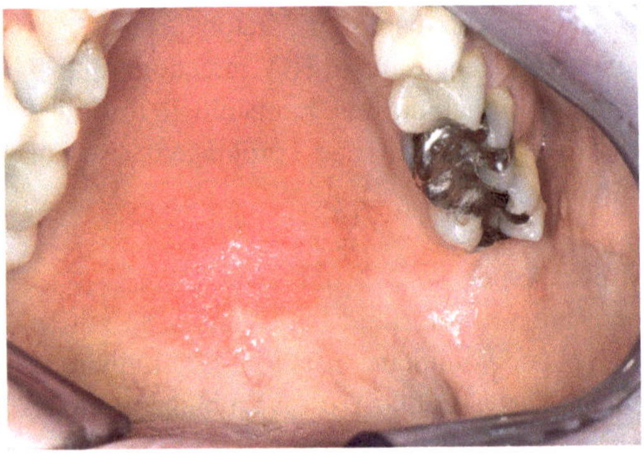

Fig. 2.45 Erythematous candidiasis of the palate; bilateral distribution

The *hyperplastic type* is characterized by a white patch that cannot be scraped off, occurring particularly in the corners of the mouth and on the dorsal surface of the tongue; some clinicians regard these lesions as Candida-associated leukoplakias.

The mucocutaneous type is caused by an underlying immune disorder and affects the oral mucosa, the skin, and nails. This rare entity will not be discussed here any further.

In most instances, the diagnosis "candidiasis" is a clinical one, either based on the clinical presentation or on a positive response to antifungal treatment.

Laboratory Studies

Exfoliative examination applying KOH may be considered but can in most cases be omitted. Culturing *C. albicans* is not very common as a routine procedure either.

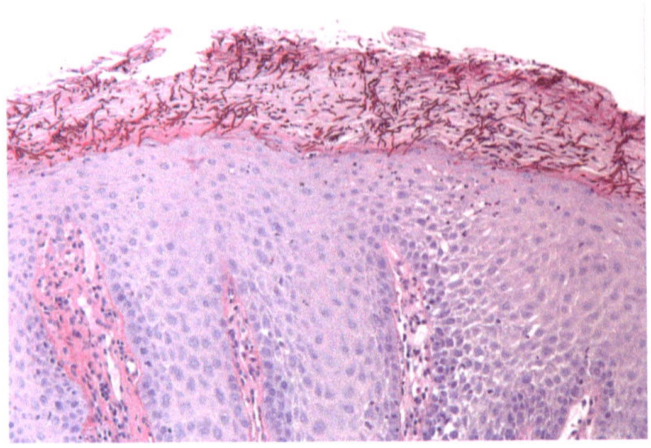

Fig. 2.46 Hyphae of *C. albicans* penetrating the superficial layer of the epithelium (PAS stain)

In the hyperplastic type, one may consider to perform a biopsy. In such event hyperplastic, parakeratotic epithelium can be observed with hyphae penetrating the epithelium (Fig. 2.46); in the superficial epithelium, microabscesses may be encountered. There may be varying degrees of chronic inflammation in the subepithelial connective tissue and sometimes also presence of neutrophils in the epithelium.

Treatment

Treatment is mainly indicated in symptomatic cases and should primarily be directed at elimination of predisposing factors, if any. In many cases, topical antifungal treatment for a few weeks is sufficient; only in persistent cases, systemic antifungal treatment is indicated.

2.8 Hemangioma and Hemangioma-Like Lesions

2.8.1 Angina Hemorrhagica Bullosa

Definition

Angina hemorrhagica bullosa is the Latin term for a painful blood blister.

Etiology

Unknown; some patients report that the lesion arose after eating hard food substances.

Epidemiology
Rather rare event; mainly in adults and probably more often in women.

Clinical Aspects
The blister suddenly appears and is often associated with pain. The palate, buccal mucosa, and the borders of the tongue are the sites of preference (Fig. 2.47). The blister ruptures soon after its development, leaving a superficial erosion of the mucosa behind (Fig. 2.48a, b).

Treatment
Treatment is rarely required since the blister ruptures soon after its development. Further healing takes place without scar formation.

Recurrence
Some patients will experience repeated recurrences. Unfortunately, no preventive measures can be taken.

2.8.2 Phlebectasia ("Varicosity")

Definition
Local dilatation of a small vein.

Etiology
Is most likely an aging phenomenon and is the result of local weakness of the vascular wall. Is not a sign of cardiopulmonal disease.

Epidemiology
Common phenomenon in middle-aged and elderly people.

Clinical Aspects
Solitary or multiple bluish swellings ranging from a few millimeters up to a centimeter (Fig. 2.49). The borders and the ventral aspect of the tongue and also the lips are the sites of preference. Phlebectasias are asymptomatic otherwise. There is rarely a need for histopathologic confirmation.

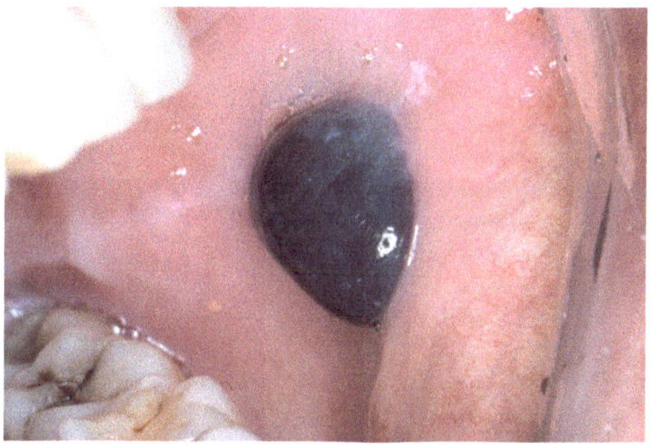

Fig. 2.47 Angina hemorrhagica bullosa in the cheek

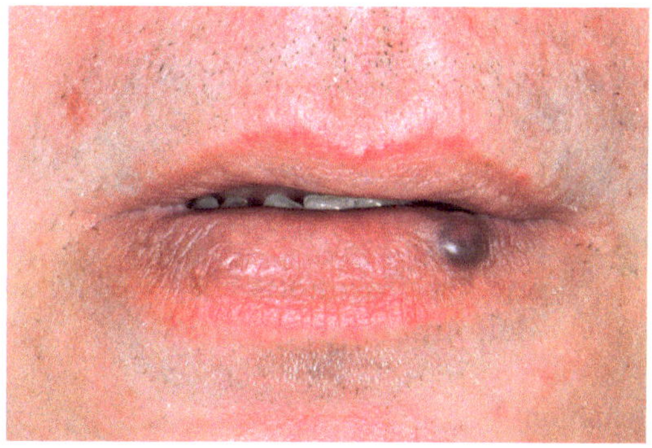

Fig. 2.49 Phlebectasia on the lower lip

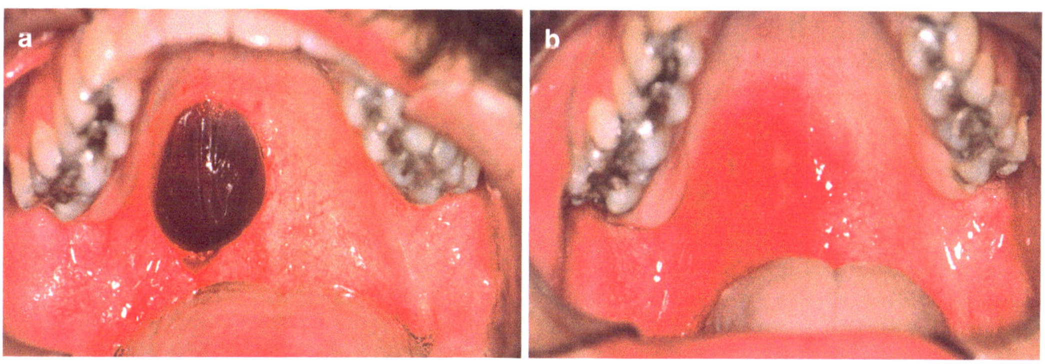

Fig. 2.48 (**a**) Angina hemorrhagica bullosa on the palate. (**b**) Clinical aspect after rupture of the blister

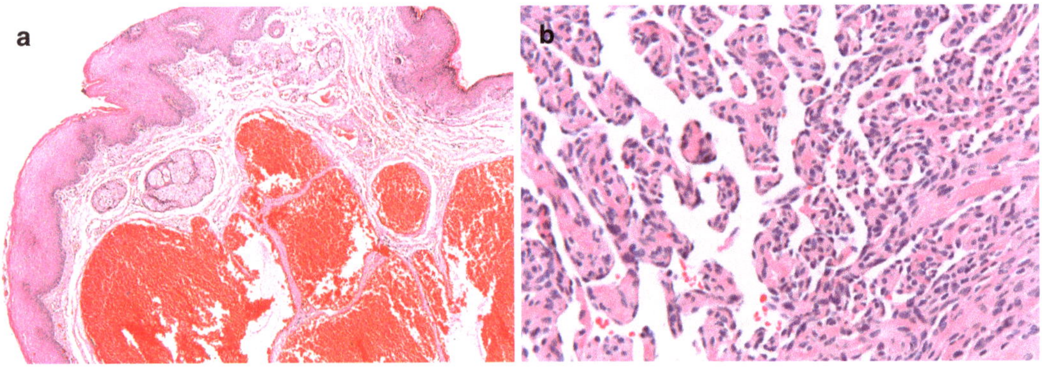

Fig. 2.50 (**a**) Low-power view of phlebectasia. (**b**) Intravascular papillary endothelial hyperplasia of the lower lip

Histopathology

Vascular spaces filled with erythrocytes (Fig. 2.50a). Thrombus formation may occur, sometimes accompanied by intravascular papillary endothelial hyperplasia. In such instance, the term "Masson tumor" has been used in the past; this benign lesion can be misdiagnosed as an angiosarcoma (Fig. 2.50b).

Treatment

Not required, although patients occasionally ask for removal because of esthetic reasons.

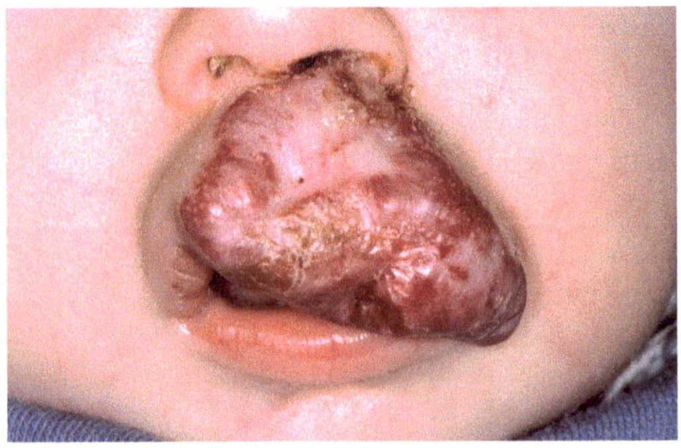

Fig. 2.51 True, fast-growing hemangioma in a 1-year-old

2.8.3 Hemangioma and Arteriovenous Malformations

Definition

The majority of the so-called hemangiomas of the oral mucosa and soft tissues are present already at birth or shortly thereafter and represent a malformation of blood vessels or lymphatic vessels (lymphangioma) rather than a neoplasm. There is, however, a rare "true" hemangioma that arises shortly after birth, showing rapid proliferation followed by spontaneous involution during childhood (Fig. 2.51). The present text focusses on the arteriovenous malformations.

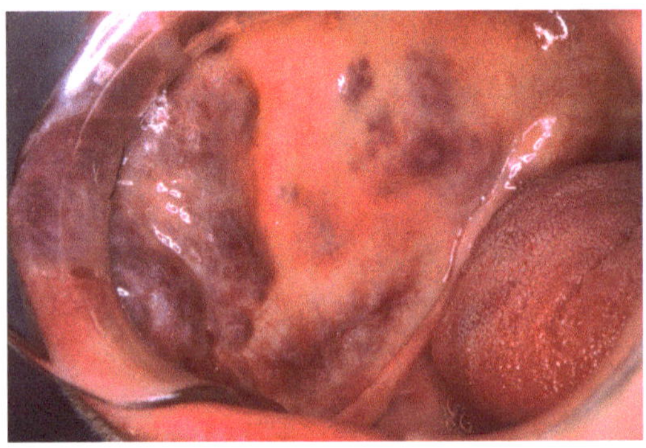

Fig. 2.52 Venous malformation in an adult, present from early childhood

Clinical Aspects

Red or bluish swelling of the oral mucosa, with or without pulsations, being usually asymptomatic otherwise. Only in arterial malformations repeated and severe spontaneous bleeding may occur. The lips, the tongue, and the buccal mucosa are the sites of preference (Fig. 2.52). Occasionally, calcified structures may be observed on a plain radiograph due to calcifications of thrombosed tissue; these are referred to as phleboliths (Fig. 2.53).

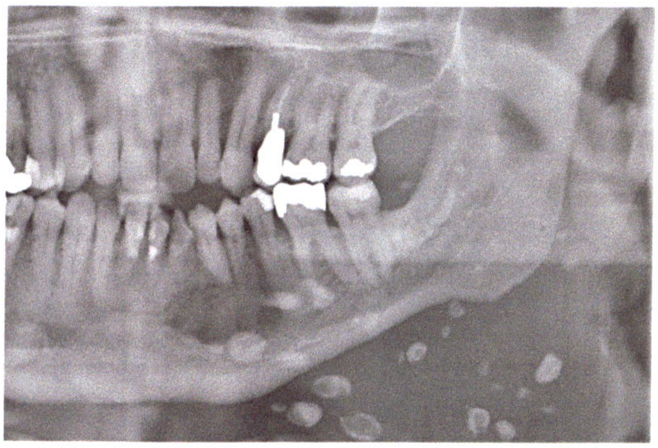

Fig. 2.53 Multiple phleboliths in a venous malformation of the left side of the neck

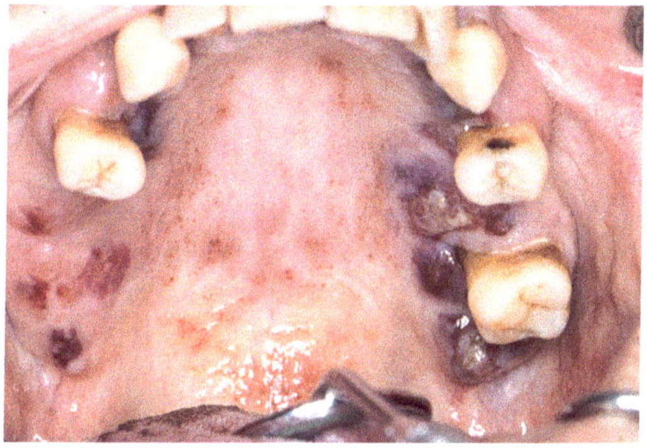

Fig. 2.54 Petechiae in a patient with thrombocytopathy

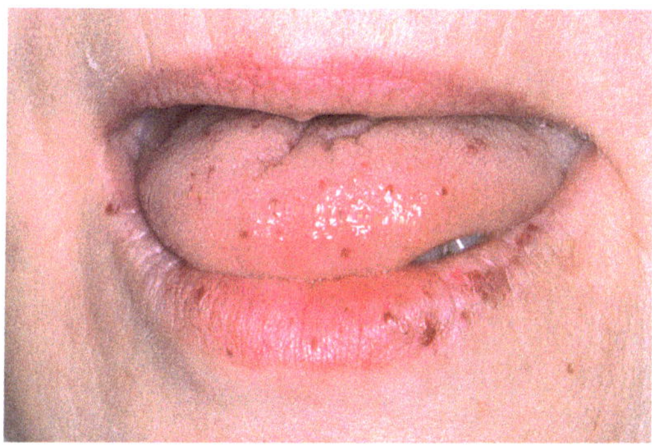

Fig. 2.55 Telangiectasias of the tongue and the lower lip in a patient suffering from Rendu-Osler-Weber disease

Differential Diagnosis

The differential diagnosis includes cystic salivary gland tumor, ecchymosis, petechiae due to thrombocytic disease (Fig. 2.54), manifestation of Rendu-Osler-Weber disease (Fig. 2.55), and Sturge-Weber syndrome (Fig. 2.56).

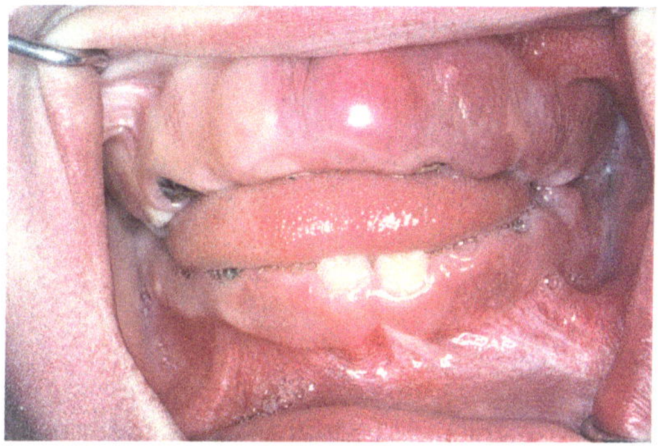

Fig. 2.56 Patient affected by Sturge-Weber syndrome. The gingival swelling may have been induced by the use of anticonvulsant drugs

Imaging

Imaging by ultrasound or MRI may be helpful in determining the extent of the malformation. In case of a suspected arterial component, arteriography should be performed (see Chap. 7).

Treatment

Arteriovenous malformations follow the normal growth of the individual and do not regress. If causing symptoms, venous malformations may successfully be managed by intralesion injections of sclerosing agents. Sometimes repeated interventions are necessary to control the anomaly. In arterial malformations, artificial embolization followed by surgery within 24–48 h may be successful.

2.8.4 Kaposi Sarcoma, AIDS Related

Definition

Inflammatory-like disease of the skin and the mucosa. It is not a true neoplasm in spite of the term "sarcoma."

Classification

There are several types of Kaposi sarcoma, being:

- "Classic" Kaposi sarcoma occurring in elderly men in the Mediterranean region
- Endemic Kaposi sarcoma in certain regions of Africa

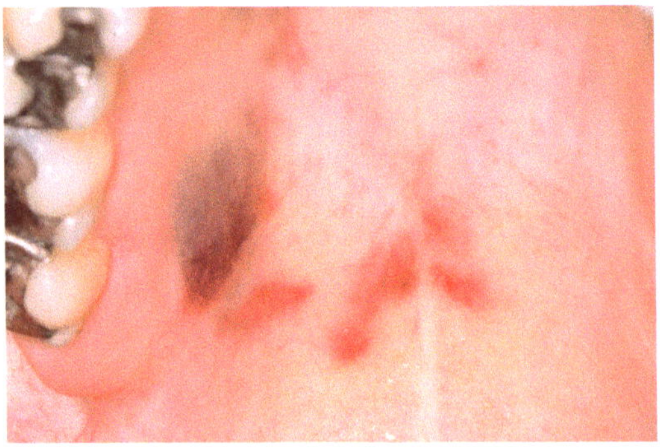

Fig. 2.57 Early presentation of Kaposi sarcoma

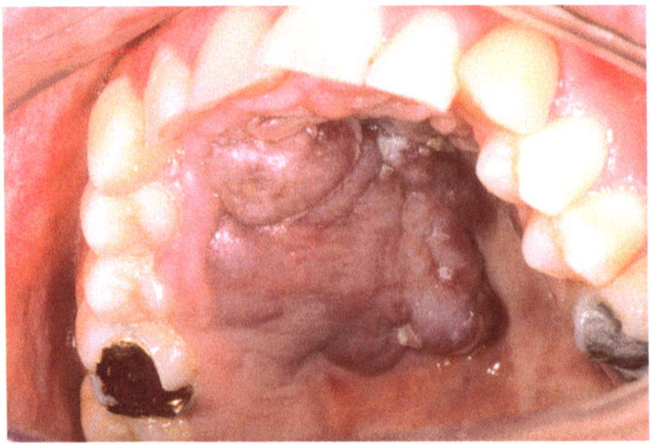

Fig. 2.58 Large Kaposi sarcoma in an AIDS patient

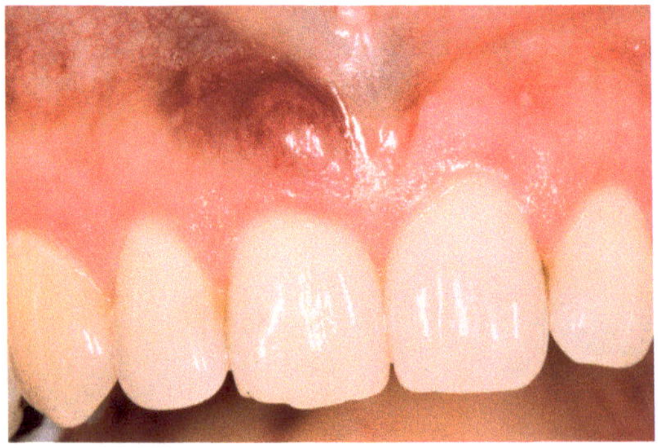

Fig. 2.59 Abscess-like Kaposi sarcoma of the gingiva

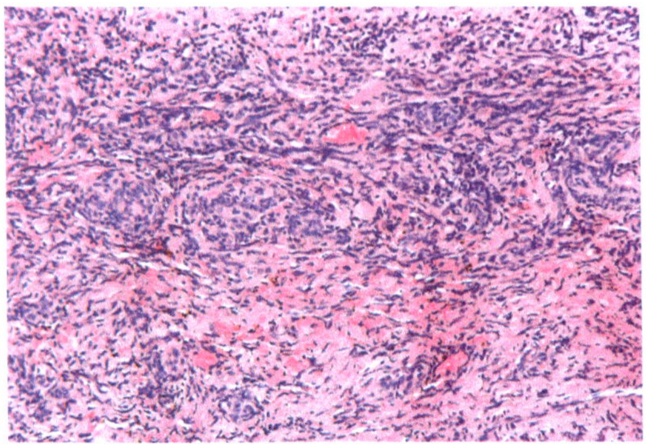

Fig. 2.60 Inflammatory-like aspect of Kaposi sarcoma

- Epidemic, AIDS-related Kaposi sarcoma
- Kaposi sarcoma caused by the prolonged use of immunosuppressive drugs

Etiology

The AIDS-related Kaposi sarcoma is linked with the human herpesvirus type 8 (HHV-8). The exact etiopathogenesis of AIDS-related Kaposi sarcoma is unknown.

Clinical Aspects

Kaposi sarcoma of the oral mucosa can be the first manifestation of HIV infection. The early manifestation may be a flat, somewhat reddish or brownish discoloration of the mucosa. At a later stage, solitary or multiple swellings may arise, being asymptomatic otherwise. The palate, the gingiva, and the tongue are the sites of preference (Figs. 2.57, 2.58, and 2.59).

Particularly in an unidentified, not-yet-HIV-tested patient, a biopsy is required to establish the diagnosis. Otherwise, the diagnosis can often be made on clinical grounds alone.

Differential Diagnosis

In the nodular stage, the clinical differential diagnosis mainly includes a non-Hodgkin lymphoma and a salivary gland tumor.

Histopathology

The histopathologic features are usually diagnostic although the inflammatory aspects may be misdiagnosed as a chronic inflammatory lesion (Fig. 2.60). The diagnosis Kaposi sarcoma can be further supported by the immunohistochemical demonstration of HHV-8 positivity.

Treatment

Treatment is only indicated in case of symptoms and may consist of local excision or, in extensive lesions, intralesional injection with certain drugs or low-dose radiotherapy.

2.9 Leukoplakia and Allied Lesions, Including Lichen Planus

2.9.1 Alveolar Ridge Keratosis

Definition

White changes of the retromolar region or the alveolar mucosa where teeth have been extracted. Most authors only use of the term "keratosis" when a biopsy has shown the presence of hyperkeratosis at histopathologic examination and avoid the clinical use of the term keratosis. Some authors suggest that alveolar ridge keratosis has no tendency to become malignant and, therefore, do not consider this phenomenon as a subtype of leukoplakia, being potentially malignant (see Sect. 2.9.6).

Etiology

Direct irritation from food that is crushed against the edentulous ridge by opposing teeth.

Clinical Aspects

The clinical aspect is just a white, homogeneous discoloration of the mucosa, being asymptomatic otherwise. The mucosa of an edentulous part of the alveolar ridge and the retromolar region are the sites of preference (Fig. 2.61).

When one believes this phenomenon to be benign, the taking of a biopsy may not be required. On the other hand, the use of "keratosis" to designate a non-biopsied lesion is somewhat debatable as has been mentioned before.

Histopathology

Hyperkeratosis and acanthosis without epithelial dysplasia.

Treatment

If one accepts that this phenomenon is benign, then no treatment or follow-up would be required. However, it seems safe practice to follow the patient at least once a year for possible changes of the clinical aspect (see Sect. 2.9.6).

2.9.2 Aspirin Burn

Definition

Superficial etching or burning of the oral mucosa due to repeated local application of aspirin for the alleviation of dental pain; may also be caused by application of paracetamol tablets. Aspirin burn is a benign lesion and should not be regarded a leukoplakia.

Clinical Aspects

Whitish, non-wipeable discoloration of the mucobuccal fold, the buccal mucosa, or the borders of the tongue (Figs. 2.62 and 2.63a, b). Only in case of doubt, the taking of a biopsy may be considered.

Histopathology

Hyperkeratosis without specific diagnostic aspects. Absence of epithelial dysplasia.

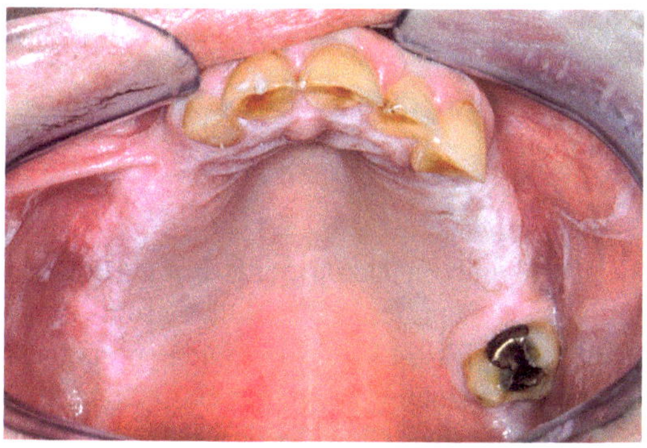

Fig. 2.61 White changes of the alveolar ridge; the patient is not wearing a denture ("alveolar ridge keratosis")

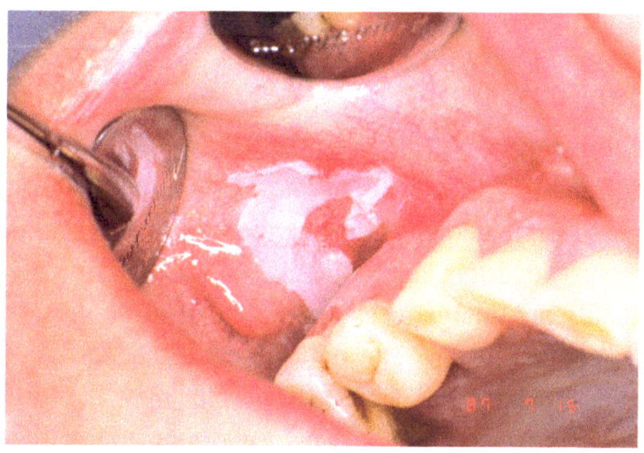

Fig. 2.62 Leukoplakia-like aspirin burn

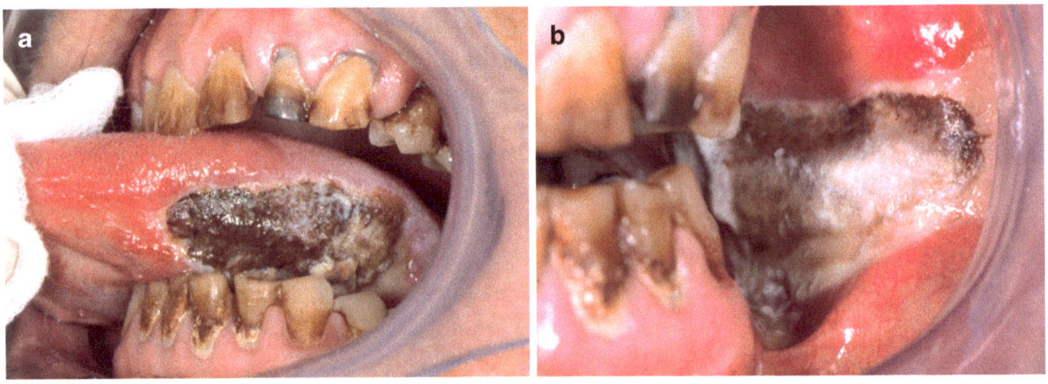

Fig. 2.63 (**a**) Extensive ulceration due to the prolonged use of aspirin in a heavy female smoker. (**b**) The buccal mucosa shows the more common whitish appearance of an aspirin burn

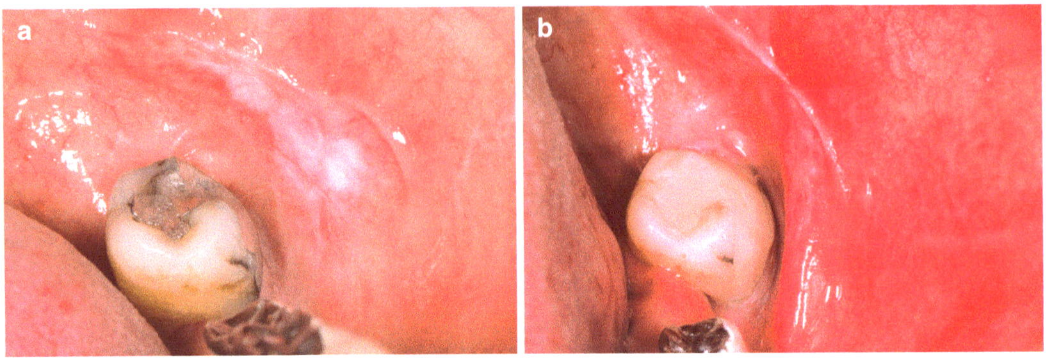

Fig. 2.64 (**a**) Leukoplakic lesion possibly due to contact with a buccal amalgam restoration ("contact lesion"). (**b**) Same patient 2 months after replacement of the amalgam restoration

Treatment

Cessation of the application of the drug should result in healing of the lesion within a week or so; this should be monitored.

2.9.3 Contact Lesion

Definition

A benign whitish, sometimes erythematous or mixed white and red lesion of the oral mucosa due to chronic, direct contact with a dental restoration, usually an amalgam restoration. A firm diagnosis of "contact lesion" can only be established when the lesion has disappeared after replacement of the amalgam restoration. In case of doubt about the diagnosis of a whitish lesion, it should be provisionally diagnosed as leukoplakia.

Etiology

It is often discussed as whether a contact lesion is caused by mechanical irritation ("frictional lesion") or by a delayed type IV allergy to mercury; some recommend to do allergy testing for mercury and amalgam. Another suggested, but difficult to proof, etiologic factor is galvanism due to the use of various metals of dental restorations.

Clinical Aspects

The buccal mucosa and the borders of the tongue are the sites of preference. Contact lesions may have a leukoplakia-like or lichenoid appearance, sometimes producing symptoms (Fig. 2.64a, b). In case of doubt of the diagnosis, one should take a biopsy before replacing the (amalgam) restoration.

Histopathology
Hyperkeratosis, no epithelial dysplasia. Occasionally, a lichenoid aspect can be observed. There is no epithelial dysplasia.

Treatment
After replacement of the amalgam regression or even complete disappearance of the lesion may be expected within a few months. A follow-up visit within 2–3 months after replacement of the amalgam restoration is mandatory in order to confirm the provisional diagnosis of a contact lesion.

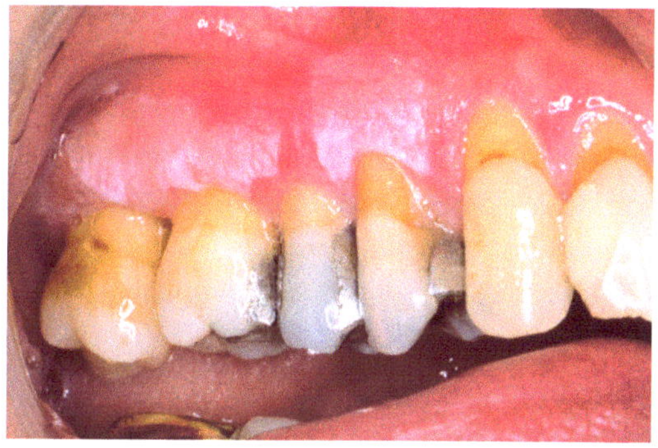

Fig. 2.65 Frictional lesion or leukoplakia of the gingiva and alveolar mucosa

2.9.4 Frictional Lesion ("Frictional Keratosis")

Definition
The term frictional lesion (some use the term "frictional keratosis") refers to a supposedly benign white lesion that is caused by mechanical irritation or friction. A firm diagnosis of "frictional lesion" can only be made retrospectively when the lesion has disappeared after elimination of the mechanical irritation.

Etiology
A frictional lesion may be located on the border of the tongue, being caused by a broken-down dental restoration. A more common location is the attached gingiva and the alveolar mucosa where vigorous toothbrushing habits or masticatory forces exerted on the oral mucosa are supposed to be the causative factors.

Clinical Aspects
Frictional lesions usually present as homogeneous white, flat lesions of the attached gingiva (Fig. 2.65), often present in all four quadrants of the dentition, being asymptomatic otherwise. In case of doubt about the diagnosis of a whitish lesion, it should be provisionally diagnosed as leukoplakia and managed as such (see Sect. 2.9.6).

Histopathology
From a practical point of view – there are often multiple sites of involvement – the taking of a biopsy is not always warranted; if taken, the histopathology will show hyperkeratosis without epithelial dysplasia.

Treatment
After changing the causative factor, e.g., vigorous brushing habits, regression may take place in some patients within a few months; complete disappearance is rare. If one accepts that a frictional lesion is benign, then no treatment or follow-up would be required. However, it seems safe practice to follow the patient once a year.

2.9.5 Leukoedema

Definition
Benign, whitish lesion of the oral mucosa; some authors regard the lesion a prestage of leukoplakia ("preleukoplakia").

Etiology
Tobacco use seems the main contributory factor.

Epidemiology
Rather rare phenomenon; occurs mainly in adults, often dark skinned.

Clinical Aspects
Veil-like appearance, bilateral, of the buccal mucosa, being asymptomatic otherwise (Fig. 2.66a, b). In view of the rather characteristic clinical aspect, there is rarely a need for a biopsy.

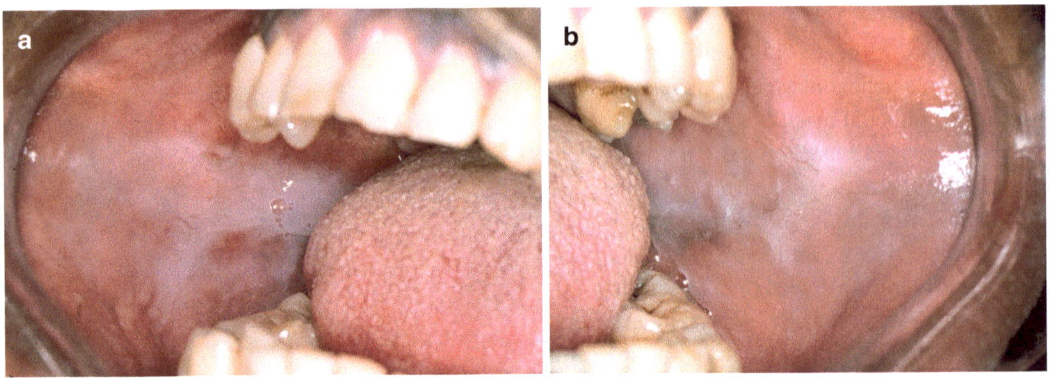

Fig. 2.66 (**a**) Veil-like appearance of leukoderma of the buccal mucosa. (**b**) Same patient as shown in **a**

Histopathology
Hyperplastic epithelium that may show intracellular edema; no epithelial dysplasia.

Treatment
Advise quitting of possible smoking habits; it is actually unknown whether the lesion then will regress or disappear.

2.9.6 Leukoplakia

Definition
Predominantly white lesion or condition of the oral mucosa that clinically and histopathologically cannot be recognized as any other well-defined lesion or condition, e.g., pseudomembranous candidiasis, morsicatio, or lichen planus. In fact, the previous definition, provided by the World Health Organization, is one by exclusion.

Leukoplakia is a premalignant, precancerous, or potentially malignant lesion or condition, which means that there is an increased risk of future malignant transformation into a squamous cell carcinoma either at the site of the leukoplakia or elsewhere in the oral cavity or the head and neck region.

Etiology
Much more common in smokers than in nonsmokers. Smokeless tobacco may result in leukoplakia-like lesions ("snuff dipper's lesions"), e.g., of the labial mucosa of the upper lip in Swedish patients using "snus." Smokeless tobacco-induced lesions may have a malignant potential depending on the type of tobacco that has been used.

The role of the use of alcohol in the etiology of leukoplakia is actually unknown. Human papillomaviruses (HPV) do not seem to play an important role.

Epidemiology
The estimated prevalence is approximately 0.1 %. There is no distinct gender preference. Leukoplakia occurs mainly above the age of 30–40 years.

Clinical Aspects
Pain or itching at the site of a leukoplakia is an ominous sign and may indicate the presence of a squamous cell carcinoma.

There are various clinical presentations (Figs. 2.67, 2.68, 2.69, and 2.70):

- *Homogeneous*: uniform *flat*, *thin*, and white
- *Nonhomogeneous*: nodular or flat with a mixed white and red discoloration ("erythroleukoplakia"); verrucous, probably often misdiagnosed as homogeneous type because of its homogeneous white color and its homogeneous verrucous appearance. A variant is *proliferative verrucous leukoplakia* (PVL), characterized by recurrences after removal and development of new leukoplakias with a widespread distribution throughout the oral cavity; in fact, the diagnosis PVL can only be

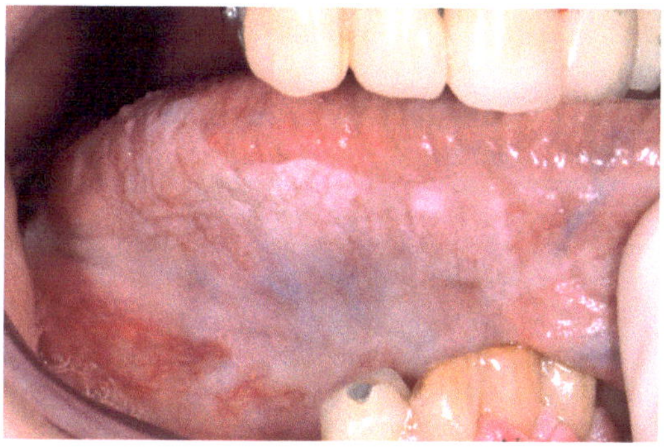

Fig. 2.67 Leukoplakia, homogeneous clinical type

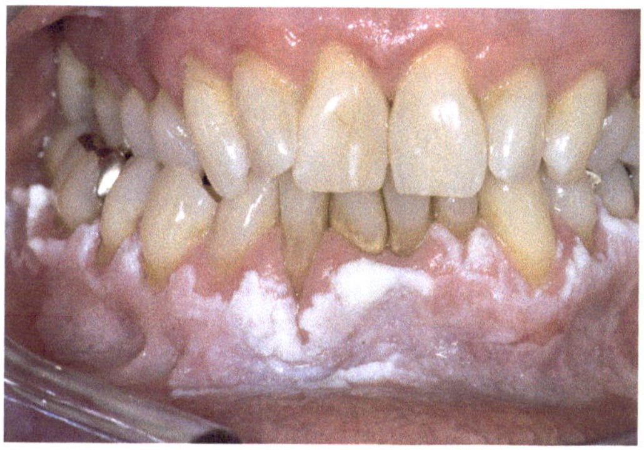

Fig. 2.68 Partly homogeneous and partly nonhomogeneous (verrucous) leukoplakia

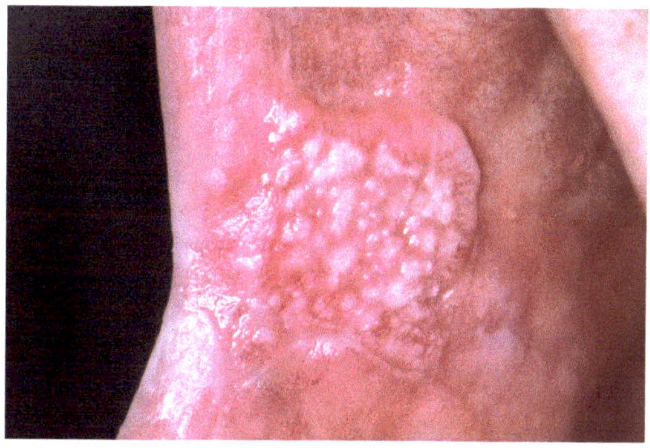

Fig. 2.69 Leukoplakia, nonhomogeneous (nodular) type

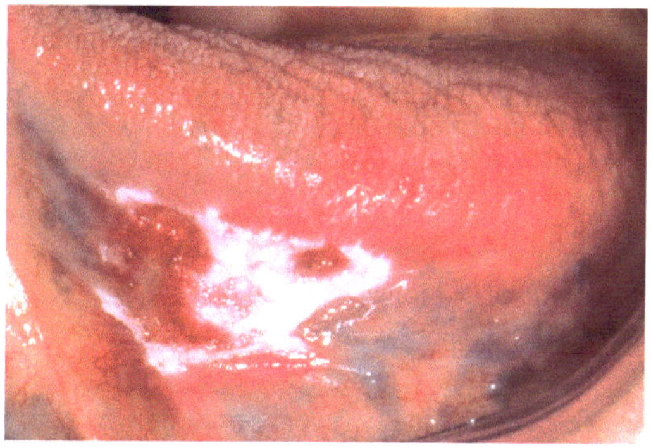

Fig. 2.70 Nonhomogeneous leukoplakia (erythroleukoplakia)

made in retrospect. Unfortunately, there are many confusing publications about this entity. Furthermore, verrucous leukoplakia and verrucous carcinoma may be clinically indistinguishable from each other.

Homogeneous leukoplakia is usually asymptomatic otherwise, while nonhomogeneous leukoplakias, particularly erythroleukoplakias, often cause a burning sensation. Leukoplakias may occur everywhere in the mouth and the lips, either solitary or in a multiple or widespread fashion. Occurrence in the floor of the mouth, the commissures, and the palate is almost exclusively seen in smokers. The clinical differential diagnosis includes:

- Alveolar ridge "keratosis"
- Aspirin burn
- Candidiasis, hyperplastic type
- Contact lesion
- Darier-White disease
- Frictional lesion
- Hairy leukoplakia in HIV infection (see Chap. 4)
- Leukoedema
- Lichen planus, plaque type and erythematous type
- Lichen sclerosus
- Linea alba
- Lupus erythematodes
- Morsicatio (cheek biting or tongue biting)
- Pachyonychia congenita
- Papilloma and allied lesions
- Skin graft
- Squamous cell carcinoma
- Syphilis, second stage ("plaques muqueuses") (Fig. 2.71)
- Tobacco-induced lesions such as nicotinic stomatitis (see Chap. 6), snuff dippers lesions,

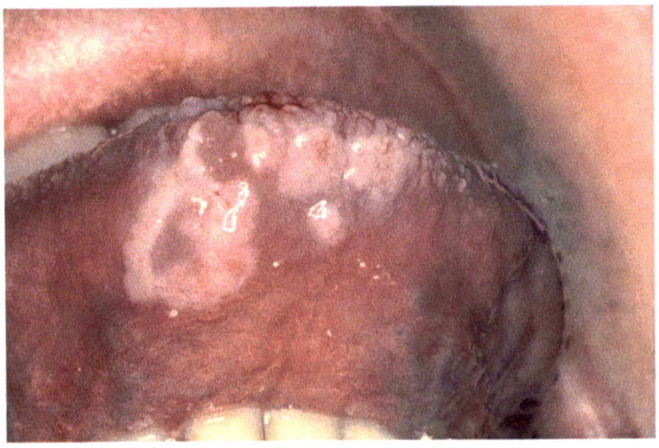

Fig. 2.71 “Plaques muqueuses” in second stage of syphilis

and palatal lesions due to reverse smoking (see Chap. 6)
- Verrucous carcinoma
- White sponge nevus

In case of a clinical diagnosis of leukoplakia, the taking of a biopsy is recommended to rule other lesions, such as mentioned before, and to assess the presence and degree of epithelial dysplasia or, occasionally, even carcinoma in situ, frank squamous cell carcinoma, or verrucous carcinoma.

The biopsy should be taken at the clinically most suspicious area, if any, or at the site of symptoms, if present. In leukoplakias up to 2–3 cm, an excisional biopsy may be performed. In larger leukoplakias, the taking of multiple biopsies should be considered (“field mapping”).

Histopathology

The histopathologic features of leukoplakia may vary from hyperkeratosis with or without epithelial dysplasia to various degrees of epithelial dysplasia, carcinoma in situ, and even invasive squamous cell carcinoma (Fig. 2.72a–c). Other features that may be encountered are verrucous hyperplasia or verrucous carcinoma; because of the highly specialistic histopathologic aspects of verrucous hyperplasia and verrucous carcinoma, these entities will not be discussed here in detail.

Malignant Transformation

The annual malignant transformation of untreated oral leukoplakia, all types together, is 2–3 % (Fig. 2.73a, b). Predicting factors of malignant transformation are, statistically:

- Female gender
- Nonsmoking
- Seize of ≥200 mm^2
- Location in the floor of the mouth or the tongue
- Presence and degree of epithelial dysplasia
- Molecular markers, such as DNA ploidy, loss of heterozygosity, suprabasal expression of p53

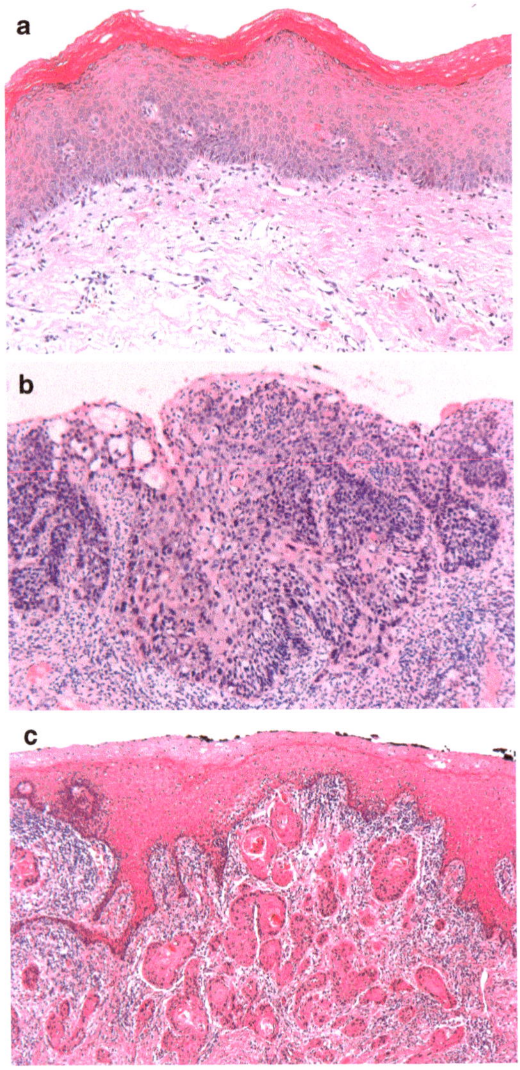

Fig. 2.72 (**a**) Hyperkeratosis, no epithelial dysplasia. (**b**) Severe epithelial dysplasia or carcinoma in situ. (**c**) Well-differentiated squamous cell carcinoma

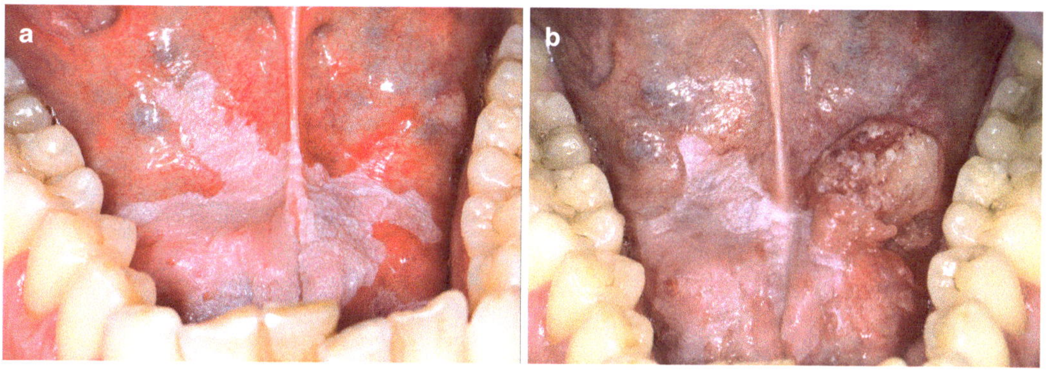

Fig. 2.73 (**a**) Homogeneous leukoplakia of the floor of the mouth; no treatment instituted. (**b**) Four years later, a squamous cell carcinoma developed on the left side

Table 2.2 Diagnosis and management of oral leukoplakia (Provisional clinical diagnosis)

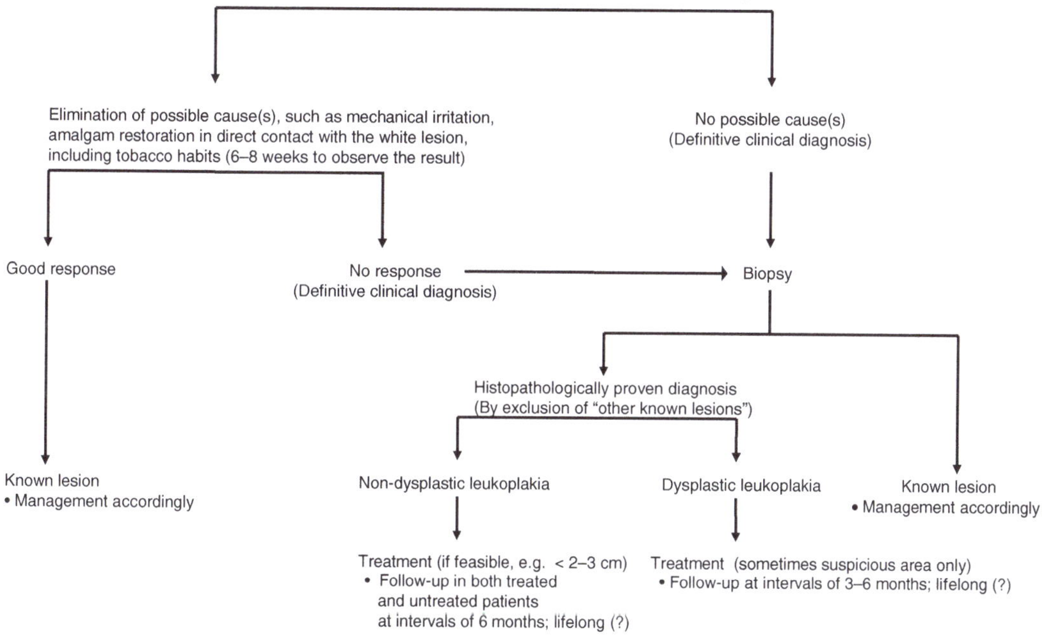

At present there is no single marker or set of markers that accurately predicts malignant transformation in an individual patient.

Treatment

A biopsy should always be taken in case of symptoms, irrespective of the clinical aspect of the lesion. In otherwise asymptomatic leukoplakias, possible etiologic factors, including smoking habits, should be eliminated. It is safe practice to wait for the result of this elimination for a period of 6–8 weeks (Table 2.2). If unchanged, one or more biopsies should be taken, depending on the extent of the leukoplakia and its clinical presentation.

If feasible, each oral leukoplakia should be excised, although the effectiveness of such removal with regard to recurrence and malignant transformation has never been proven. Removal should preferably be performed by surgical excision (including laser excision) since this treatment modality will provide a surgical specimen for (additional) histopathologic examination. Nevertheless, in some cases, particularly in case of involvement of the floor of the mouth, the cheek, and the alveolar ridges, laser evaporation may result in less morbidity. In widespread leukoplakias, there may be an indication for systemic photodynamic treatment. Yet, another option is to limit the treatment to the area of clinical suspicion, if any.

Nonsurgical treatment modalities are, in general, not effective in preventing possible malignant transformation either and may carry adverse side effects.

In all instances, patients with oral leukoplakia, being treated or not, should be followed-up at intervals of no longer than 3–6 months, lifelong, although the effectiveness of such follow-up program with regard to better survival in case of malignant transformation has never been shown.

Prognosis
In spite of whatever type of treatment, the risk of development of a squamous cell carcinoma either at the site of the leukoplakia or elsewhere in the oral cavity or the upper aerodigestive tract, seems to remain unchanged.

It is well taken that some types of leukoplakia, particularly the much debated proliferative verrucous leukoplakia, will probably always become malignant. However, this may take more than 10 years which for this particular patient population would result in an annual transformation rate of 10 %.

2.9.7 Lichen Planus and Lichenoid Lesions

Definition
Inflammatory-like mucocutaneous disease. Oral lichen planus is by some regarded as a premalignant condition, the annual malignant transformation rate being less than 0.5 %.

Etiology
Probably based on T-cell autoimmunity. Lichen planus-like lesions, usually referred to as lichenoid lesions or lichenoid reactions, may be caused by certain drugs (Table 2.3) or by direct anatomic contact with large amalgam restorations (see Sect. 2.9.3) and may also represent a chronic graft-versus-host reaction after allogenic stem cell transplantation.

Table 2.3 Drugs possibly causing lichenoid lesions

Antihypertensives (e.g., ACE inhibitors)
Oral hypoglycemics (e.g., tolbutamide)
Non-steroidal anti-inflammatory drugs
Second line antiarthritics (gold; penicillamine)
Xanthine oxidase inhibitors (allopurinol)
Psychoactive drugs (e.g., tricyclic antidepressants)
Diuretics (e.g., furosemide)
Antiparasitic drugs
Antimicrobial agents, including mouthrinses (e.g., tetracycline)
Miscellaneous drugs (e.g., iodides, quinidine)

Rice PJ, Hamburger J. Dent Update 2002;29:442–7

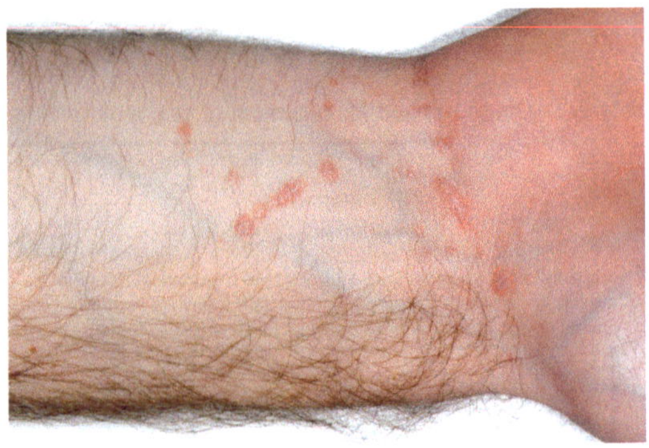

Fig. 2.74 Cutaneous lichen planus in patient also suffering from oral lichen planus

Epidemiology
The estimated prevalence of oral lichen planus is approximately 0.1 %. Oral lichen planus mainly affects middle-aged people and is more common among women than in men.

Clinical Aspects
Lichen planus of the skin and of the oral mucosa or other mucosas, such as of the vulva or vagina (vulvovaginal-gingival syndrome), may occur together but probably do more often so separately (Fig. 2.74).

Oral lichen planus has various clinical manifestations, such as *reticular* (characterized by

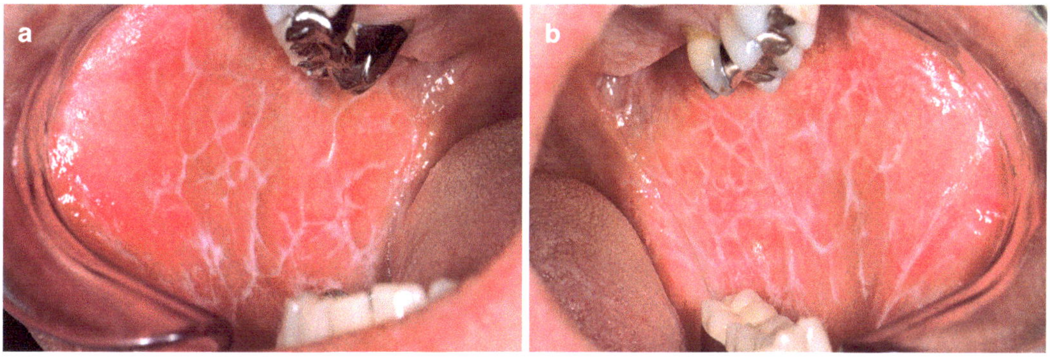

Fig. 2.75 (**a**) Lichen planus, reticular type. (**b**) Same patient; other side

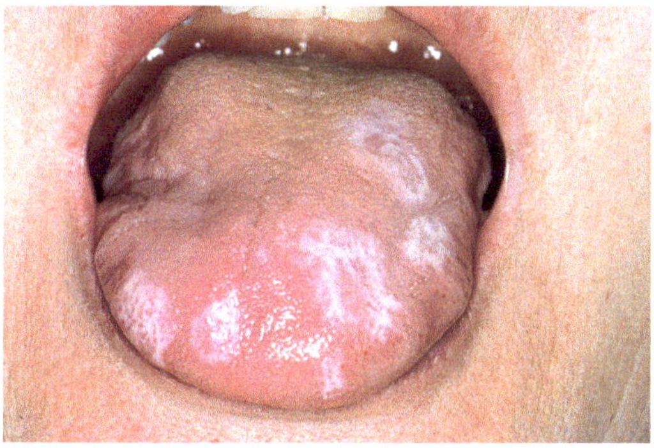

Fig. 2.76 Lichen planus of the tongue, reticular type

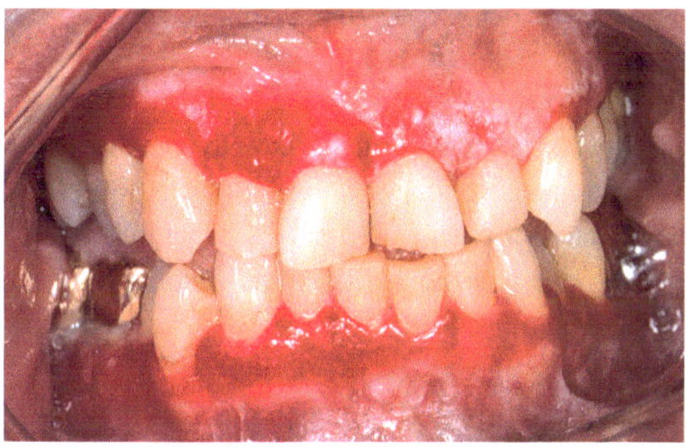

Fig. 2.77 Erosive lichen planus of the gingiva

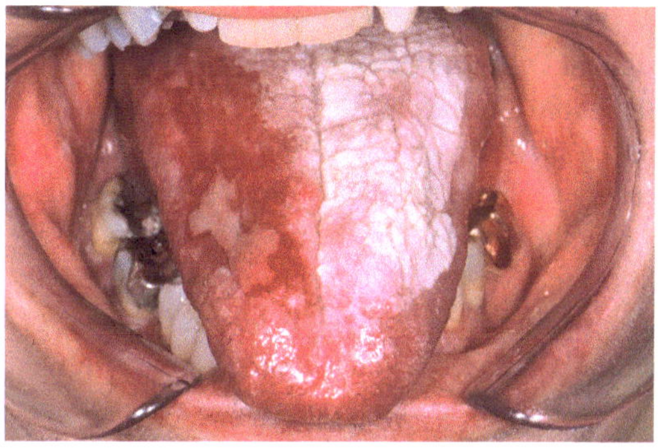

Fig. 2.78 Lichen planus, partly erosive/ulcerative and partly plaque type

white striae, also referred to as "Wickham's striae"), *erythematous*, *plaque type* (resembling leukoplakia), *ulcerative,* and *bullous* type (Figs. 2.75a, b, 2.76, 2.77, and 2.78). There is nearly always a bilateral, more or less symmetrical distribution. The buccal mucosa, the gingiva, and the dorsal surface of the tongue are the sites of predilection. Occurrence in the floor of the mouth and the palate is rare.

Particularly the erythematous type may cause symptoms, such as pain and, in case of gingival involvement, severe bleeding during toothbrushing. Patients affected by oral lichen planus usually do not tolerate spicy food. When the gums are involved, patients may complain about the esthetic aspect of their gums. In involvement of the gingiva, the presence of the "vulvovaginal-gingiva syndrome" should be considered.

The course of oral lichen planus is characterized by remissions and exacerbations with intervals of several weeks or months of both the clinical signs and the symptoms.

Because of the chronicity of the disease, some clinicians will always do a biopsy, while others take a biopsy only in case of doubt about the clinical diagnosis.

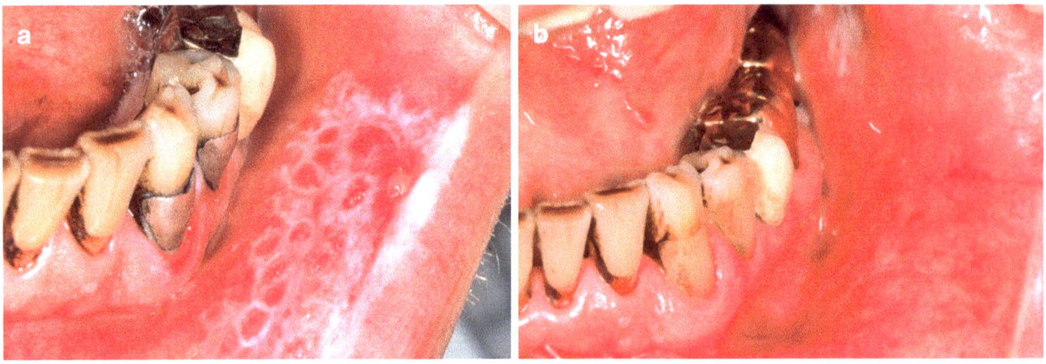

Fig. 2.79 (**a**) Lichenoid lesion possibly due to prolonged contact with amalgam restorations. (**b**) Result 2 months after replacement of the amalgam restorations

Clinical Differential Diagnosis, Including Lichenoid Lesions

Lichen planus resembling (lichenoid) lesions or reactions may be caused by direct anatomic contact with a large (amalgam) restoration ("see Sect. 2.9.3") (Fig. 2.79a, b) or may be induced by the use of certain drugs; in contrast to drug-induced cutaneous lichenoid lesions, drug-induced oral lichenoid lesions are extremely rare. Furthermore, lichenoid lesions may occur in chronic graft-versus-host disease, being clinically sometimes indistinguishable from "idiopathic" lichen planus.

At times, it may be difficult, if not impossible, to clinically distinguish oral lichen planus not only from lichenoid lesions but also from leukoplakia, lupus erythematodes, linear IgA disease, mucous membrane pemphigoid, and some other white or red lesions of the oral mucosa. In some of these cases, the medical history or other clinical features may be helpful in establishing the correct diagnosis. Unfortunately, a biopsy is not always helpful in such cases.

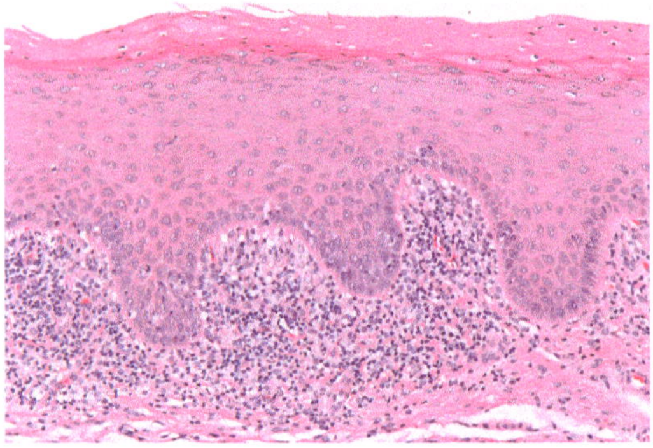

Fig. 2.80 Low-power view compatible with but not diagnostic of lichen planus

Histopathology

In case of a distinct clinical diagnosis of lichen planus, the histopathologic features are usually quite characteristic (Fig. 2.80). However, when the clinical diagnosis is not that clear, the histopathologic aspects are usually not that clear either.

Histopathologically, no distinction can be made between lichen planus and the various lichenoid lesions. Epithelial dysplasia is by most pathologists not accepted as compatible with a histopathologic diagnosis of lichen planus. Some pathologists use the term "lichenoid dysplasia" when reporting on leukoplakic lesions that show a subepithelial band-like lymphocytic infiltrate in the presence of epithelial dysplasia. The use of this term may erroneously be interpreted by the clinician as the presence of dysplastic changes in lichen planus.

Treatment

Oral lichen planus may last for many years, if not lifelong. There is no cure for oral lichen planus. Treatment can only be symptomatic and most commonly consists of topical corticosteroids.

The issue of premalignancy is still under debate in the literature. At present, it seems safe practice to check the patient annually.

2.9.8 Lichen Sclerosus

Definition
Benign chronic mucocutaneous disease characterized by flat, pale, or whitish changes of the skin or mucosa, particularly of the vulva.

Etiology
Unknown.

Epidemiology
Rather rare disease that may occur already at a young age. Involvement of the oral mucosa is extremely rare.

Clinical Aspects
Oral lichen sclerosus presents with a whitish, atrophic discoloration of the mucosa of the upper or lower lip and, rarely, of the tongue or the corners of the mouth (Fig. 2.81). Lichen sclerosus is usually asymptomatic otherwise. In the majority of cases of oral involvement, the disease has already been diagnosed based on cutaneous or vulval manifestation; in such instances, there is no need for a biopsy.

Histopathology
Depending on the stage of the disease, rather typical histopathologic features are encountered, although the disease has various stages. A subepithelial hyalinized aspect of the connective tissue, somewhat mimicking amyloid deposition, with or without signs of inflammation, is the hallmark of lichen sclerosus (Fig. 2.82).

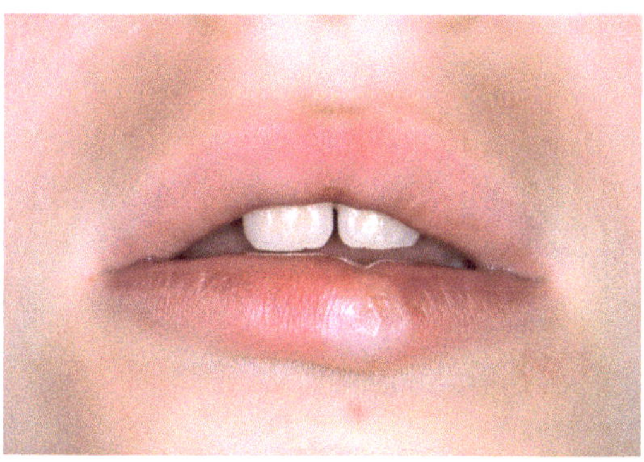

Fig. 2.81 Lichen sclerosus of the lower lip in a 10-year-old boy

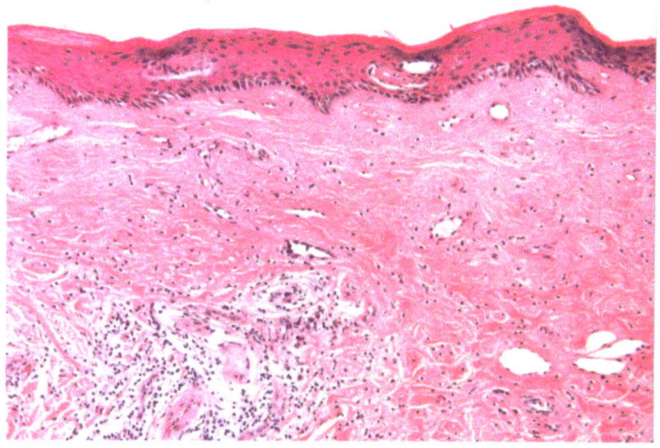

Fig. 2.82 Low-power view of lichen sclerosus

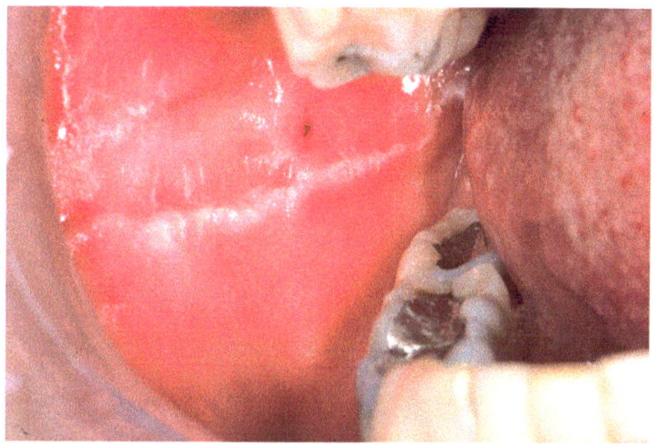

Fig. 2.83 Linea alba on the buccal mucosa

Treatment
There is no cure for lichen sclerosus; in some cases, the lesions regress spontaneously.

2.9.9 Linea Alba

Definition
Benign whitish line on the buccal mucosa at the line of occlusion.

Etiology
Linea alba is caused by mechanical friction from the (pre)molars.

Epidemiology
The estimated prevalence in adults is approximately 1 %.

Clinical Aspects
Always bilateral distribution; is asymptomatic otherwise (Fig. 2.83). A biopsy is only required in case of doubt about the diagnosis.

Histopathology
Histopathologic examination will show hyperkeratosis without signs of epithelial dysplasia.

Treatment
One may look for sharp edges of the teeth, but in general no treatment is required nor is there a need for follow-up.

2.9.10 Lupus Erythematodes, Discoid Type

Definition
Immunologically mediated mucocutaneous disease characterized by scaly, somewhat erythematous patches of the skin (Fig. 2.84) and, in case of oral involvement, lichenoid lesions of the mucosa.

Systemic lupus erythematodes will not be discussed here.

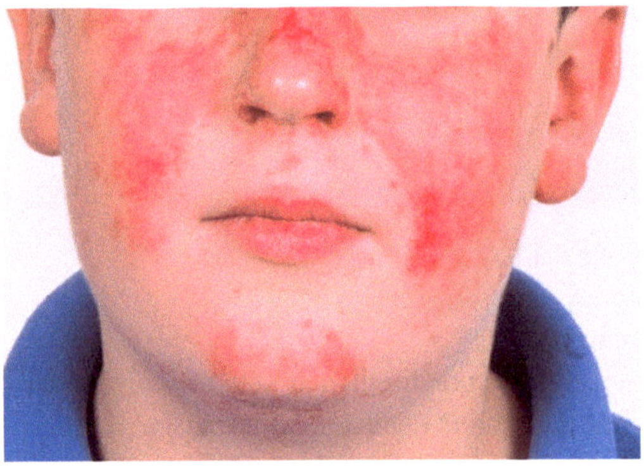

Fig. 2.84 Butterfly appearance of the face in a boy affected by lupus erythematodes

Etiology
The exact etiopathogenesis is unknown.

Epidemiology
May occur already in children; more often in women.

Clinical Aspects
The oral lesions may have a lichenoid appearance or present as tiny reddish nodules, particularly when occurring on the palate. The lesions are often painful and have a bilateral distribution and mainly occur on the buccal mucosa and the palate (Fig. 2.85a, b). Oral lesions rarely occur in the absence of cutaneous lesions.

Clinical Differential Diagnosis
The differential diagnosis includes lichen planus, erythematous candidiasis – particularly when located on the palate – and erythroplakia.

Histopathology
The histopathologic features resemble those of lichen planus, although the lymphocytic subepithelial infiltrate is not that well delineated as in lichen planus and is often located around blood vessels (Fig. 2.86).

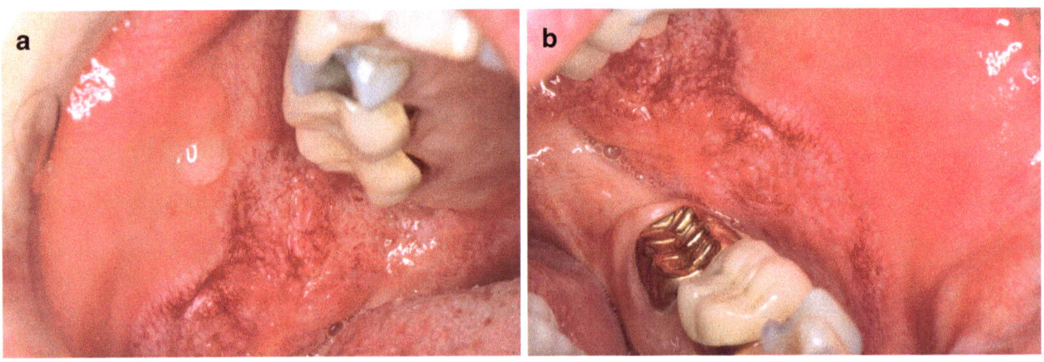

Fig. 2.85 (**a**) Lupus erythematodes of the buccal mucosa. (**b**) The other side of the same patient

Treatment
Topical application of corticosteroids.

2.9.11 Morsicatio

Definition
Benign whitish-yellowish lesion of the oral mucosa caused by habitual biting or chewing.

Epidemiology
Rather common phenomenon; occurs mainly in adults.

Clinical Aspects
Almost always bilateral presentation (Fig. 2.87a, b); may occur on the buccal mucosa but also on the borders of the tongue and on the lips. Whitish-yellowish scaly appearance, asymptomatic otherwise. Usually, a clinical diagnosis. The clinical differential diagnosis includes:

- Candidiasis, hyperplastic type
- Hairy leukoplakia (most likely caused by underlying HIV infection) bilaterally on the borders of the tongue
- Leukoplakia
- Pachyonychia congenita (Fig. 2.88a–d); see also Chap. 4
- White sponge nevus

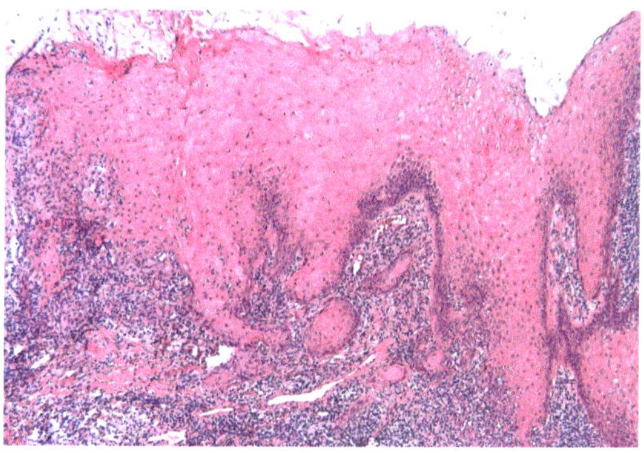

Fig. 2.86 Low-power view of lupus erythematodes

Histopathology
In case of a biopsy, the histopathology will show some acanthosis. There is no epithelial dysplasia. On the surface, a rather characteristic layer of microorganisms is often present (Fig. 2.89).

Treatment
There is no need for treatment, although the patient may want to eliminate his or her habit. In case of bruxism, an occlusal splint may be prepared for wearing at night.

2.9.12 White Sponge Nevus

Definition
Benign autosomal dominant hereditary disorder of the mucosa due to a defect in the process of keratinization related to keratin 4 and keratin 13.

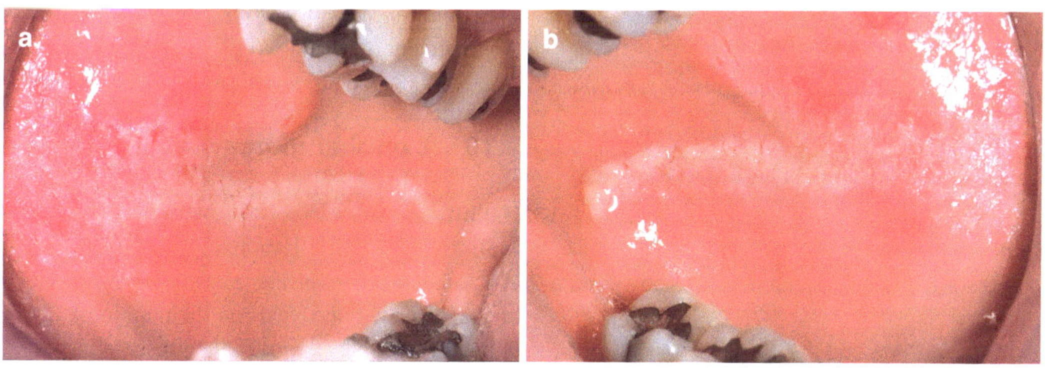

Fig. 2.87 (**a**) Morsicatio of the right cheek. (**b**) Morsicatio of the left cheek in the same patient

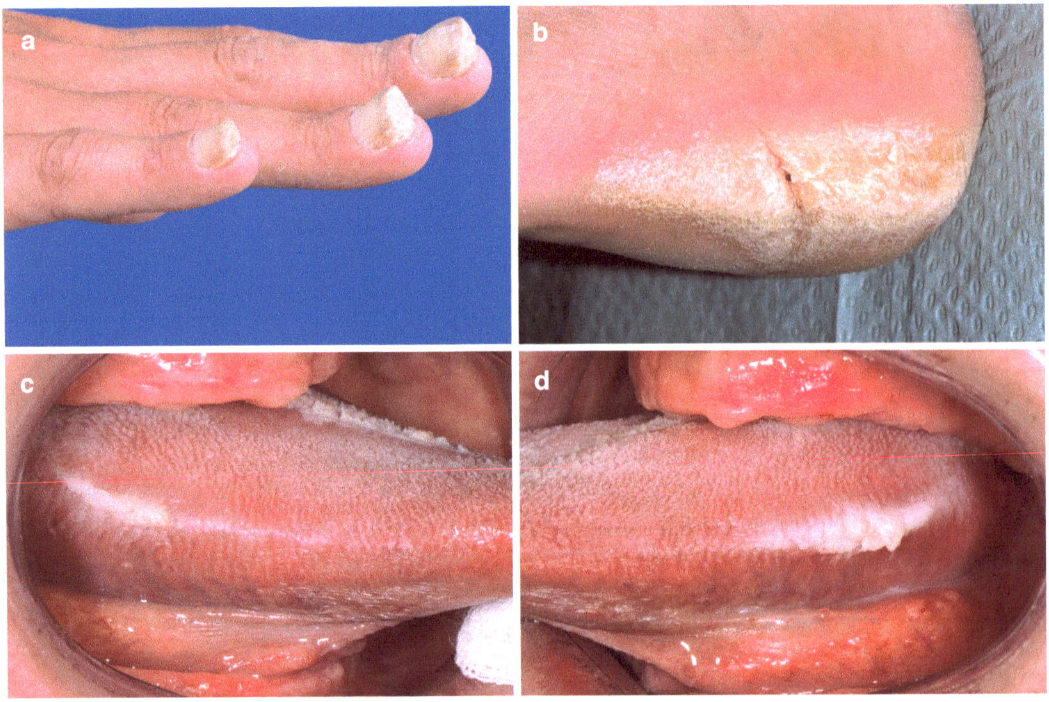

Fig. 2.88 (**a**) Pushed-up nails in a patient suffering from pachyonychia congenita. (**b**) Hyperkeratosis of the heel. (**c**) Morsicatio-like aspect of the right border of the tongue. (**d**) Left side of the tongue of the same patient

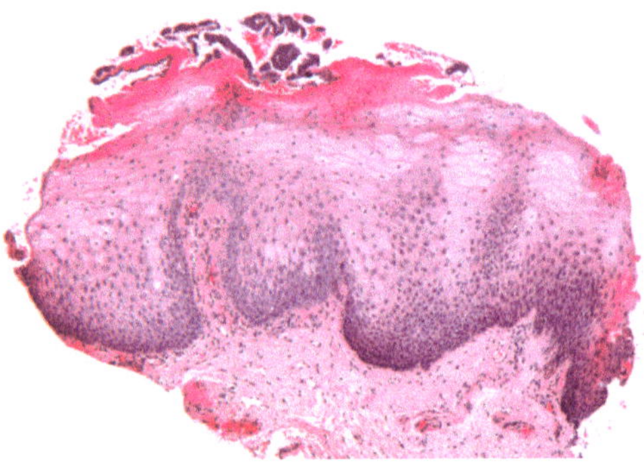

Fig. 2.89 Low-power view of a biopsy from morsicatio; notice the rather characteristic layer of microorganisms on the surface

Epidemiology
Rare disorder; becomes manifest already during childhood.

Clinical aspects
White, thickened mucosa, usually bilateral, of the buccal mucosa and the borders of the tongue (Fig. 2.90a, b). White sponge nevus is primarily a clinical diagnosis for which a biopsy is rarely indicated. The differential diagnosis mainly includes pachyonychia congenita and morsicatio.

Histopathology
There may be hyperkeratosis and acanthosis with distinct vacuolization of the epithelium (Fig. 2.91). These features are not pathognomonic of the disease.

Treatment
No treatment or follow-up is required.

2.10 Lymphangioma

Definition
Malformation of lymphatic vessels, usually becoming manifest already shortly after birth (see also the text on hemangioma and hemangioma-like lesions in the present chapter).

Clinical Aspects
Usually multiple, grapelike small swellings, grayish, of the mucosa, often being traumatized

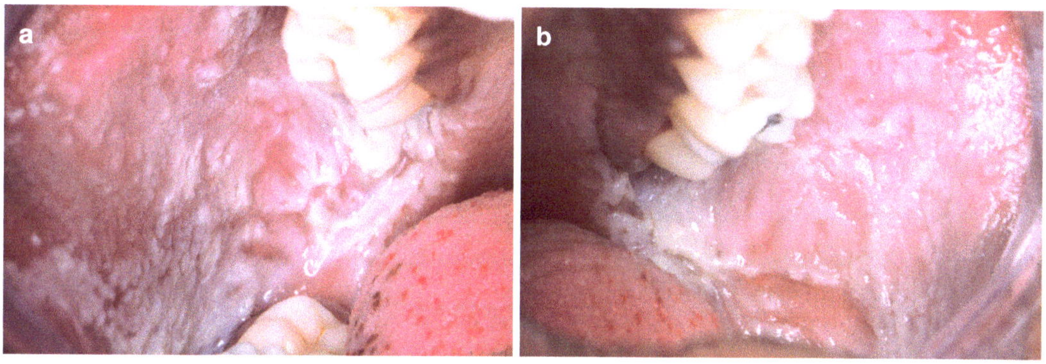

Fig. 2.90 (a) White sponge nevus of the buccal mucosa in a 16-year-old boy. (b) The other side in the same patient

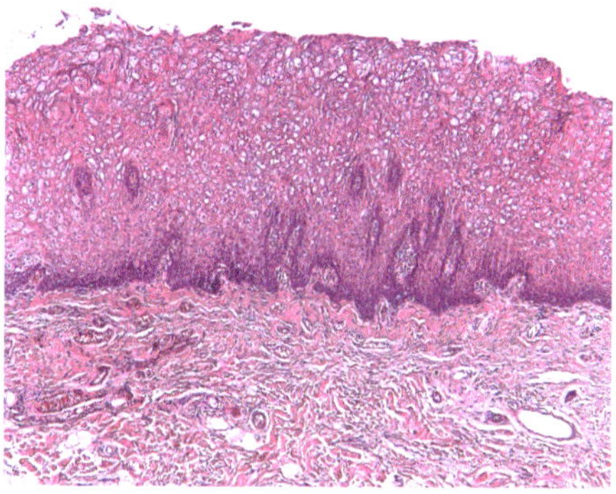

Fig. 2.91 Low-power view of white sponge nevus; notice the vacuolization of the epithelium

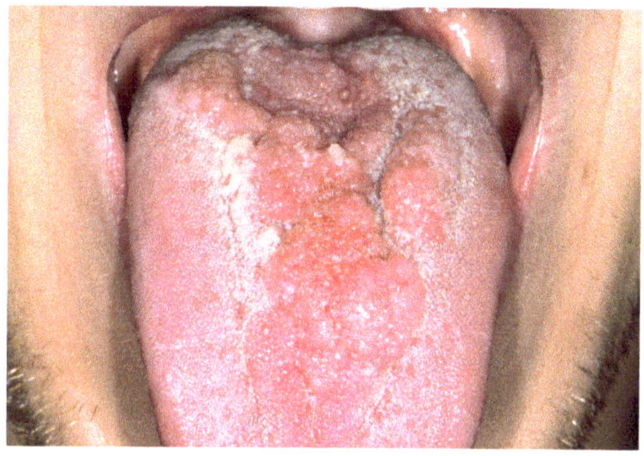

Fig. 2.92 Lymphangioma of the tongue

(Fig. 2.92). Sites of preference are the tongue, floor of mouth, and the cheeks. Secondary infection may lead to recurrent and painful swelling, often resembling a hemangioma-like lesion. In the majority of cases, the diagnosis of intraoral lymphangioma can be made on clinical grounds. Nevertheless, some clinicians prefer to have their clinical diagnosis confirmed by a biopsy.

Imaging

Imaging by MRI and ultrasound examination may be helpful to visualize the extent of the lesion.

Histopathology

Histopathologic examination will reveil widened lymphatic spaces (Fig. 2.93); occasionally, it may be difficult to distinguish lymphatic vessels from blood vessels ("angiomatosis").

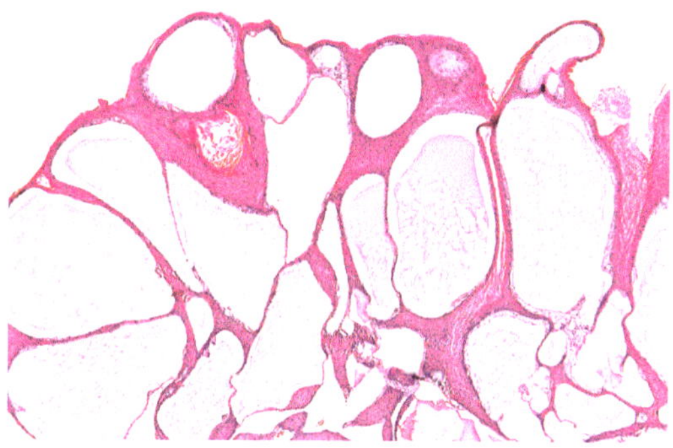

Fig. 2.93 Low-power view of lymphangioma

Treatment

Because of the poor delineation, it is rarely possible to excise a lymphangioma completely. There may be some advantage in excising part of the lesion, e.g., when occurring on the tongue. Laser evaporation may also be useful to somewhat reduce the size of the lesion. In some cases, there may be a role for injection with sclerosing agents. In secondary infection, the administration of antibiotics and corticosteroids may be helpful.

2.11 Metastases, Soft Tissues

Definition
Metastases to the oral soft tissue from a neoplasm located elsewhere in the body.

Epidemiology
Rare phenomenon; mainly in the elderly. The prevalence of the various types of oral metastases correlates with the prevalence of the common tumor sites, such as the breast, lung, prostate, and kidney.

Clinical Aspects
The clinical presentation of a metastasis in the oral soft tissues is usually that of a swelling with or without ulceration (Fig. 2.94). The palatal mucosa and the gingiva are the sites of preference; the tongue and floor of the mouth are rarely involved.

Occasionally, the oral metastasis is the first and only metastasis at that time. In rare cases, the primary cannot be identified.

Treatment
Before treatment is considered, dissemination studies are required to detect the possible presence of metastases at other body sites. In the majority of cases, no curative treatment can be instituted.

2.12 Papillomatous Lesions

2.12.1 Multifocal Epithelial Hyperplasia

Definition
Benign disease of the oral mucosa caused by certain viruses.

Etiology
Caused by the human papillomaviruses type 13 and 32. The exact route of transmission is unknown. Malnutrition may be a predisposing factor.

Epidemiology
Occurs mainly in children but may also affect adults.

Clinical Aspects
Slightly elevated whitish or pinkish papules of the oral mucosa; usually in a multiple fashion, being asymptomatic otherwise. The lips, the borders of the tongue, and the buccal mucosa are the sites of predilection (Figs. 2.95 and 2.96). In general, the diagnosis can be made on the clinical aspects alone, not requiring a biopsy.

Histopathology
Characterized by acanthosis and clubbing of the rete ridges (Fig. 2.97). Occasionally, nuclear inclusion bodies in the upper epithelial layer are observed, sometimes mimicking mitotic activity ("mitosoïds").

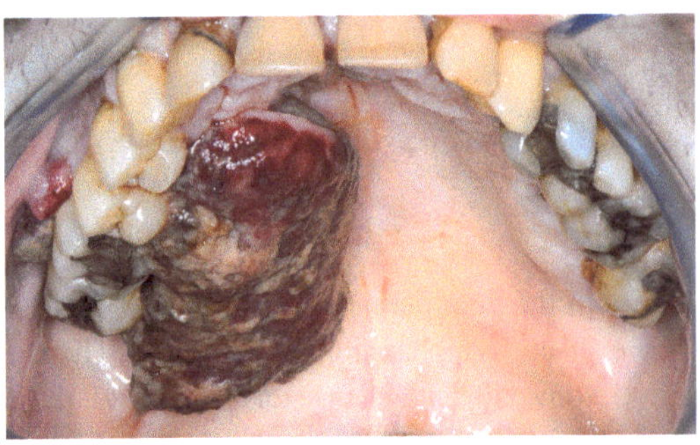

Fig. 2.94 Metastasis from a carcinoma of the lung

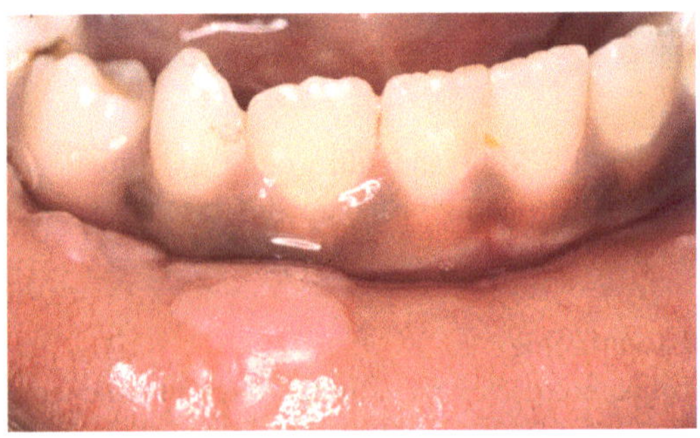

Fig. 2.95 Multifocal epithelial hyperplasia

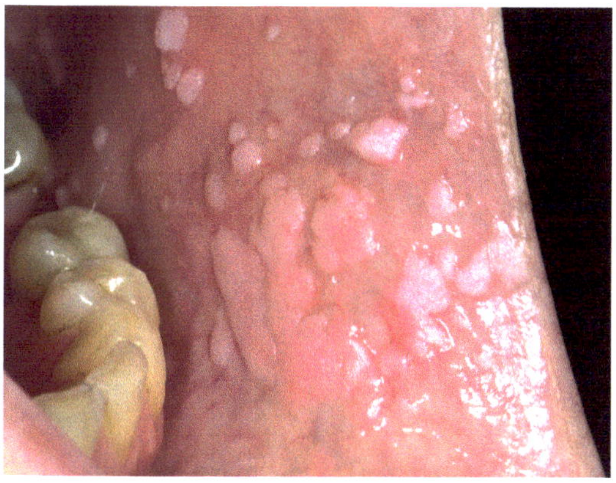

Fig. 2.96 Multifocal epithelial hyperplasia in the buccal mucosa

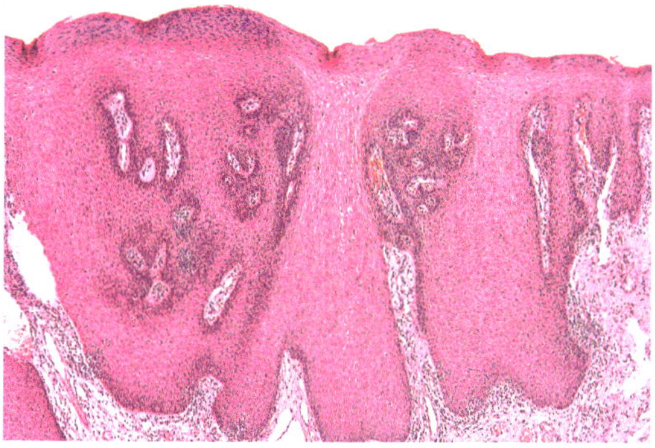

Fig. 2.97 Low-power view of multifocal epithelial hyperplasia; rather diagnostic features

Treatment

Usually spontaneous regression within a few years; some patients insist on surgical excision or laser evaporation.

2.12.2 Papilloma (Squamous Papilloma)

Definition

Benign epithelial neoplasm; counterpart of verruca vulgaris of the skin.

Etiology

Caused by a human papillomavirus, most commonly types 6 and 11; the exact way of transmission is unknown.

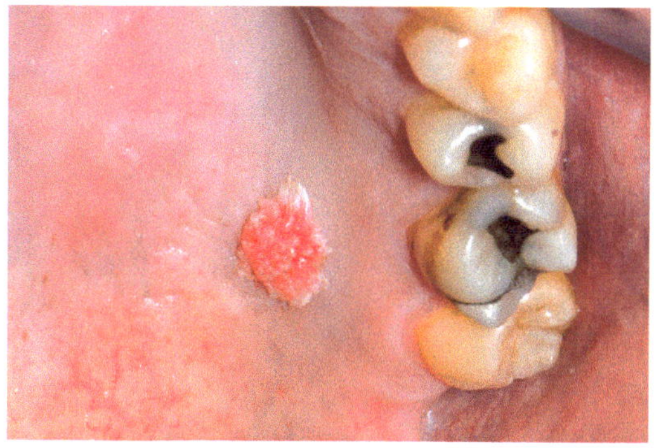

Fig. 2.98 Papilloma of the hard palate. It may be difficult to distinguish this lesion from a sexually transmitted condyloma acuminatum

Epidemiology

More common among children but may also occur in adults; no reliable prevalence rates are available. May occur in HIV-infected patients.

Clinical Aspects

Whitish or pinkish, pedunculated cauliflower-like appearance (Fig. 2.98). The tongue and the soft palate are the sites of preference. There may be a solitary or multiple presentation, being asymptomatic otherwise.

The differential diagnosis relates particularly to the viral-induced (several HPV types may be involved) condyloma acuminatum ("venereal wart") that is sexually transmitted and that may occur in the anogenital region and the mouth. The clinical and histopathologic aspects may mimic a papilloma. Because the lesion is contagious, oral condyloma should be excised.

Histopathology

Proliferation of stratified epithelium arranged in finger-like projections (Fig. 2.99).

Treatment

A papilloma may regress spontaneously; conservative excision may nevertheless be considered. A papilloma rarely recurs.

2.12.3 Verruciform Xanthoma

Definition

Benign wart-like proliferation of the skin and the oral mucosa, characterized by accumulation of

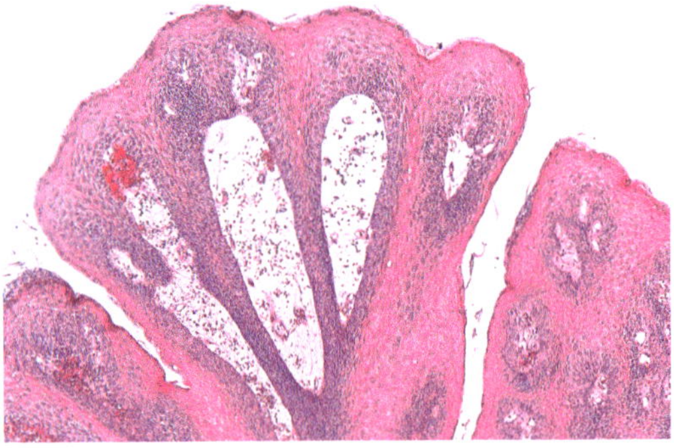

Fig. 2.99 Low-power view of papilloma

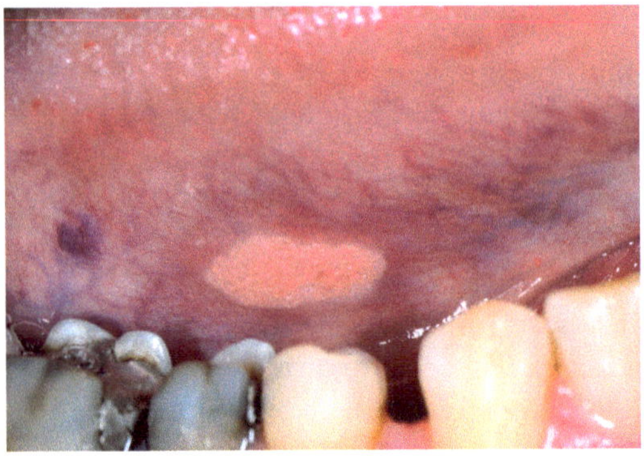

Fig. 2.100 Verruciform xanthoma of the tongue

lipid-laden histiocytes in the subepithelial connective tissue.

Etiology
The cause is actually unknown, although trauma has been suggested to play a role.

Epidemiology
Rare oral lesion.

Clinical Aspects
Slightly elevated, yellowish lesion with a papillary surface, being asymptomatic otherwise (Fig. 2.100). May occur anywhere in the oral cavity.

Histopathology
Histopathologically, elongated rete ridges can be observed showing macrophages with foamy cytoplasm in the lamina propria (Fig. 2.101).

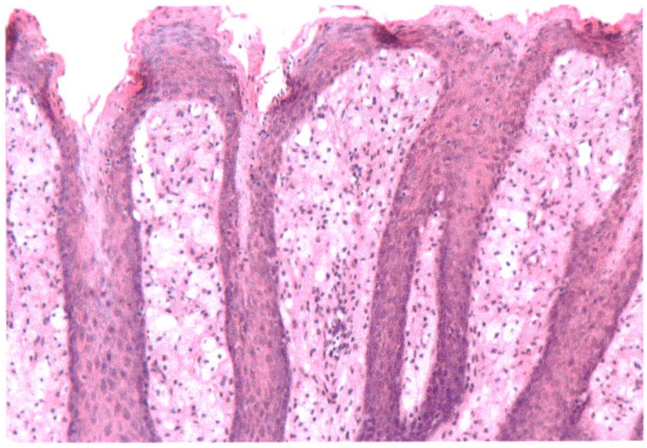

Fig. 2.101 Low-power view of verrucous xanthoma

Treatment
Conservative excision; recurrence is rare.

2.13 Pigmented Lesions

2.13.1 Pigmentation Caused by Amalgam (Amalgam Tattoo) or Other Metals

Definition
Pigmentation of the gingiva or oral mucosa caused by fragments or particles of amalgam ("amalgam tattoo") or other metals.

Etiology
During a tooth extraction, fragments of an amalgam restoration may become inserted in the oral mucosa resulting in a bluish pigmentation or may be entrapped in the alveolus, being detected as a radiopaque spot on a radiograph. Metal particles of a dental bur can also penetrate the oral mucosa.

A rare cause of metal pigmentation of the gingiva is the one caused by prolonged exposition to lead dust, for instance, in painters using lead-containing paint (see Chap. 5); this bluish line is referred to as Burton line.

In some parts of the world, there is the tradition of tattooing the gingiva (see Chap. 5). Furthermore, it is not uncommon today to encounter all kinds of "recreational" tattoos in the oral mucosa.

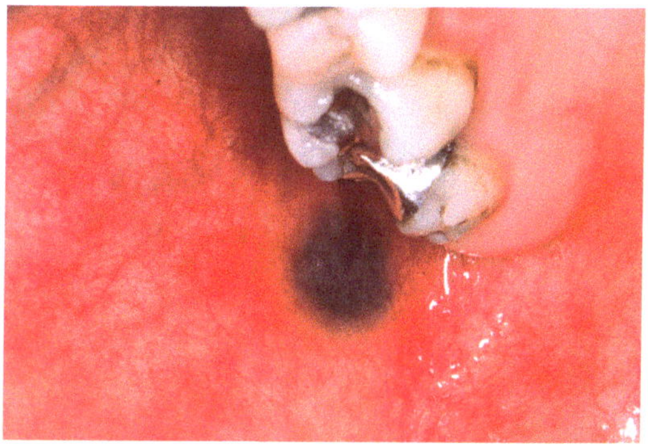

Fig. 2.102 Amalgam tattoo of the buccal mucosa

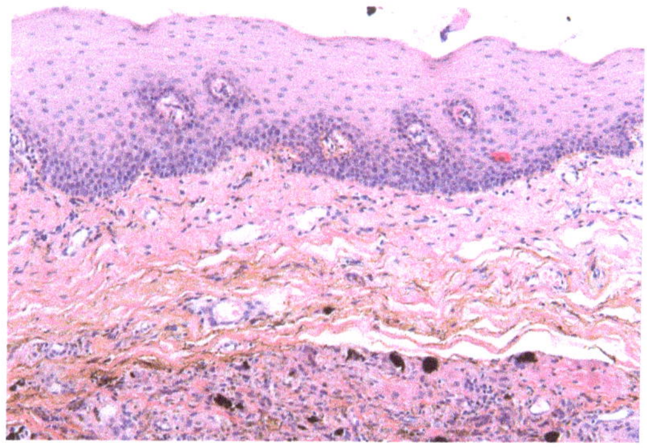

Fig. 2.104 Low-power view of numerous amalgam particles in the connective tissue

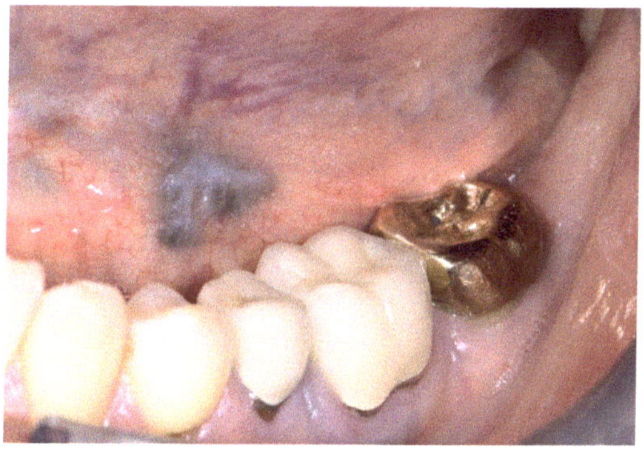

Fig. 2.103 Amalgam tattoo in the floor of the mouth

Epidemiology
Amalgam tattoo is rather common.

Clinical Aspects
Bluish or bluish-grayish flat pigmentation, more or less circumscribed, occurring particularly on the gingiva, the buccal mucosa, and the floor of the mouth (Figs. 2.102 and 2.103). Is asymptomatic otherwise; remains unchanged, lifelong. The differential diagnosis includes:

- Melanin pigmented lesions, such as a nevus nevocellularis and melanoma, may resemble metal pigmentation.
- Hemochromatosis (systemic diseases in which there is an increased iron content of the serum, resulting in discoloration of the skin and the mucosas)
- Pigmentation on the palate due to the use of certain drugs, e.g., antimalarian drugs that may also be used for rheumatic disease

In the majority of cases, the diagnosis of amalgam tattoo can be made on clinical ground alone. In case of doubt, a biopsy should be taken.

Histopathology
Metal particles can usually easily be identified as such at histopathologic examination (Fig. 2.104), but the exact type of metal requires additional examing techniques, if of relevance.

Treatment
Treatment or follow-up is not indicated.

2.13.2 Melanin Pigmentation

Definition
Pigmentation caused by deposition of melanin in the oral mucosa.

Etiology
Physiologic phenomenon in the dark-skinned population, often referred to as racial pigmentation, particularly occurring on the gingiva but also on other sites, such as buccal the mucosa, tongue, and palate (Fig. 2.105).

Although not much discussed in the literature, melanin pigmentation seems to be part of the aging process like it occurs in the skin.

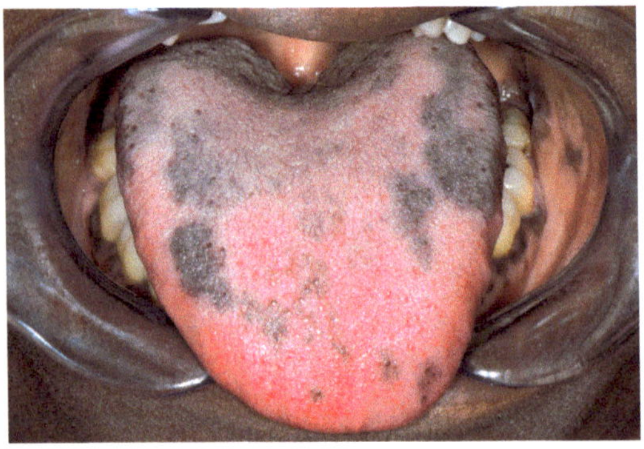

Fig. 2.105 Racial pigmentation of the tongue

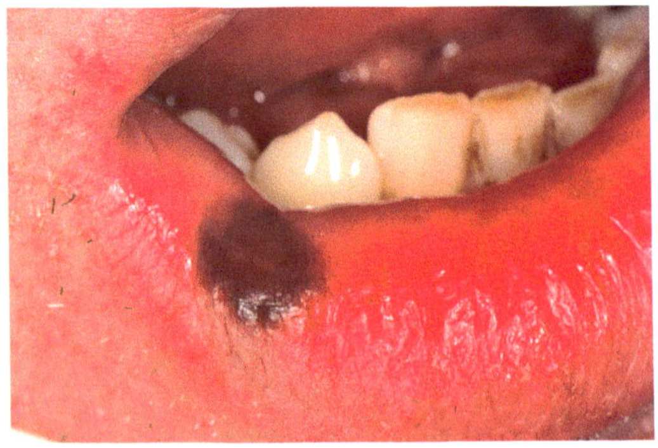

Fig. 2.107 Smokers' melanosis of the lower lip

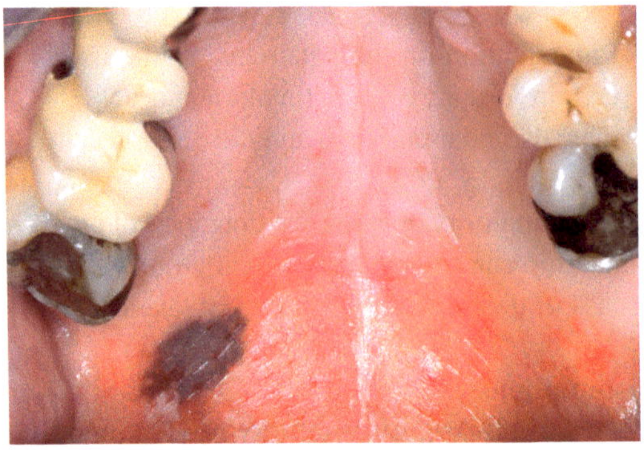

Fig. 2.106 Melanosis, asymptomatic. Excision recommended for histopathologic verification

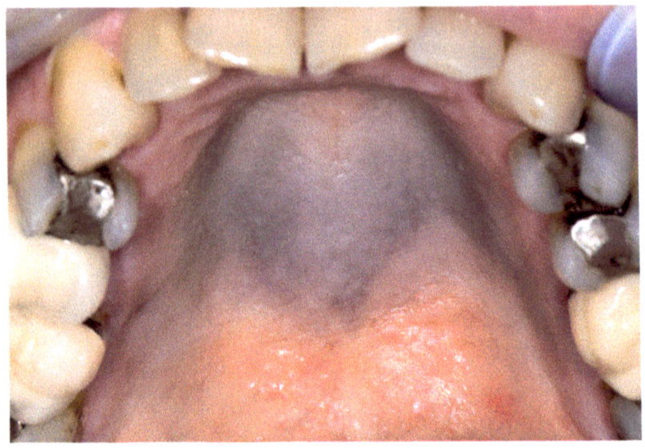

Fig. 2.108 Pigmentation of the palatal mucosa due to the use of hydroxychloroquine

In case of idiopathic melanin pigment deposition, one may be dealing with a prestage of melanoma (Fig. 2.106).

Another cause of melanin pigmentation consists of excessive smoking habits (smokers' melanosis), particularly in the anterior part of the mouth but also on the buccal mucosa. After cessation of the smoking habits, the pigmentation will disappear in some months (Fig. 2.107).

Side effect of certain drugs, e.g., hydroxychloroquine, particularly on the palate (Fig. 2.108); it is a harmless phenomenon, and there is no need to change the medication.

Adrenal insufficiency, as is the case in Addison disease, may result in generalized brownish discoloration of the skin and mucosas; when treating the underlying disease, the discoloration will disappear in a matter of a few months (Fig. 2.109a, b).

Melanin pigmentation can also be a manifestation of the hereditary Peutz-Jeghers syndrome, particularly occurring around the eyes and the lips and also often affecting the buccal mucosa (Fig. 2.110a, b). Genetic counseling is important and patients should be aware of having an increased risk of developing intestinal neoplasms and neoplasms, benign or malignant, at other sites, e.g., the breast.

Clinical Aspects

Idiopathic melanin pigmentation may occur as a localized, small lesion ("melanotic macule") but also as a large, poorly circumscribed lesion, usually flat and asymptomatic otherwise. Such lesion may occur everywhere in the oral cavity. Particularly in case of dark brown-black discoloration or in case of a thickened texture, one may be dealing with a pigmented nevus or a melanoma.

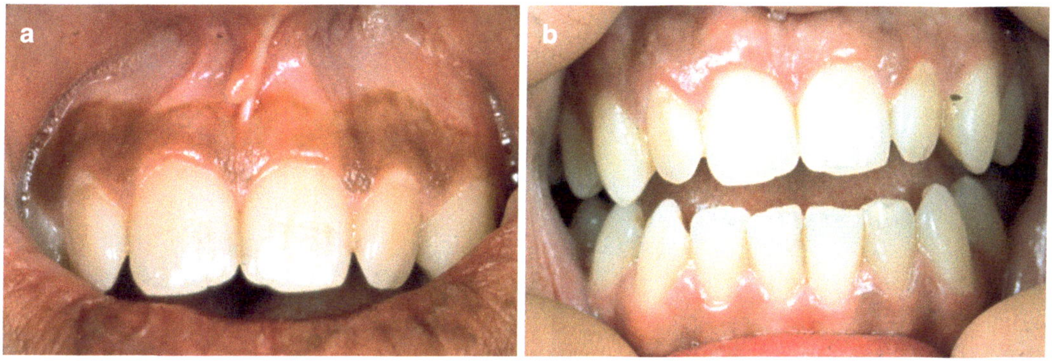

Fig. 2.109 (**a**) Melanin pigmentation in a patient affected by Addison disease. (**b**) Disappearance of the pigmentation a few months after treatment of Addison disease

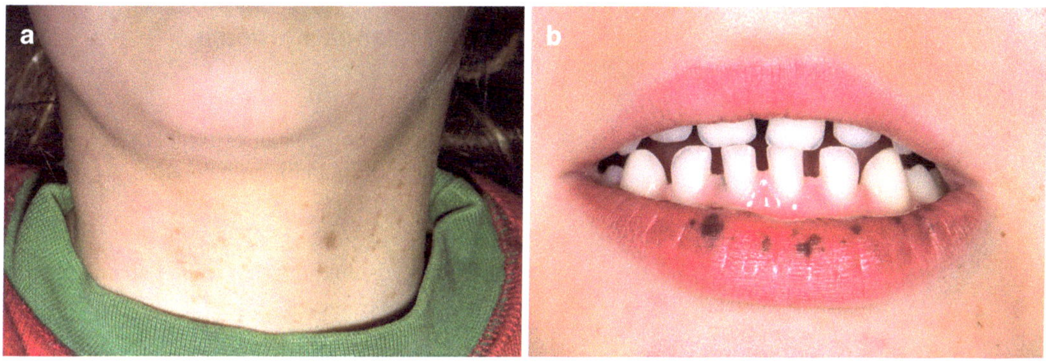

Fig. 2.110 (**a**) A 6-year-old girl with Peutz-Jeghers syndrome. (**b**) Multiple pigmented spots on the lower lip

Histopathology

In case of idiopathic melanin pigmentation, the histopathology will usually show only some increase of melanin pigment in the basal cell layer of the epithelium without atypia of the melanocytes; some refer to this finding as "melanosis." Such lesion may be a precursor lesion of melanoma, particularly when occurring on the palate or the upper or lower gingiva. Unfortunately, there are no markers to predict possible malignant transformation.

Treatment

Idiopathic melanin pigmentation may be removed, if feasible, although it is actually unknown whether such removal will decrease the low risk of future melanoma development. In case of large or multiple idiopathic melanin pigmentations, follow-up, e.g., twice a year, is recommended in order to detect any possible clinical changes.

2.13.3 Nevus, Pigmented

Definition

Benign neoplasm of melanin-producing nevus cells. There is no evidence that oral nevi are premalignant.

Etiology

Unknown.

Epidemiology

Intraoral nevi are rare and may become manifest already at an early age.

Clinical Aspects

Usually a solitary, slightly elevated lesion on the palate, the buccal mucosa or the gingiva.

The color may vary from blue to brown or even black (Fig. 2.111). The size may vary from a few millimeters up to a few centimeters; a nevus

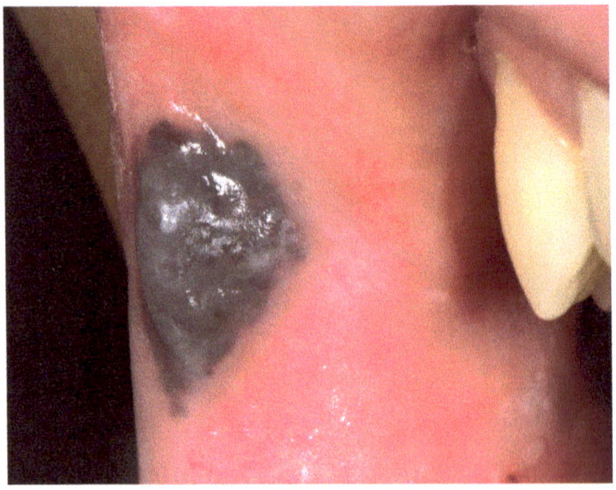

Fig. 2.111 Pigmented nevus in the corner of the mouth; present since early childhood

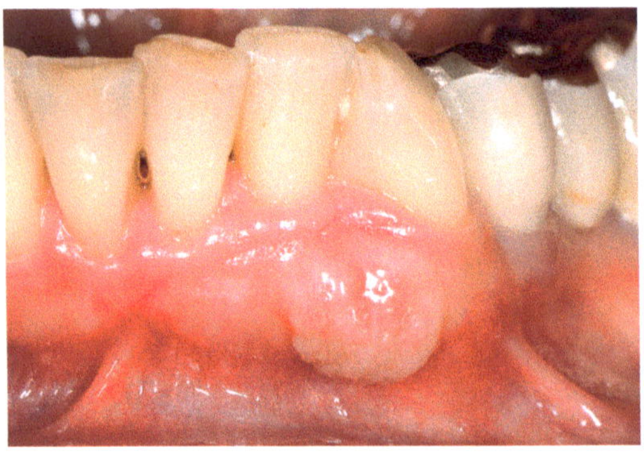

Fig. 2.112 Nonpigmented nevus of the gingiva

is asymptomatic otherwise. An oral nevus may clinically strongly resemble melanoma; therefore, a biopsy is required to establish the diagnosis. Occasionally a nevus is not pigmented (Fig. 2.112).

Histopathology
Based on the location and level of the nevus cells, several subtypes are recognized, such as blue nevus, compound nevus, intramucosal nevus (Fig. 2.113), and junctional nevus. This classification does not have much clinical relevance.

Treatment
A biopsy is required to establish the diagnosis; there is no tendency for recurrence.

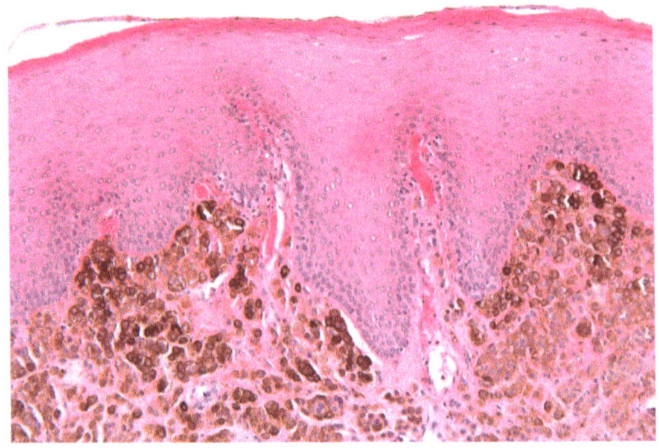

Fig. 2.113 Low-power view of an intramucosal nevus; abundant presence of melanin pigment

2.13.4 Melanoacanthoma

Definition
A melanoacanthoma is an extremely rare benign reactive type of melanin pigmentation.

Etiology
The etiology is unknown. In some patients, there is a history of trauma.

Epidemiology
Mainly occurs in dark-skinned people, particularly in adult women.

Clinical Aspects
Usually a solitary, flat brownish pigmentation. The buccal mucosa is the site of predilection. Symptoms of burning have been reported. Since a melanoacanthoma may mimic a melanoma, a biopsy is required to establish a firm diagnosis.

Histopathology
The hallmark is the distribution of dendritic cells throughout the epithelium and acanthosis of the epithelium.

Treatment
Once the diagnosis has been established, there is no need for treatment. Occasionally, regression occurs in time.

2.13.5 Melanoma

Definition
Malignant proliferation of melanocytes.

Etiology
In contrast to melanomas of the skin, where excessive sun exposure is an important etiologic factor, no etiologic factors are known for oral melanoma.

Epidemiology
Of all melanomas that may arise in the body, less than 1 % arises in the oral mucosa. Oral melanomas usually affect patients above 40 years.

Clinical aspects
Brownish-bluish or even black discoloration of the oral mucosa, sometimes plaque-like or ulcerative. In rare cases, there is absence of clinical visible pigmentation ("amelanotic melanoma") (Figs. 2.114, 2.115, and 2.116). A melanoma may be preceded for several years by pigmentation without histopathologic signs of melanocytic atypia. The palate and gingiva of the mandible and maxilla are the sites of preference. In some cases, melanomas are asymptomatic otherwise, while in other cases, pain or increased mobility of teeth in case of gingival involvement is present.

In very rare instances, an oral melanoma is a metastasis from a melanoma located elsewhere in the body.

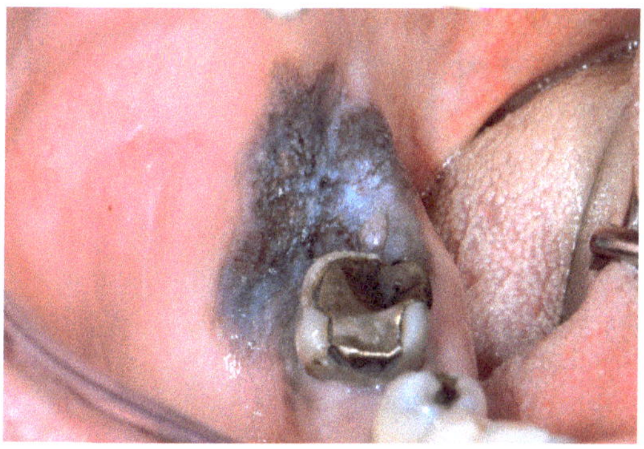

Fig. 2.114 Melanoma in the trigonum region, initially mistaken for amalgam tattoo

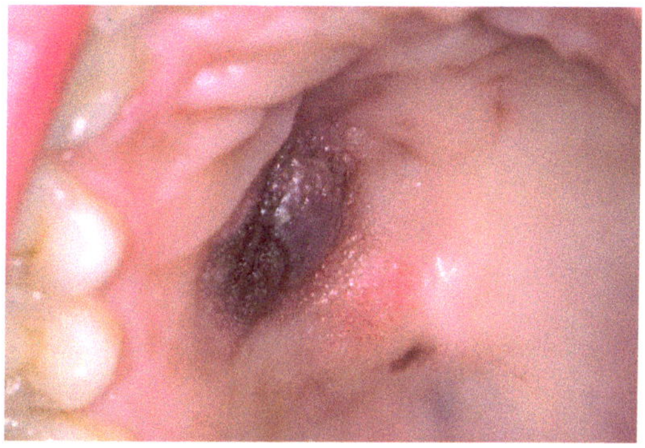

Fig. 2.115 Melanoma of the palate in a 33-year-old woman

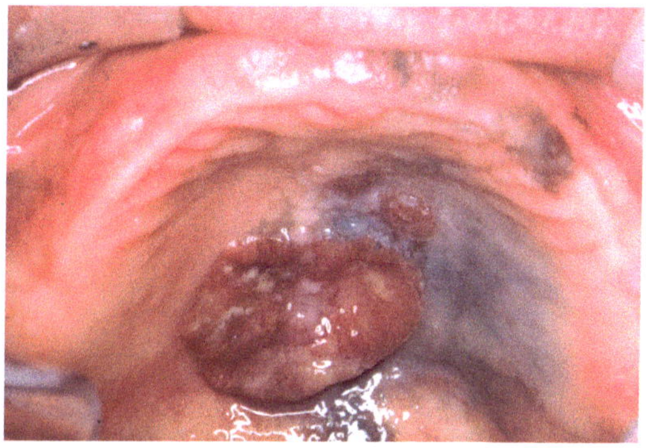

Fig. 2.116 Melanoma of the palate; notice the surrounding mucosal pigmentation

There is an ongoing debate about the question whether an incisional biopsy of a melanoma will enhance the risk of metastatic spread. An excisional biopsy of an oral melanoma is rarely feasible because of anatomic limitations.

Histopathology
There is wide histologic variety of melanomas, such as spindle cell type and clear cell type (Fig. 2.117).

Treatment
Wide surgical removal. Radiotherapy is not effective and there is as yet no adequate chemotherapy or immunotherapy available, although in recent years some promising results have been obtained

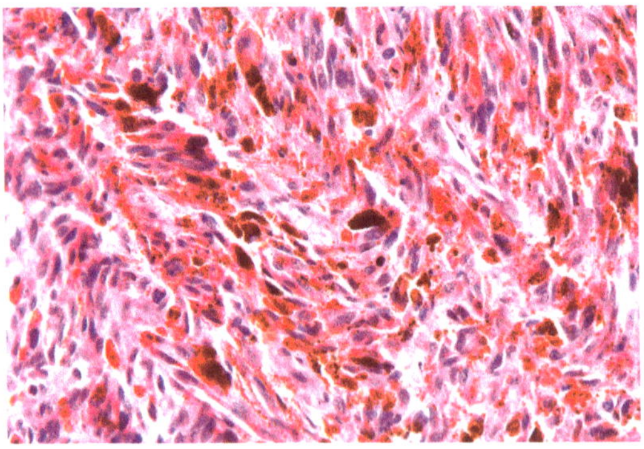

Fig. 2.117 Abundant melanin pigment in melanoma

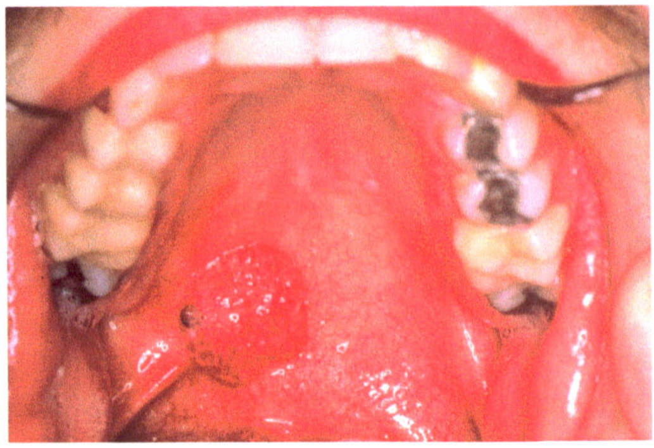

Fig. 2.118 Rhabdomyosarcoma of the palate in a 26-year-old man

with immunotherapy, at least in cutaneous melanomas. The prognosis of oral melanoma is rather poor, the 5-year survival being some 20 %, mainly due to local recurrence and metastatic spread either through the lymph vessels or the blood vessels.

2.14 Sarcomas of the Soft Tissues

Definition
Malignant neoplasm of mesenchymal tissues.

Epidemiology
Of all cancers that may arise in the oral cavity, approximately 1 % represents soft tissue sarcomas. The estimated incidence is one per million population per year. Oral sarcomas may occur at all ages.

Clinical Aspects
Non-characteristic swelling of the oral soft tissues, usually without ulceration (Fig. 2.118).

Metastatic spread mainly occurs through the blood vessels.

Histopathology
There is a wide variety of soft tissue sarcomas, such as fibrosarcoma, liposarcoma, rhabdomyosarcoma, leiomyosarcoma, and neurosarcoma. Quite often the pathologist needs a panel of immunohistochemical stains to arrive at the proper subtype of a soft tissue sarcoma.

Treatment
In general, radical surgery is the preferred treatment modality, sometimes in combination with chemotherapy or radiotherapy. The prognosis depends on the radicality of the surgical excision and the presence or absence of hematogenous spread.

2.15 Stomatitis

Definition
Stomatitis is a general term for inflammatory changes of the oral mucosa. In case of inflammatory changes caused by irradiation or chemotherapy, the term mucositis is used.

Nicotinic stomatitis is a separate entity and will be discussed in Chap. 6.

Etiology
There is a wide variety of causative factors, such as poor oral hygiene in patients wearing a denture, resulting in denture stomatitis of the palate ("stomatitis prothetica") (Fig. 2.119).

Venereal diseases such as gonorrhea may present as stomatitis, e.g., on the palate (Fig. 2.120). Furthermore, some medications, e.g., azathioprine, may cause stomatitis, with or without ulceration, usually in a bilateral pattern (Fig. 2.121a, b).

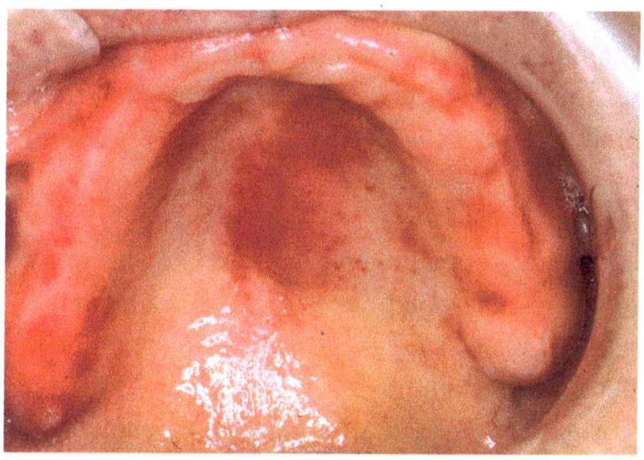

Fig. 2.119 Denture stomatitis

Herpes simplex infection, erythema multiforme, anemia, uremia, and irradiation of the oral cavity are other sources of stomatitis (Fig. 2.122).

Clinical Aspects

Fiery red, sometimes ulcerative aspect of the oral mucosa, and presenting in a bilateral distribution; also the gingiva may be involved ("gingivostomatitis").

Laboratory Examination

The indication for laboratory examination depends on the provisional diagnosis.

Treatment

Depends on the type of stomatitis.

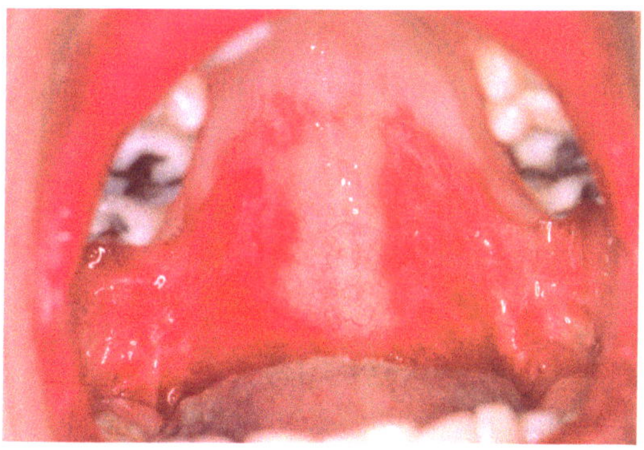

Fig. 2.120 Gonococcal stomatitis

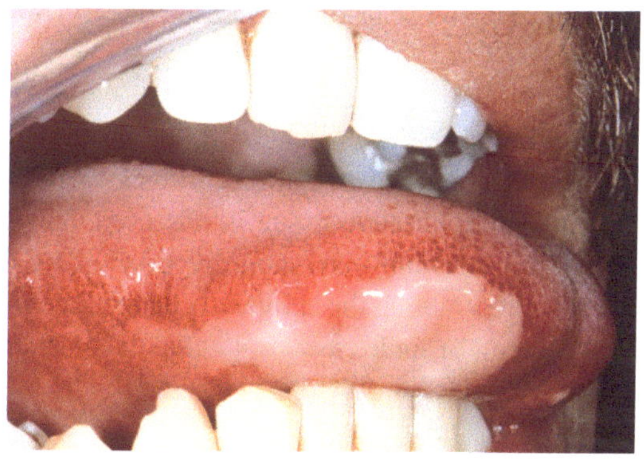

Fig. 2.122 Radiation mucositis of the tongue

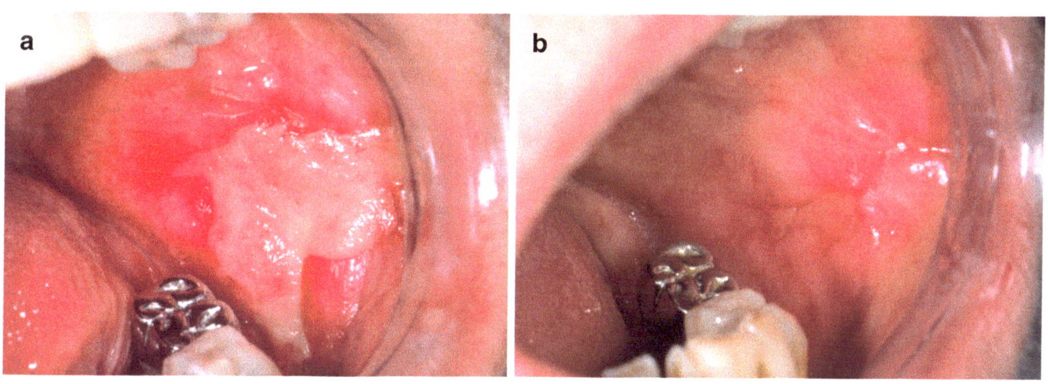

Fig. 2.121 (**a**) Drug stomatitis due to the use of azathioprine. (**b**) Same patient 2 weeks after withdrawal of the drug

2.16 Submucous Fibrosis

Definition

Scarring of the submucosa of the oral epithelium caused by chewing betel quid, consisting of a.o. areca nut, being often mixed with tobacco products. There is an increased risk of squamous cell carcinoma development (potentially malignant disorder).

Etiology

Chronic chewing of betel quid and smoking. Mainly occurs in people originating from Southeast Asia.

Clinical Aspects

Bleaching, pale aspect of the oral mucosa, particularly of the buccal mucosa and the palate (Fig. 2.123). The scarring may result in severe trismus.

Histopathology

On histopathologic examination, fibrosis of the subepithelial connective tissue is observed. The overlying epithelium may show hyperkeratosis, somewhat resembling the epithelial changes seen in morsicatio. In some cases, epithelial dysplasia may be encountered.

Treatment

Cessation of the chewing quid habit will not readily result in improvement of the oral condition.

2.17 Ulcers

2.17.1 Aphthous Ulcers

Definition

Inflammatory-like, painful, recurrent disease of the oral mucosa, also referred to as recurrrent aphthous stomatitis (RAS).

Etiology

The exact etiopathogenesis is unknown; stress has been mentioned as a possible predisposing factor. Other suggested etiologies comprise allergy for certain food substances.

After cessation of smoking habits, some people may become affected by RAS. There is no proper explanation for this event.

Epidemiology

The estimated prevalence is approximately 10 %, which means that one out of ten persons may occasionally suffer from the disease. RAS mainly affects young adults.

Clinical Aspects

Aphthous ulcers mainly affect nonkeratinized mucosa such as the buccal mucosa and the lips (Figs. 2.124 and 2.125), either as a solitary lesion or in a multiple fashion. Aphthous ulcers are usually well circumscribed and are not indurated at palpation. There are three types of aphthous ulcerations:

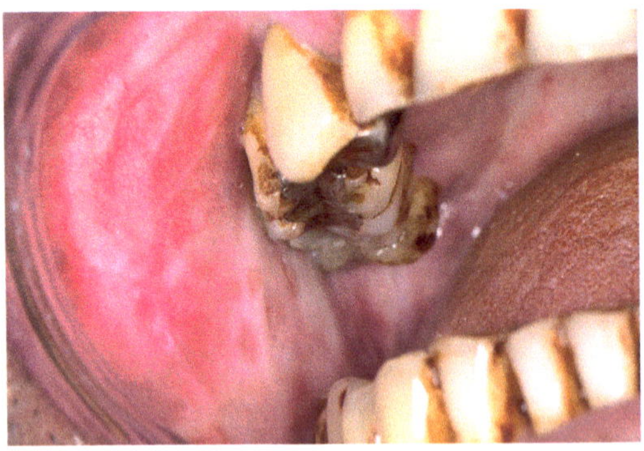

Fig. 2.123 Bleaching, pale aspect of the buccal mucosa in submucous fibrosis

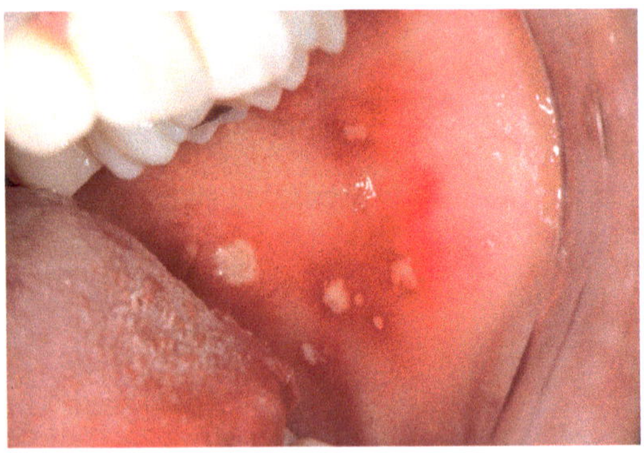

Fig. 2.124 Multiple aphthous ulcers, minor type

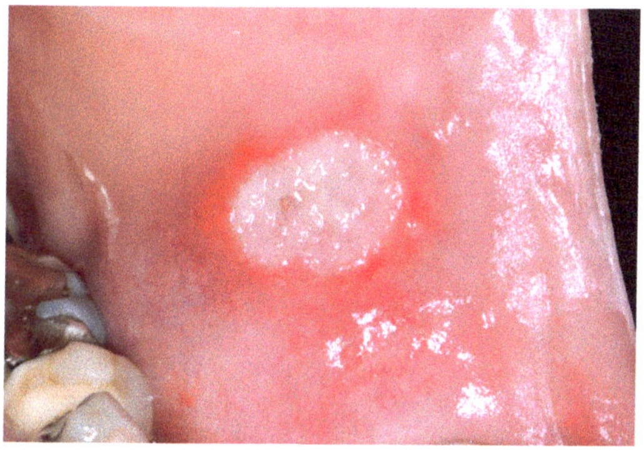

Fig. 2.125 Aphthous ulcer, major type

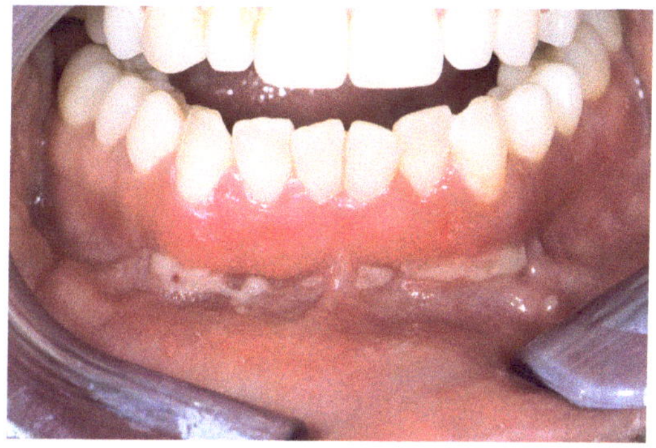

Fig. 2.126 Slit-like ulceration in the mucobuccal fold suggestive of Crohn's disease

- *Minor* type: <0.5 cm; most common type; healing takes place within a week without scarring.
- *Major* type: >0.5 cm; healing may take several weeks and often results in scarring.
- *Herpetiform* type: numerous pinpoint-sized, extremely painful ulcers; spontaneous healing within 1–2 weeks without scar formation.

Differential Diagnosis

Aphthous ulcers may be part of the rather rare Behcet's syndrome, consisting of aphthous-like ulcers on the genitals, conjunctivitis, uveitis, and erythema nodosum of the skin.

Aphthous-like ulcers may also occur in Crohn's disease in which case the biopsy may demonstrate the presence of a granuloma with the presence of multinucleated giant cells (Figs. 2.126 and 2.127), celiac disease, periodic fever-aphthous-stomatitis-pharyngitis-adenitis (PFAPA), erythema multiforme, herpes simplex/herpes zoster, hematinic deficiency (iron, folate, B12), immunodeficiency (HIV), and neutropenia.

Laboratory Examinations

In an otherwise healthy patient, there is hardly any role for laboratory studies. The histopathologic aspects of aphthous ulcers are nonspecific and just show an ulcer with signs of subacute or chronic inflammation.

Treatment

There is no effective treatment or prevention. In the early stage or prestage ("prodromal stage"), local application of corticosteroids, such as triamcinolonacetonide ointment 0.1 %, three times a day, may in some patients prevent aphthous ulcers to break through or may speed up healing.

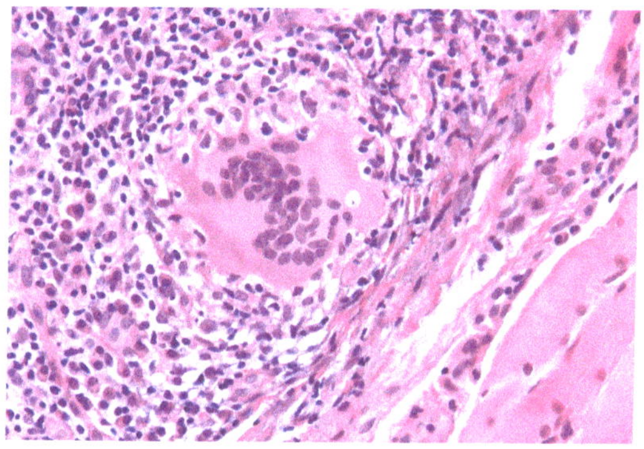

Fig. 2.127 Biopsy of oral ulcer in Crohn's disease; granuloma formation and multinucleated giant cells

Systemic corticosteroids should only be considered in severe cases (1 mg per kilogram body weight orally for 10 days).

2.17.2 Ulcers in Viral Infections

2.17.2.1 Herpes Simplex

Primary Infection

Definition

Herpes simplex infection can be primary or secondary (recurrent), affecting the skin and also the oral mucosa and the gingiva (gingivostomatitis).

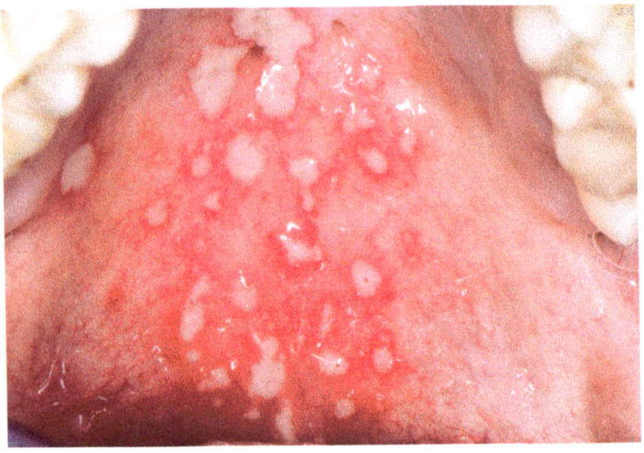

Fig. 2.128 Multiple herpetiform ulcers; notice the bilateral distribution

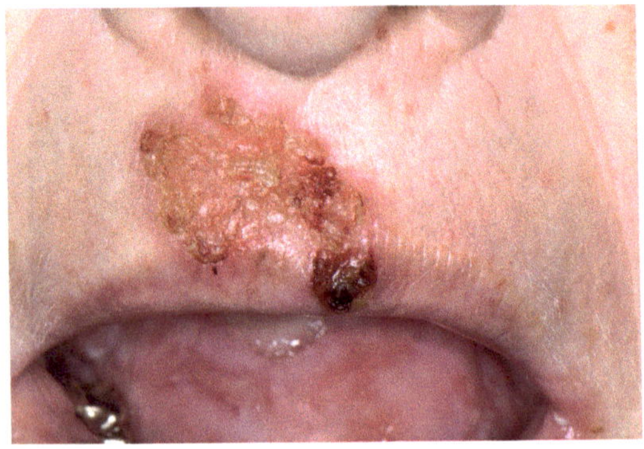

Fig. 2.129 Secondary herpes simplex infection affecting the upper lip (herpes labialis)

Etiology
Herpes simplexvirus type 1 is the most common type. Transmission takes place via saliva. After the primary infection, the virus remains dormant lifelong, being reactivated in some people.

Epidemiology
The majority of the population will become infected at an early age.

Clinical Aspects
A primary herpetic infection causes fever and general malaise. The oral lesions consist of multiple, bilateral, vesicles that easily rupture, leaving a superficial, aphthous-like, and painful ulcer behind (Fig. 2.128). Herpetiform ulcers mainly affect the keratinized mucosa such as palatal mucosa, the gingiva, and the dorsum of the tongue. The main clinical differential diagnosis includes the early stage of erythema multiforme.

Laboratory Examination
In an otherwise healthy patient, there is no role for additional laboratory examinations nor for histopathologic examination. In case of unusual clinical features, one may try to culture the content of an intact vesicle or to collect some cells from a vesicle for cytologic examination (presence of intranuclear inclusion bodies) or to look for serum values of antibodies directed against the herpesvirus.

Treatment
Spontaneous healing of the disease will take place in approximately 1 week; there is no scar formation. In an otherwise healthy patient, there is hardly any advantage in prescribing antiviral drugs. It is important to advice the patient to maintain optimum oral care. Temporary mouthrinses with chlorhexidine 0.12 % and analgesics may be prescribed.

Secondary or Recurrent Infection

Definition
Secondary or recurrent herpes simplex infection due to reactivation of the virus (see also Chap. 3).

Etiology
The exact mechanism of the reactivation is unknown. Predisposing factors may be stress, exposure to sunlight (herpes labialis), and immunosuppression.

Clinical Aspects
Less severe signs and symptoms than in primary infection; no general malaise. Usually involves the mucocutaneous junction of the lips (herpes labialis) and rarely the intraoral mucosa. The clinical presentation consists of multiple vesicles (Fig. 2.129).

Laboratory Examination
There is rarely a need for any type of laboratory examination.

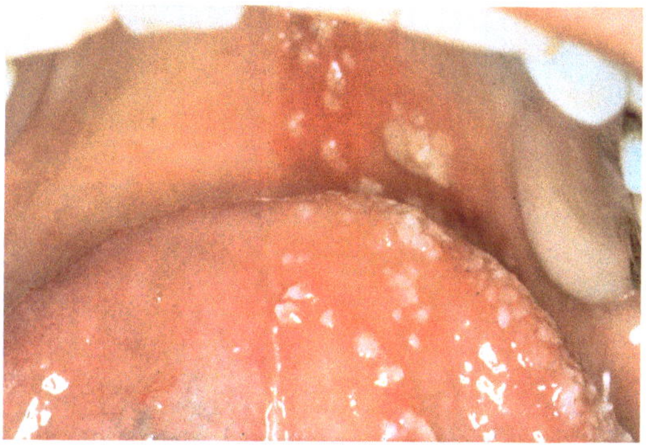

Fig. 2.130 Herpes zoster of the tongue; notice the unilateral distribution

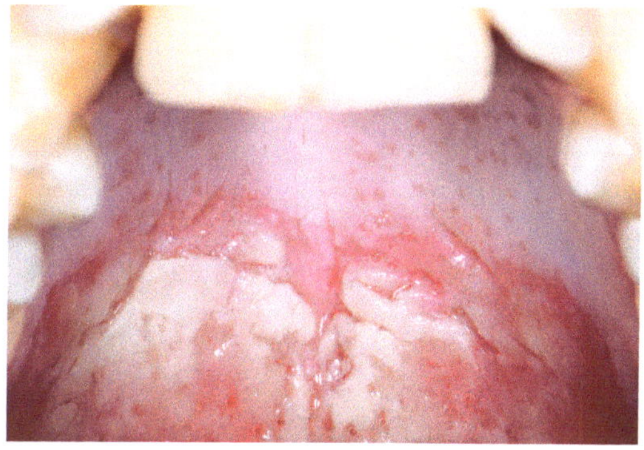

Fig. 2.131 Erythema multiforme of the palate

Treatment

In otherwise healthy patients, there is hardly an indication for antiviral treatment. Healing usually takes place within 1–2 weeks. Recurrences are not uncommon. In rare instances, one may consider to prescribe antivirals as a preventive measure.

2.17.2.2 Herpes Zoster (Shingles)

Definition

Infection caused by reactivation of varicella-zoster virus (herpesvirus type 3) that causes chickenpox during childhood.

Etiology

Immunosuppression, old age, and stress are among the possible predisposing factors.

Epidemiology

Occurs mainly in elderly people.

Clinical Aspects

Unlateral involvement of the skin or the oral mucosa; painful (Fig. 2.130). There may be a prodromal stage of some days in which the patient suffers from general malaise and fever. Some patients will develop postherpetic neuralgia.

Treatment

Systemic antiviral treatment, preferably prescribed within a few days after the onset of the vesicles.

2.17.3 Ulcers in Mucocutaneous Diseases

2.17.3.1 Erythema Multiforme

Definition

Inflammatory-like mucocutaneous disease. A severe variant is the Stevens-Johnson syndrome (involvement of the eyes and the genitals). Another, somewhat debatable, variant is the Lyell syndrome based on toxic epidermal necrolysis.

Etiology

Unknown; possibly associated with herpes simplexvirus. May also be caused by certain drugs, such as sulfonamides, penicillins, and anticonvulsant drugs. Also mycoplasma pneumoniae may play a role in the etiology.

Epidemiology

Rare disease, mainly affecting young adults.

Clinical Aspects

Associated with general malaise. The oral lesions usually become manifest before the cutaneous lesions and may have a stomatitis-like presentation. In many cases, there is crust formation on the lips (Figs. 2.131 and 2.132).

The cutaneous lesions consist of concentric erythematous rings, also referred to as bull's-eye or target lesions (fig. 2.133). In the Stevens-

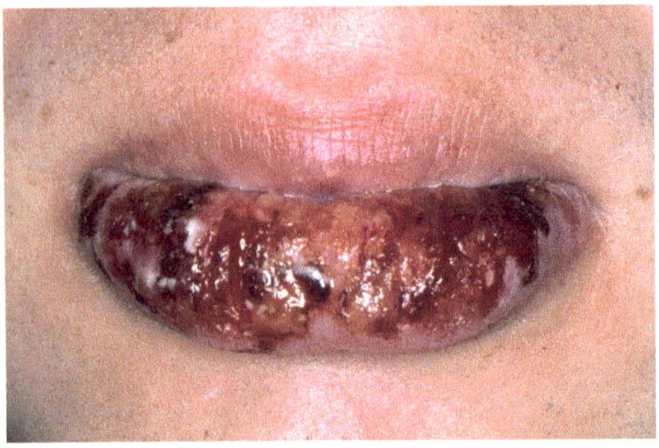

Fig. 2.132 Crust formation of the lower lip in erythema multiforme

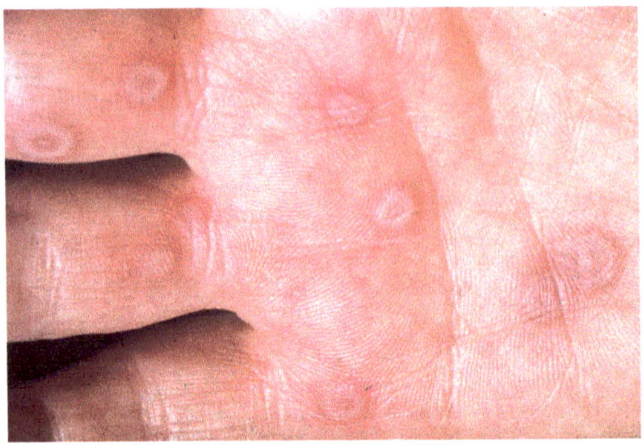

Fig. 2.133 Target or bull's-eye lesion rather typical of erythema multiforme

Johnson syndrome, also the eyes are involved (conjunctivitis) and the genitals (balanitis) (Fig. 2.134).

Histopathologic Examination

Non-characteristic intraepithelial or subepithelial bulla formation. Immunofluorescence examination is not characteristic but may be useful to exclude other vesiculobullous diseases.

Treatment

Erythema multiforme is a self-limiting disease with healing taking place within 2–6 weeks.

Treatment can only be symptomatic. The value of corticosteroids or antivirals is questionable, although there may be a place for the preventive use of antivirals in patients who experience frequent recurrences.

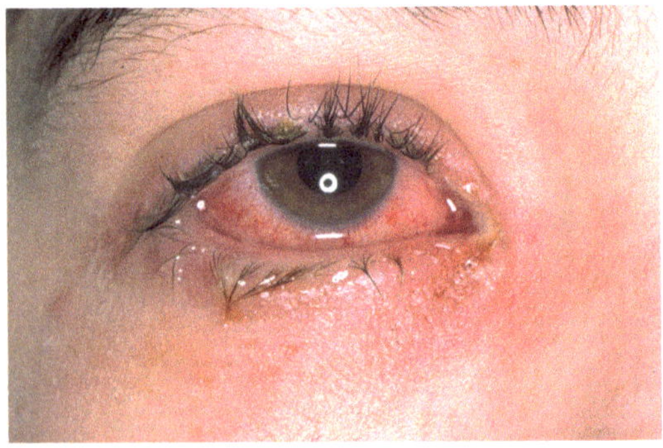

Fig. 2.134 Conjunctivitis in patient suffering from Stevens-Johnson syndrome

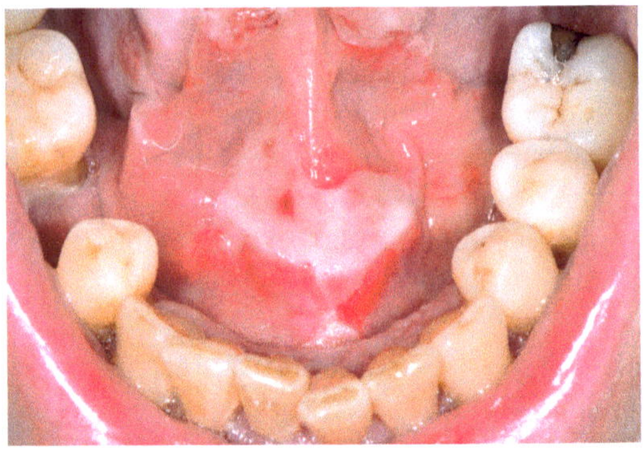

Fig. 2.135 Ulcer in the floor of the mouth caused by pemphigus vulgaris

2.17.3.2 Pemphigus Vulgaris

Definition

Vesiculobullous disease of the skin and the mucosa.

Etiology

The exact etiopathogenesis is unknown; possibly due to immunosuppression.

Epidemiology

Rare disease; more common among women. Pemphigus vulgaris mainly affects adults and elderly patients but occasionally also children.

Clinical Aspects

The mucosal lesions may precede cutaneous involvement and consist of painful blisters that easily rupture, resulting in ulceration of the mucosa and the gingiva (Fig. 2.135). There is a positive Nikolsky phenomenon (on gently rubbing the normal skin or mucosa at a distance of at least 0.5 cm distance from an ulcer, the epithelium will easily separate from the underlying tissue). The clinical differential diagnosis includes erythema multiforme, mucous membrane pemphigoid, drug stomatitis, ulcerative lichen planus, and linear IgA disease. Occasionally, pemphigus vulgaris represents a paraneoplastic phenomenon of an underlying malignant diseases, e.g., a non-Hodgkin lymphoma.

Histopathology

A biopsy taken from perilesional tissue will show suprabasilar bulla formation of the epithelium due to acantholysis of the epithelial cells (Fig. 2.136). On direct immunofluorescent examination, there is positivity for IgG around the epithelial cells ("fishnet pattern"). Indirect immunofluorescent examination will show the presence of circulating antibodies in the serum.

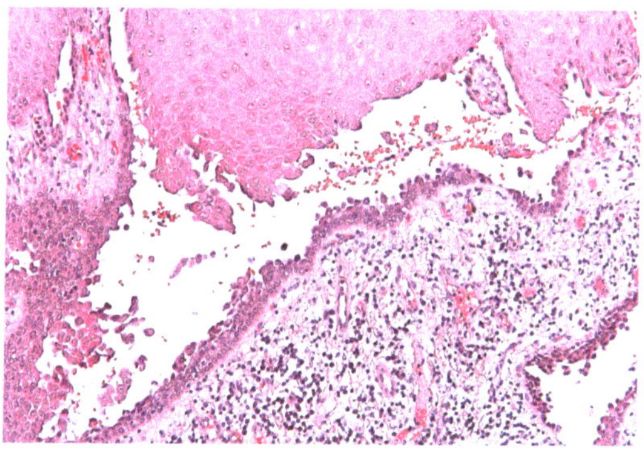

Fig. 2.136 Suprabasilar cleft in the epithelium, suggestive of pemphigus vulgaris; direct IF is required

Treatment

Local, and often systemically, administered corticosteroids, with or without corticosteroids sparing drugs.

2.17.3.3 Mucous Membrane Pemphigoid

Definition

Vesiculobullous disease of the mucosa.

Etiology

Unknown; possibly autoimmune related.

Epidemiology

Mainly occurs in women; usually at an older age.

Clinical Aspects

Usually symmetrical bulla formation and ulceration, painful. May affect all oral subsites, including the gingiva (Fig. 2.137a, b). The clinical differential diagnosis includes erythema multiforme, pemphigus vulgaris, ulcerative lichen planus, and linear IgA disease.

Histopathology

Subepithelial bulla formation (Fig. 2.138). On direct immunofluorescent examination, a band-like positivity of the basement membrane with complement C3 is seen.

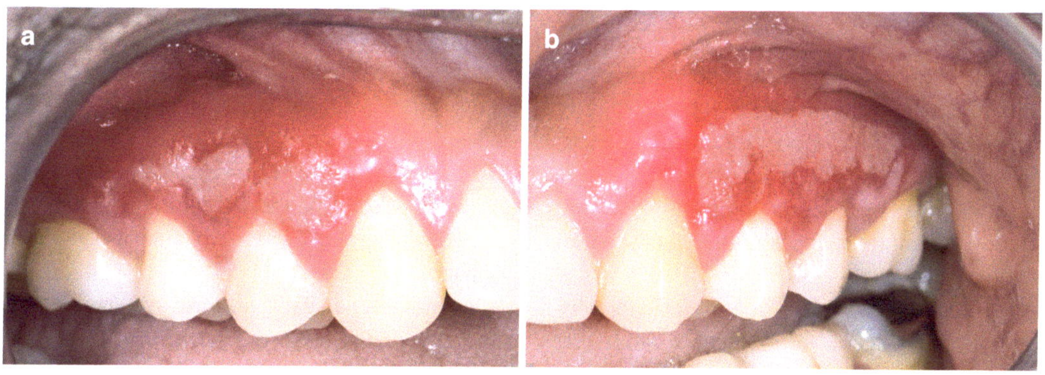

Fig. 2.137 (**a**) Mucous membrane pemphigoid of the alveolar mucosa. (**b**) Other side in the same patient

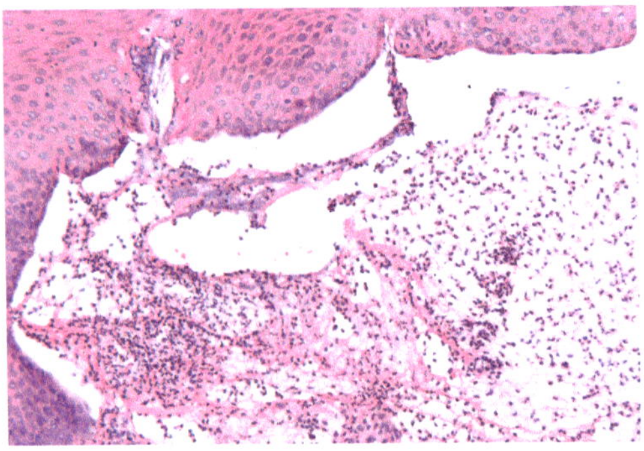

Fig. 2.138 Subbasilar cleft compatible with mucous membrane pemphigoid; direct IF is required

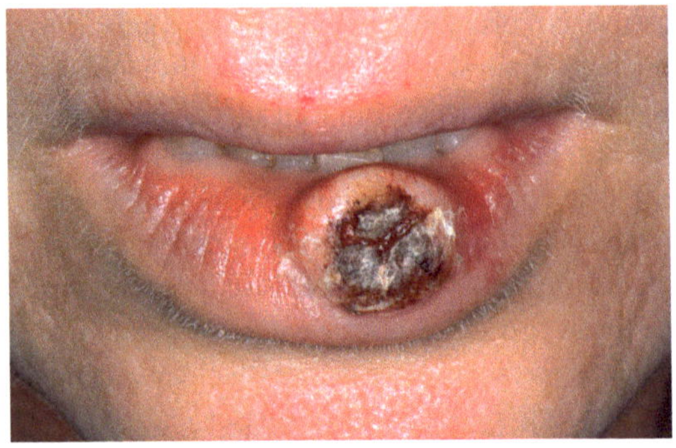

Fig. 2.139 Squamous cell carcinoma of the lower lip

Treatment
Local or systemic corticosteroids.

2.17.4 Ulcer in Squamous Cell Carcinoma

Definition
An oral squamous cell carcinomas (OSCCs) is a malignant neoplasm derived from squamous epithelium of the mucosal surface.

Etiology
Tobacco use and alcohol are the most important etiologic factors. Human papillomavirus (HPV) type 16 may play a role in a small subset of patients with oral cancer. Other factors, such as the use of alcohol-containing mouthrinses, poor oral hygiene, or ill-fitting dentures, do not seem to play a major role. Excessive sun exposure may play a role in the etiology of lower lip cancer.

Immunosuppressed patients, e.g., by the prolonged use of immunosuppressive drugs as in solid organ transplantation, have a slightly increased risk of developing oral cancer, particularly of the lower lip. There are some rare conditions, such as xeroderma pigmentosum and Fanconi's anemia, that predispose to the development of oral cancer.

Some oral cancers arise from preexisting leukoplakia and perhaps also, but much less frequent than in leukoplakia, from preexisting lichen planus.

Epidemiology
The incidence of OSCC differs in different parts of the world and may vary from 3 to 6 per 100,000 population per year. Most OSCCs occur in people above the age of 40 years. In general, men are more often affected than women. The gender distribution is also related to the specific subsite. For instance, lower lip cancer mainly occurs in men and is rare, indeed, in women.

Clinical Aspects
A solitary, sometimes painful ulcer is the most common clinical manifestation of OSCC. There is usually induration at palpation. Occasionally, OSCC presents as a non-ulcerative fibroma-like swelling or wart-like proliferation. An OSCC may also present itself as leukoplakia or erythroplakia.

The lower lip, the borders of the tongue, the floor of the mouth, and the lower alveolar ridge are the sites of predilection (Figs. 2.139, 2.140, 2.141, and 2.142). The anterior part of the hard palate is a very rare site for oral cancer (Fig. 2.143). Occasionally, multiple OSCCs are present simultaneously in the oral cavity or the head and neck region.

In rare instances, a second primary is present outside the head and neck region, particularly related to the lungs, the bladder, and the esophagus.

Occasionally, an OSCC causes referred pain at the side of the cancer; e.g., an OSCC of the right lateral border of the tongue may cause a right-sided ear ache. Another rare presentation is

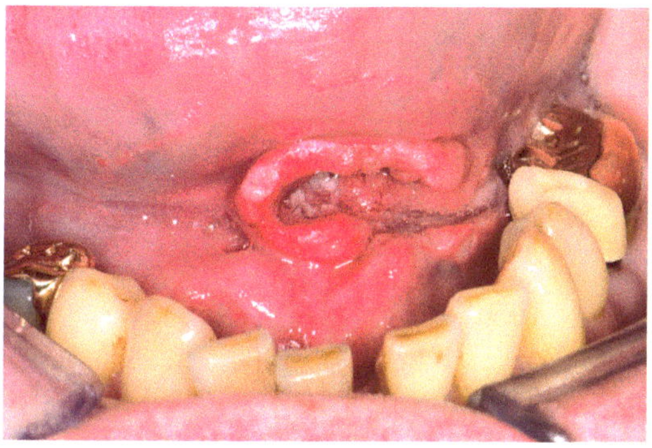

Fig. 2.140 Squamous cell carcinoma of the floor of the mouth

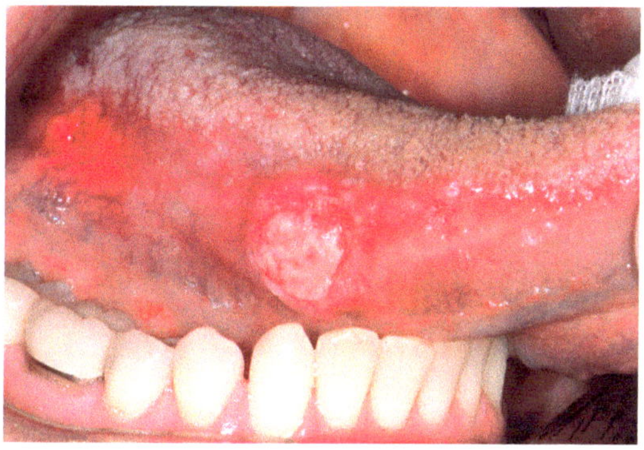

Fig. 2.141 Squamous cell carcinoma of the border of the tongue

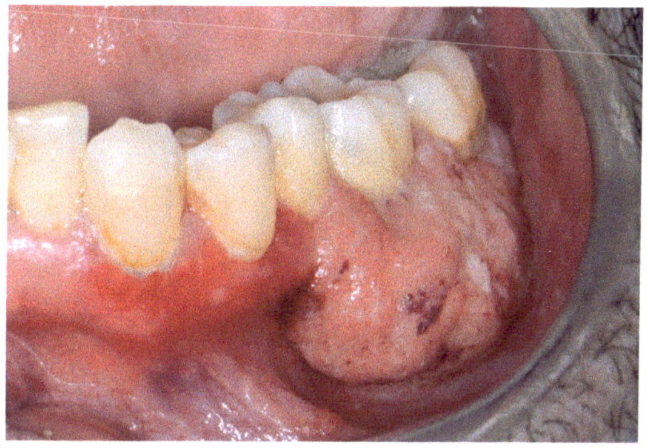

Fig. 2.142 Squamous cell carcinoma of the gingiva

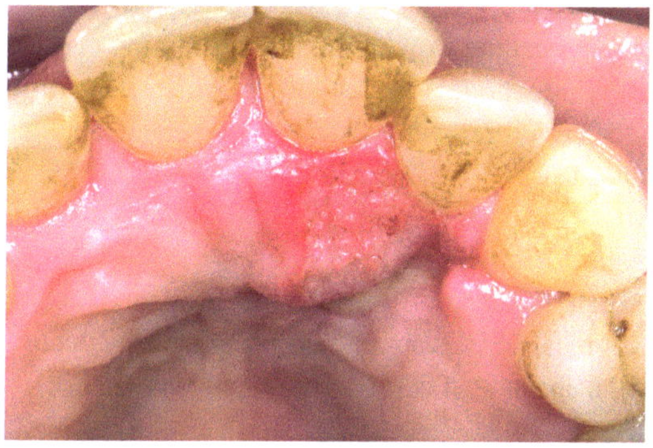

Fig. 2.143 Squamous cell carcinoma of the papilla incisiva; extremely rare oral subsite for cancer involvement

recurrent, painful swelling of the submandibular gland during meals, mimicking sialoadenitis, what can be explained by cancerous obstruction of the orificium of the submandibular gland by an OSCC in the anterior part of the floor of the mouth. In rare instances, a lymph node in the neck is the first presenting symptom of OSCC.

There are numerous benign ulcerative lesions that clinically may mimic OSCC. There are various adjunct techniques that can be used in case of a suspicious oral ulcer, e.g., exfoliative cytology, brush biopsy, fluorescent techniques, and vital staining with toluidine blue. However, the gold standard is histopathologic examination. For various reasons, it is rarely justified to perform an excisional biopsy in case of a suspicious oral ulcer.

An oral ulcer that is not recognized as a benign lesion and that does not disappear after elimination of a possible causative factor within 1–2 weeks should raise suspicion of cancer.

Cervical Lymph Node Metastases

Oral SCCs may metastasize to the regional lymph nodes of the neck, either at the homolateral or heterolateral side or to both sides simultaneously.

The risk of lymphatic spread increases with the size of the primary tumor and is also related to the oral subsite of the cancer. For instance, an OSCC of the lower lip has a lower risk of metastatic spread than a similar-sized OSCC of the tongue or floor of the mouth.

There are various methods to assess the status of the neck, varying form manual palpation to imaging, e.g., by CT scans or MRI. In many oncologic centers, ultrasound examination is used in combination with fine-needle aspiration cytology. Yet, another technique is the sentinel

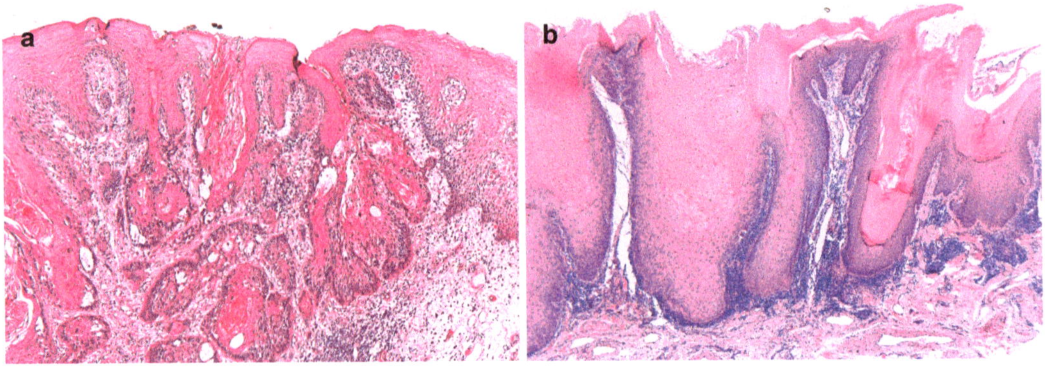

Fig. 2.144 (**a**) Low-power view of well-differentiated squamous cell carcinoma. (**b**) Low-power view of verrucous carcinoma; pushing rather than infiltrating borders

node procedure in which the first draining cervical lymph node is removed and histologically assessed for the possible presence of a metastasis.

Distant Metastases

Distant metastases, outside the head and neck region, in OSCCs are late events and rarely occur in the absence of cervical lymphatic spread.

Histopathology

Most OSCCs are well differentiated (Fig. 2.144a). In rare instances, one may be dealing with a verrucous carcinoma, being a subvariant of squamous cell carcinoma (Fig. 2.144b). A verrucous carcinoma is occasionally histopathologically misinterpreted as a benign hyperplastic epithelial lesion. Another rare variant of OCSS is the spindle cell carcinoma, also referred to as carcinosarcoma (Fig. 2.145). These two entities will not be discussed here in detail.

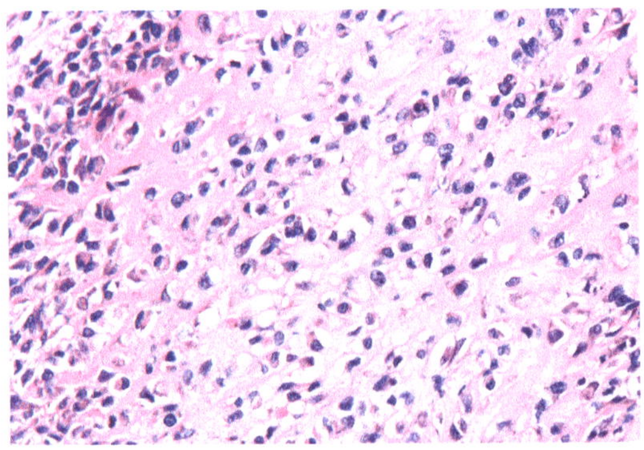

Fig. 2.145 Spindle cell variant of a squamous cell carcinoma; can be mistaken for an osteosarcoma

Staging

OSCCs are staged with the use of the international TNM staging system (T=tumor size, N=(regional) lymphnode metastases, M=metastatic spread beyond the regional lymphnodes, usually referred to as distant metastases) (Table 2.4).

Treatment

In relatively small tumors (T1, T2), surgery is the preferred treatment, usually performed in dedicated head and neck cancer centers. Radiotherapy may be administered postoperatively on indication, e.g., in case of irradicality of the surgical margins or in case of the presence of more than one positive cervical lymph node. In large tumors, a combination of radiotherapy and chemotherapy (chemoradiation) may be used instead of surgery.

Prognosis

The prognosis is largely dependent on the stage at admission. Unfortunately, worldwide some 50 % of patients suffering from OSCC present with stage III and IV disease. Stage I has a 5-year survival rate of approximately 80–85 %, while the percentage for patients presenting with stage IV disease drops to some 20 % (Fig. 2.146).

Table 2.4 TNM classification of oral squamous cell carcinoma (UICC 2009[a])

T	Primary tumor
TX	Primary tumor cannot be assessed
T0	No evidence of primary tumor
Tis	Carcinoma in situ
T1	Tumor 2 cm or less in greatest dimension
T2	Tumor more than 2 cm but not more than 4 cm in greatest dimension
T3	Tumor more than 4 cm in greatest dimension
T4a	*(Lip)* Tumor invades through cortical bone, inferior alveolar nerve, floor of mouth, or skin (chin or nose)
T4a	*(Oral cavity)* Tumor invades through cortical bone, into deep/extrinsic muscle of tongue (genioglossus, hyoglossus, palatoglossus, and styloglossus), maxillary sinus, or skin of face
T4b	*(Lip and oral cavity)* Tumor invades masticator space, pterygoid plates, or skull base or encases internal carotid artery
Note: superficial erosion alone of bone/tooth socket by gingival primary is not sufficient to classify a tumor as T4	
N	Regional lymph nodes
NX	Regional lymph nodes cannot be assessed
N0	No regional lymph node metastasis
N1	Metastasis in a single ipsilateral lymph node, 3 cm or less in greatest dimension
N2	Metastasis in a single ipsilateral lymph node, more than 3 cm but not more than 6 cm in greatest dimension; or in multiple ipsilateral lymph nodes, none more than 6 cm in greatest dimension; or in bilateral or contralateral lymph nodes, none more than 6 cm in greatest dimension
N2a	Metastasis in a single ipsilateral lymph node, more than 3 cm but not more than 6 cm in greatest dimension
N2b	Metastasis in multiple ipsilateral lymph nodes, none more than 6 cm in greatest dimension
N2c	Metastasis in bilateral or contralateral lymph nodes, none more than 6 cm in greatest dimension
N3	Metastasis in a lymph node more than 6 cm in greatest dimension
M	Distant metastasis
MX	Distant metastasis cannot be assessed
M0	No distant metastasis
M1	Distant metastasis

Stage grouping:

Stage 0	Tis	N0	M0
Stage I	T1	N0	M0
Stage II	T2	N0	M0
Stage III	T1, T2	N1	M0
	T3	N0, N1	M0
Stage IVA	T1, T2, T3	N2	M0
	T4a	NO, N1, N2	M0
Stage IVB	Any T	N3	M0
	T4b	Any N	M0
Stage IVC	Any T	Any N	M1

[a]Ref.: L.H. Sobin, M.K. Gospodarowicz, Ch. Wittekind (eds). TNM Classification of Malignant Tumours. Seventh edition, 2009. UICC International Union against Cancer. John Wiley & Sons Ltd. New York. ISBN 978-1-4443-3241-4

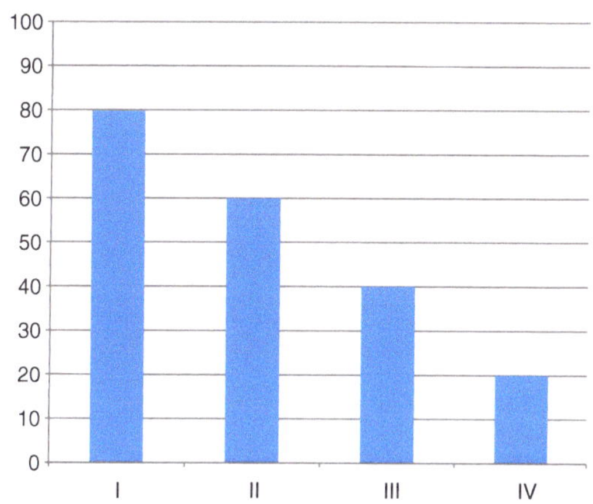

Fig. 2.146 The 5-year survival rate of oral squamous cell carcinoma per tumor stage (I–IV)

2.17.5 Traumatic Ulcer

Definition of Traumatic Ulcer

Superficial ulceration of the mucosa caused by mechanical irritation.

Etiology

Mechanical irritation may consist of a sharp edge of a broken-down tooth (Fig. 2.147a, b) or a broken-down dental restoration; also the edge of a denture may be the irritating factor. Occasionally, a traumatic ulcer is based on automutilation (Fig. 2.148). In babies, an erupting lower incisor may cause an ulcer of the ventral aspect of the tongue (Riga-Fede disease; see Chap. 4) (Fig. 2.149).

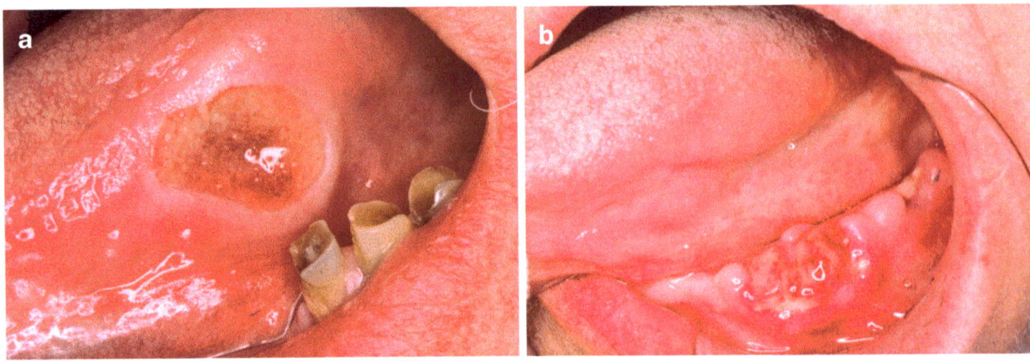

Fig. 2.147 (a) Traumatic ulcer caused by sharp edges of the teeth. (a) Complete healing within 2 weeks after the teeth have been extracted

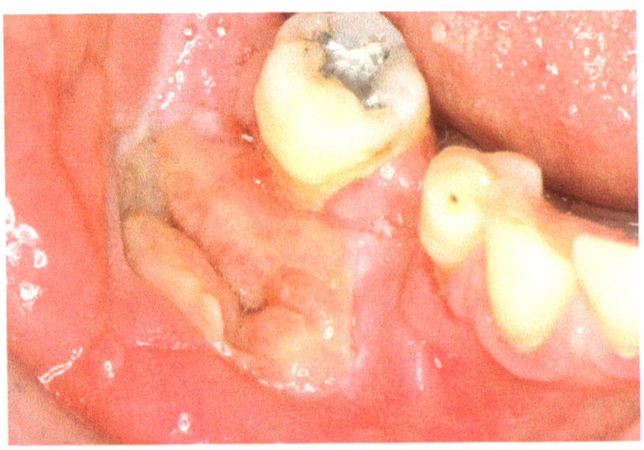

Fig. 2.148 Ulcer in the mucobuccal fold due to automutilation

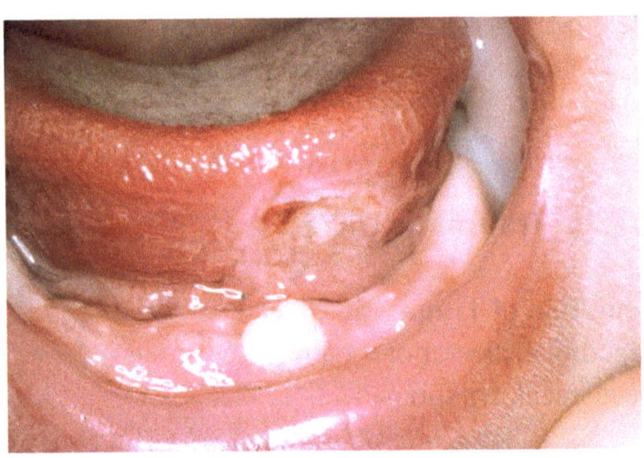

Fig. 2.149 Ulcer at the ventral aspect of the tongue during eruption of a lower incisor (Riga-Fede disease)

Clinical Aspects

Usually, a traumatic ulcer is painful and has a sharp border. In general, a traumatic ulcer is not indurated. Particularly in ulcers of the tongue and the lower lip, one should be alert for the presence of a squamous cell carcinoma.

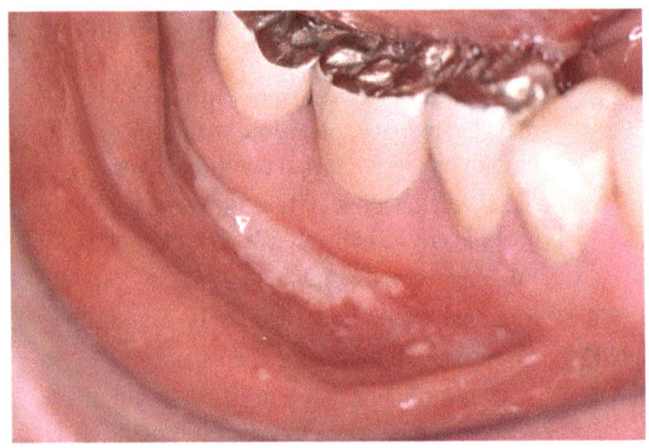

Fig. 2.150 Cotton roll ulcer in the mucobuccal fold

Histopathologic Examination

A traumatic ulcer does not have any characteristic histopathologic features.

Treatment

After elimination of the causative factor, a traumatic ulcer should heal within 1–2 weeks; if not, further evaluation is indicated, particularly focussing on the possible presence of a malignancy. In rare cases (traumatic?), ulcers may recur several times after excision, particularly when located at the borders of the tongue. Such behavior cannot be properly explained.

2.17.6 Ulcers, Miscellaneous Etiologies

The prolonged use of a cotton roll during dental treatment may result in a harmless but painful cotton roll ulcer (Fig. 2.150). Another cause of

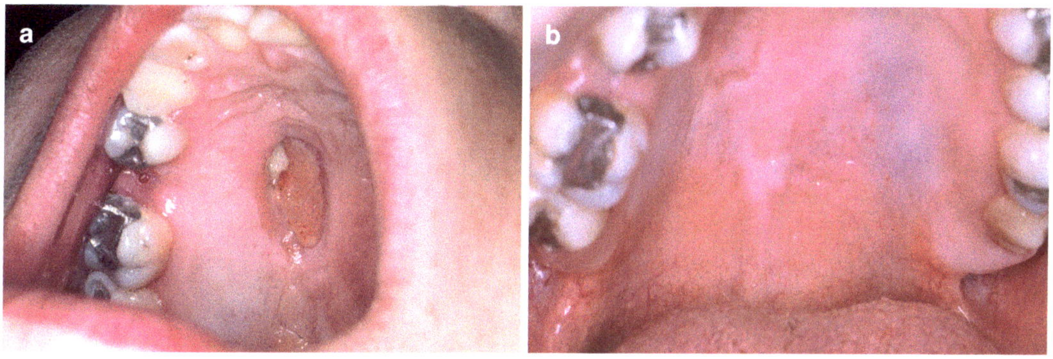

Fig. 2.151 (**a**) Palatal ulcer a few days after the administration of local anesthesia for extraction of 16. (**b**) Spontaneous healing within 3 weeks

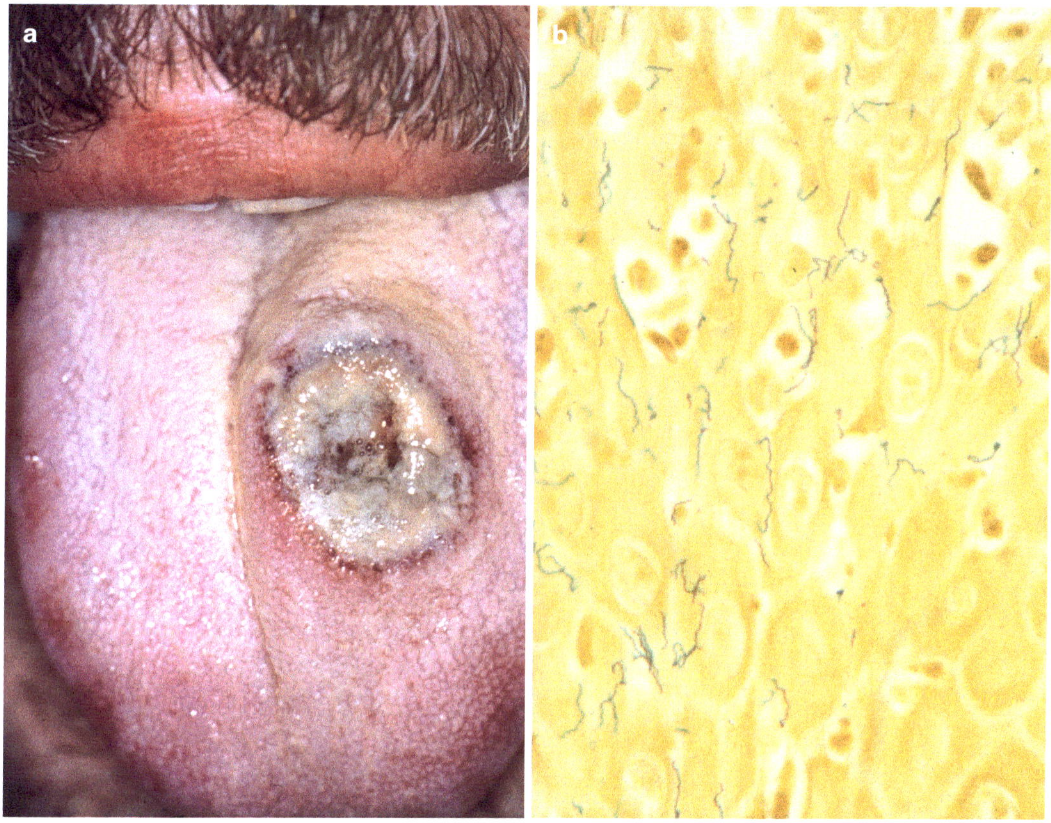

Fig. 2.152 (**a**) Ulcer in first stage Syphilis; (**b**) Spirochetes made visible in a special stain

ulceration may be the use of palatal infiltration anesthesia (Fig. 2.151); a biopsy of such ulcer may show a misleading histologic picture of necrotizing sialometaplasia. This phenomenon can occasionally be misdiagnosed by the pathologist as squamous cell carcinoma or mucoepidermoid carcinoma (see also Chap. 6).

The benign eosinophilic granuloma, more or less limited to the tongue, can clinically mimic an ulcerative squamous cell carcinoma and may histopathologically be misdiagnosed as a non-Hodgkin lymphoma (see Chap. 4).

An oral ulcer may also be the result of a specific infection, e.g., tuberculosis or syphilis (Fig. 2.152).

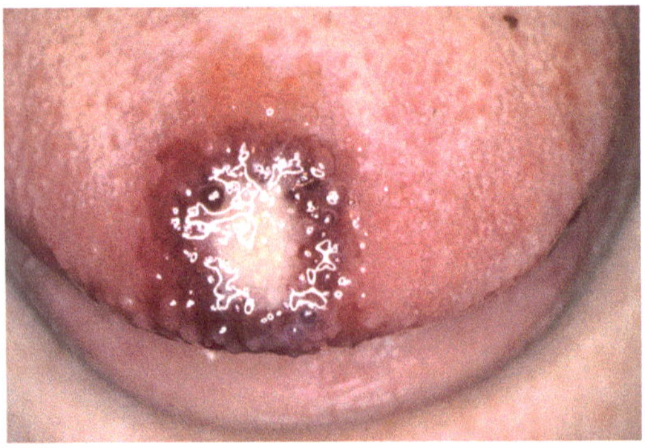

Fig. 2.153 Ulcer of the tongue as the first manifestation of acute lymphoblastic leukemia

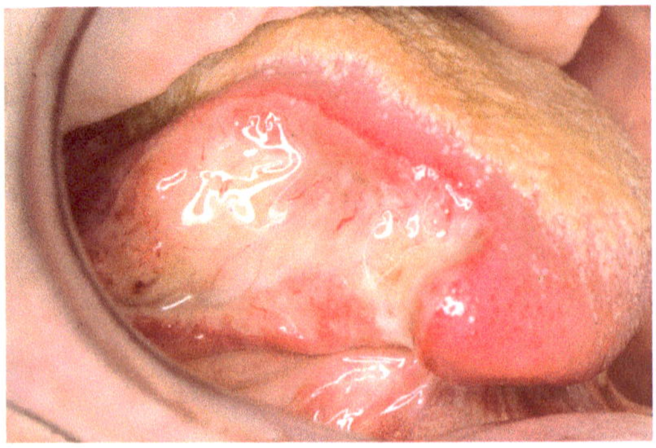

Fig. 2.154 Suddenly arising ulcer of the tongue due to lingual arteritis

Another cause of an oral ulcer may be an underlying blood disorder, e.g., leukemia (Fig. 2.153). In this event, there are usually multiple oral ulcers present, and the patient most likely will have general symptoms, such as fever or general malaise. Also non-Hodgkin lymphomas may present as an ulcerative lesion (see Chap. 6).

An oral ulcer may also be of ischemic origin as is the case in arteriitis cranialis, e.g., lingual arteritis, comparable with temporal arteritis (Fig. 2.154).

3 Diseases of the Lips

3.1 Introduction

Many diseases that affect the oral mucosa may occur on the lips as well. However, there are a number of lesions that exclusively or preferably affect the lips. Both types of lesions will be discussed in this chapter.

3.2 Acanthosis Nigricans

Definition
Pigmented papillomatous cutaneous lesion that occasionally involves the lips. Acanthosis nigricans may be a manifestation of a gastrointestinal malignant tumor.

Etiology
The etiopathogenesis is unknown.

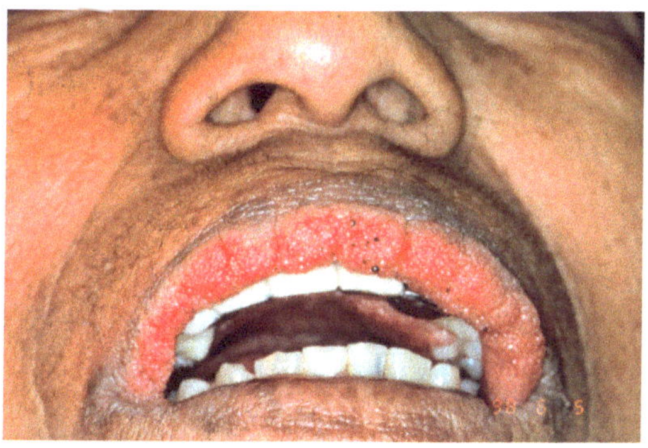

Fig. 3.1 Acanthosis nigricans of the upper lip

Epidemiology
Rare phenomenon.

Clinical Aspects
Multiple papillomatous lesions of the labial mucosa; in contrast to the cutaneous lesions, pigmentation of the labial lesions is rare (Fig. 3.1).

Treatment
It is not feasible to remove the numerous papillomatous lesions.

3.3 Cheilitis

3.3.1 Cheilitis Actinica

Definition
Inflammatory-like, premalignant disease of the lips caused by excessive exposure to sunlight. Some pathologists only report a diagnosis of cheilitis actinica when there is epithelial dysplasia.

Etiology
Apart from excessive exposure to sunlight, smoking may play a role in the etiology.

Epidemiology
Mainly in men; usually above the age of 50–60 years.

I. van der Waal, *Atlas of Oral Diseases: A Guide for Daily Practice*,
DOI 10.1007/978-3-662-48122-6_3

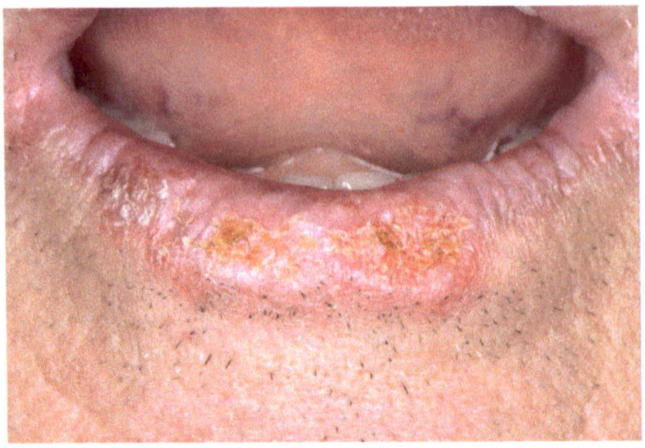

Fig. 3.2 Clinical aspect of actinic cheilitis

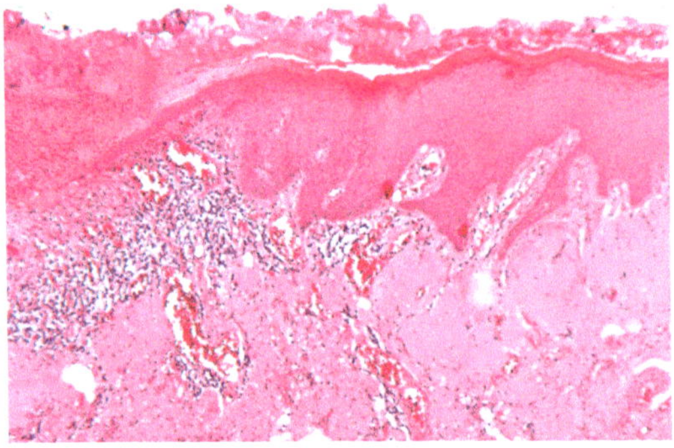

Fig. 3.3 Low-power view of actinic cheilitis

Clinical Aspects
Solitary or multiple, often recurrent but otherwise asymptomatic crusts on the vermillion border of the lower lip (Fig. 3.2); the upper lip is, indeed, rarely involved.

Clinical Differential Diagnosis
The main clinical differential diagnosis relates to a squamous cell carcinoma; in case of doubt, a biopsy should be taken.

Histopathology
Various degrees of hyperkeratosis with or without the presence of epithelial dysplasia may be observed (Fig. 3.3). In the subepithelial connective tissue, basophilic amorphic changes can be observed, referred to as actinic elastosis.

Occasionally, it may be difficult for the pathologist to render a firm diagnosis of actinic cheilitis based on a biopsy, particularly with regard to the distinction of a squamous cell carcinoma ("…most likely actinic cheilitis, but a squamous cell carcinoma cannot be ruled out"). As has been mentioned before, some pathologists use the diagnosis of actinic cheilitis only in the presence of epithelial dysplasia. In this respect, proper communication between the clinician and pathologist is essential in order to prevent any misunderstanding.

Treatment
In the absence of epithelial dysplasia, follow-up may be advised, e.g., twice a year.

In case of epithelial dysplasia or because of esthetic reasons, treatment may be instituted, e.g., by superficial surgical removal of the vermillion border ("lip shave"); also laser evaporation may be applied provided the biopsy has not shown signs of malignancy. Other treatment modalities include the topical use of trichloracetic acid and other ointments such as 5-fluorouracil.

3.3.2 Cheilitis Angularis

Definition
Inflammatory-like lesion of the commissures of the lips ("perlèches").

Etiology
The etiology is unclear; several factors may play a role, such as decreased vertical dimension of the jaws in denture wearers. Apparently, C. albicans may play a role as well. Also, the possibility of an underlying disorder, such as vitamin B deficiency or folic acid deficiency, has been mentioned as possible causative factors. In some patients, none of the aforementioned causes can be identified.

Epidemiology
Angular cheilitis occurs only in adults and elderly persons; mainly in women.

Clinical Aspects
Cracked, reddish, and atrophic changes of the mucosa of the commissures, painful; usually bilateral distribution (Fig. 3.4).

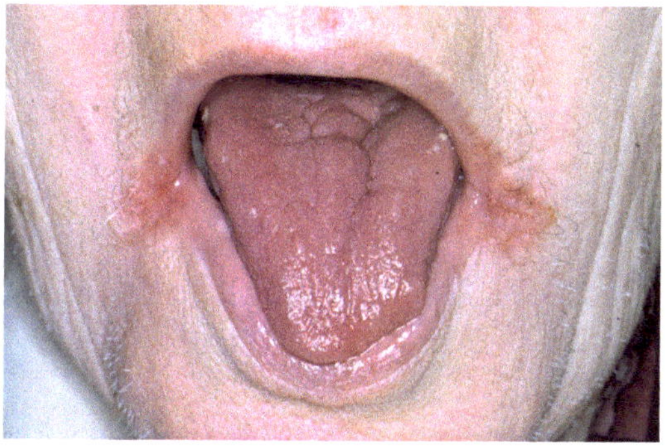

Fig. 3.4 Bilateral angularis cheilitis in an elderly woman

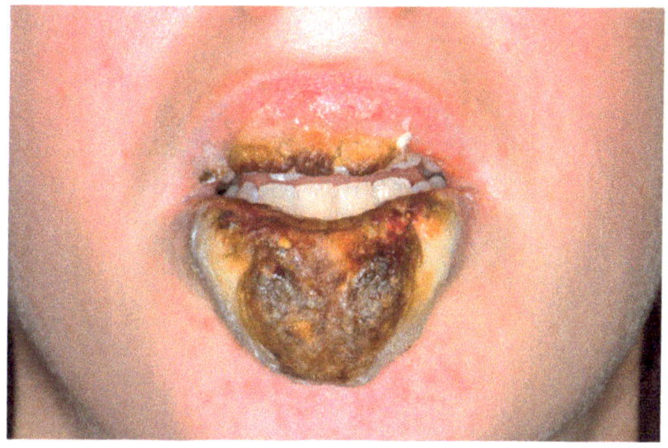

Fig. 3.5 Rather severe manifestation of exfoliative cheilitis, probably caused by automutilation

Treatment
Adjustment of the vertical height of the jaws, if applicable. Local application of antifungals may be helpful. Some advise to prescribe a mixture of antifungals and antibiotics, such as neomycin sulfate.

3.3.3 Cheilitis Exfoliativa

Definition
Inflammatory-like condition of the lips due to epithelial exfoliation.

Etiology
Habitual biting ("morsicatio") on the lips, occasionally driven by automutilation. In most instances, such habits are denied by the patient.

Clinical Aspects
Crust formation on the lower or upper lip; usually not painful (Fig. 3.5).

Treatment
It is often difficult for the patient to discontinue the habit, in spite of the often unpleasant cosmetic appearance.

3.3.4 Cheilitis Fissurata (Fissured Lip)

Definition
Fissuring of the mucosa of the vermillion border of the upper or lower lip.

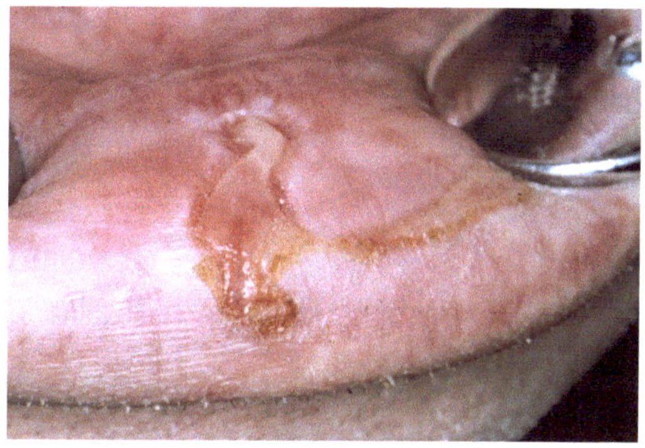

Fig. 3.6 Cheilitis fissurata of the lower lip

Etiology
The cause of the fissuring is actually unknown.

Epidemiology
Rare phenomenon, almost exclusively occurring in adults.

Clinical Aspects
Superficial, often painful fissuring of the mucosa, usually in the midline (Fig. 3.6). Absence of induration.

Histopathology
There are no pathognomic histopathological features.

Treatment
Since there is hardly any tendency for spontaneous healing, surgical correction may be considered.

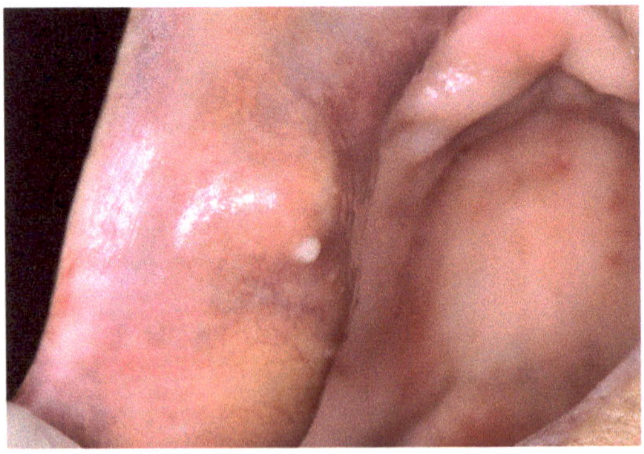

Fig. 3.7 Nodule in the upper lip caused by glandular cheilitis

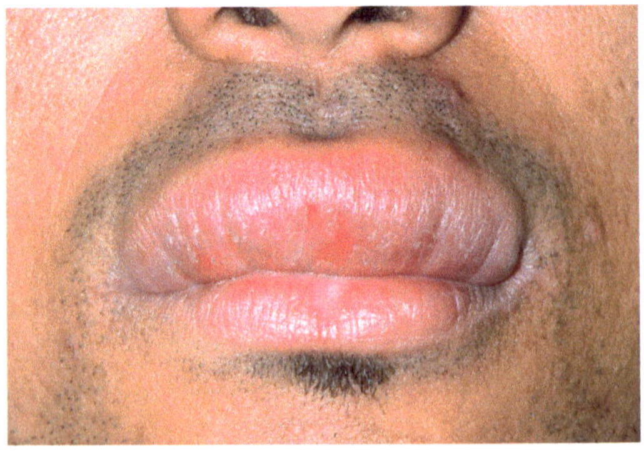

Fig. 3.8 Granulomatous cheilitis

3.3.5 Cheilitis Glandularis

Definition
Inflammation of the minor, intraoral salivary glands (see also Chap. 2).

Etiology
Most likely caused by a retrograde infection from the oral cavity.

Epidemiology
Mainly in adults.

Clinical Aspects
The clinical manifestation consists of often painful solitary or multiple painful nodules, being firm elastic on palpation. Sites of preference are the lips and the buccal mucosa. When solitary, the differential diagnosis includes a sialolith, a salivary gland neoplasm or, rarely, a foreign body reaction to cosmetic fillers (Fig. 3.7).

Histopathology
Nonspecific chronic inflammation of the salivary glands.

Treatment
In general, conservative surgical excision suffices.

3.3.6 Cheilitis Granulomatosa

Definition
Inflammatory-like swelling of the upper or lower lip. Can be a manifestation of Melkersson-Rosenthal syndrome (a combination of cheilitis granulomatosa, fissured tongue, and transient facial paralysis; this triad does not necessarily occurs simultaneously).

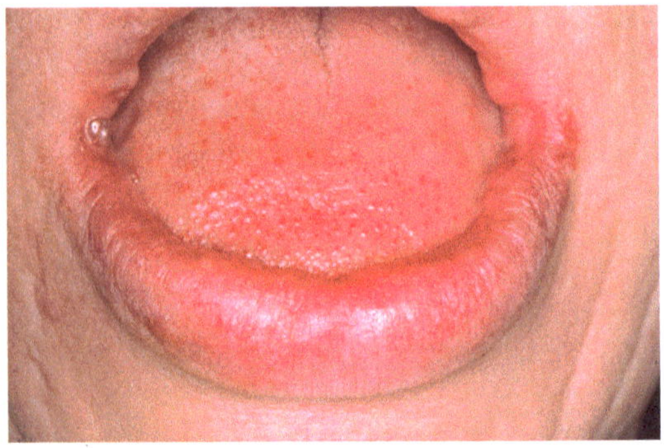

Fig. 3.9 Diffuse, slowly developing swelling of the lower lip caused by deposition of amyloid

Etiology
Unknown; in rare instances, granulomatous cheilitis is a manifestation of an underlying disease such as Crohn's disease or sarcoidosis.

Epidemiology
Mainly in adolescents and adults.

Clinical Aspects
Diffuse, slowly increasing, and sometimes painful swelling of the entire upper and/or lower lip (Fig. 3.8).

Cheilitis granulomatosa may run a recurrent clinical course. Although the diagnosis is usually made on clinical grounds alone, the taking of a biopsy should be considered in case of the slightest doubt.

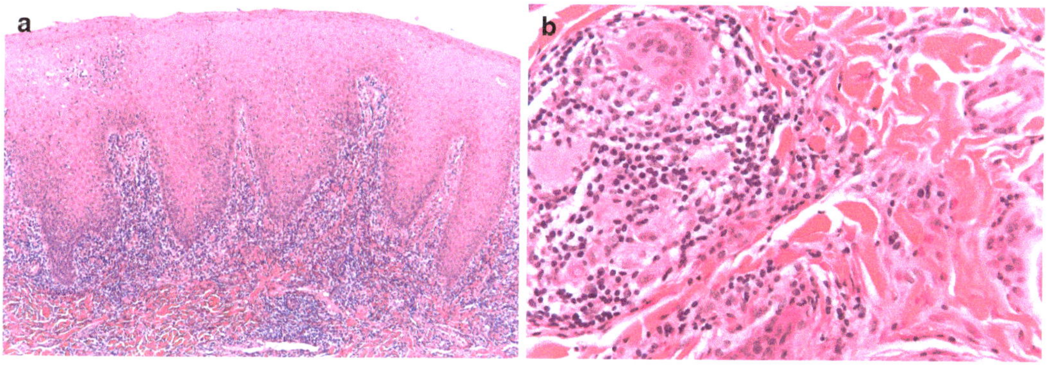

Fig. 3.10 (**a**) Low-power view of granulomatous cheilitis. (**b**) In the deep layer, granuloma formation and the presence of multinucleated giant cells can be seen

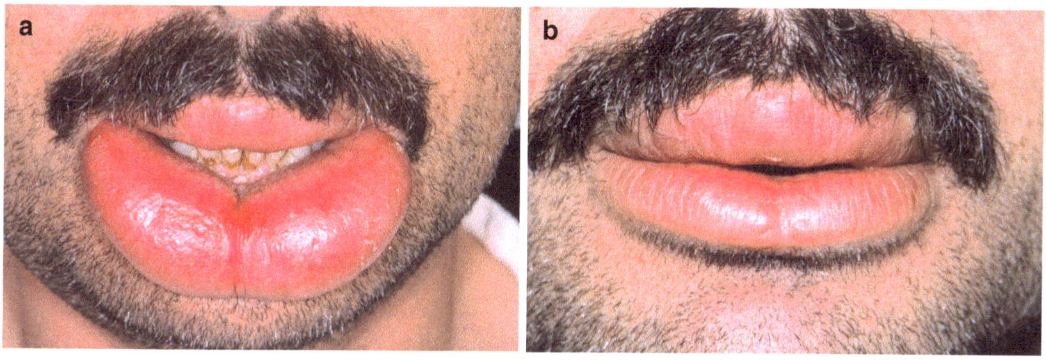

Fig. 3.11 (**a**) Severe manifestation of granulomatous cheilitis. (**b**) Result 2 months after surgical correction

Clinical Differential Diagnosis

In case of a suddenly arising swelling, the possibility of angioedema should be taken into account (see Chap. 2). A slowly growing swelling of the lower lip in an elderly patient may also be caused by deposition of amyloid (Fig. 3.9), although the tongue is a much more common location for this disorder.

Histopathology

Chronic inflammation; only if the biopsy has been taken deep enough, the presence of granulomas and multinucleated giant cells may be encountered (Fig. 3.10a, b).

Treatment

Occasionally, spontaneous regression takes place. In persisting cases, local application of corticosteroids may be considered in spite of the lack of scientific evidence for this type of treatment; the same applies to intralesional injections of corticosteroids. In severe cases, surgical correction may be indicated, but the final cosmetic result cannot be reliably predicted (Fig. 3.11a, b).

In the absence of gastrointestinal symptoms, further work-up for the possible presence of Crohn's disease is not indicated, although a few patients with cheilitis granulomatosa may develop Crohn's disease at a later stage.

3.4 Cleft Lip

Definition

Congenital cleft of the (upper) lip.

Epidemiology

Occurs in 1:650 babies; more often in boys than in girls.

Etiology

Multifactorial; cleft formation is occasionally a manifestation of a syndrome.

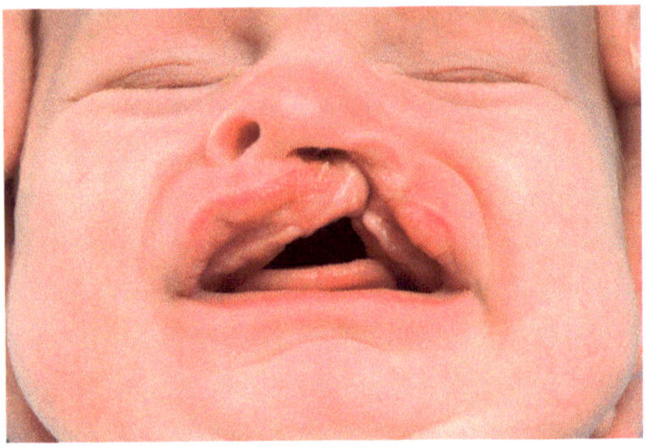

Fig. 3.12 Cheilognathopalatoschisis

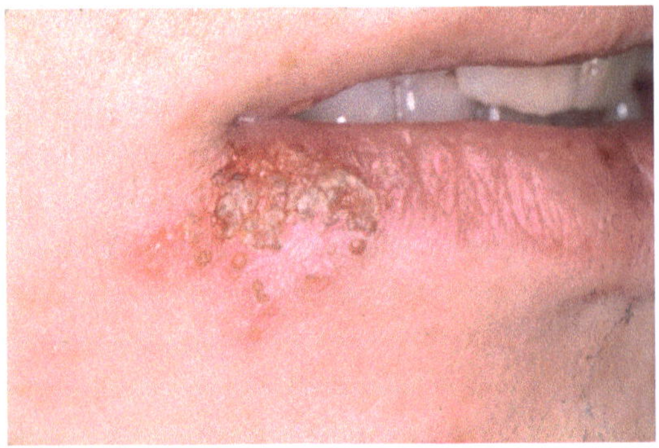

Fig. 3.13 Herpes labialis of the lower lip

Clinical Aspects
Affects almost always the upper lip. Involves more often the left side; occasionally bilateral.

May be associated with a cleft palate or maxilla (cheilognathopalatoschisis) (Fig. 3.12).

Treatment
Treatment of patients with a cleft lip is in most parts of the world concentrated in specialized, multidisciplinary units. A cleft lip is usually closed a few months after birth.

3.5 Herpes Labialis

Definition
Secondary infection with herpes simplex virus (HSV); see also Chap. 2.

Etiology
Reactivation of latent HSV in the ganglion of the trigeminal nerve, caused by a.o. sun exposure. The exact mechanism of the reactivation is unknown.

Epidemiology
Occurs in approximately 5 % of the population.

Clinical Aspects
Affects the mucocutaneous junction of the upper or lower lip. Secondary herpes simplex infection rarely occurs intraorally. The clinical manifestation consists of multiple, painful vesicles that easily rupture (Fig. 3.13). In contrast to a primary HSV infection, there are no signs of general malaise or fever. Healing takes place without scar formation.

Treatment
In an otherwise healthy patient, there is hardly any benefit from local application of antiviral ointments.

3.6 Keratoacanthoma

Definition
Benign, usually fast-growing, crust-forming lesion of the skin. Mucosal involvement is rare and is limited to the vermillion border of the lips.

Etiology
May originate from hair follicles and the associated sebaceous glands. However, the exact etiopathogenesis is unknown.

Epidemiology
Rare lesion of the lips; occurs almost exclusively in adults.

Clinical Aspects
Usually a solitary, somewhat pedunculated, often fast-growing and painful swelling with a central crater in the surface (Fig. 3.14). The main differential diagnosis relates to a squamous cell carcinoma; there are no reliable criteria to clinically distinguish a keratoacanthoma from a squamous cell carcinoma.

Histopathology

Based on a small biopsy, it is sometimes not possible to distinguish a keratoacanthoma from a well-differentiated squamous cell carcinoma. In some cases, the distinction between these two entities cannot even be made when an entire surgical specimen is available (Fig. 3.15).

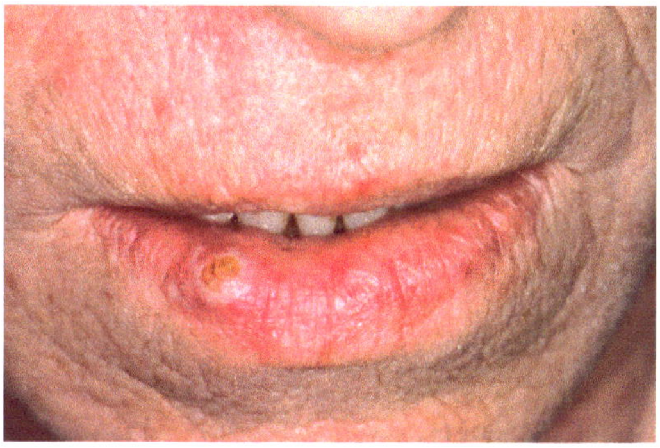

Fig. 3.14 Keratoacanthoma can strongly mimic a squamous cell carcinoma

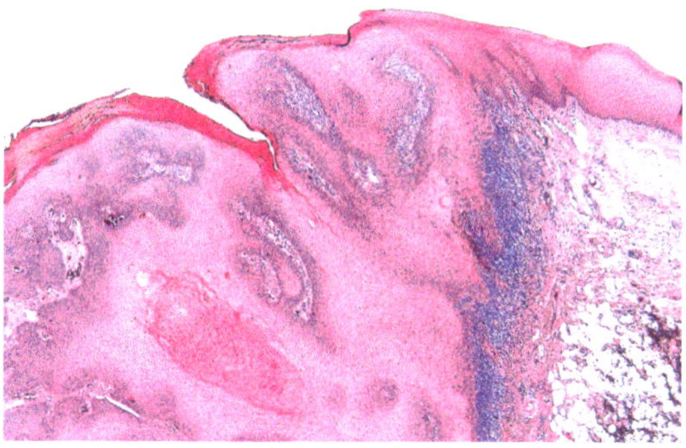

Fig. 3.15 Low-power view suggestive but not diagnostic of keratoacanthoma

Treatment

Spontaneous healing usually takes place within 4–6 months ("self-healing carcinoma") (Fig. 3.16a, b). When in doubt about the diagnosis, radical excision is advised, thereby providing a surgical specimen for additional histopathological examination.

3.7 Mucocele

Definition

Retention of mucous from the (minor) salivary glands of the oral mucosa (see also Chap. 2).

Etiology

Mucous retention is the result of traumatic injury of the orificium of the excretory ducts, causing either retention of saliva in the ductal system ("retention phenomenon") or rupture of the salivary gland duct, resulting in mucous extravasation ("extravasation phenomenon").

Epidemiology

May occur at all ages but is more common among children and adolescents.

Clinical Aspects

Mucoceles present as a bluish, solitary, otherwise asymptomatic, and often recurrent cystic swelling of the mucosa. The lower lip ("mucocele"), the floor of the mouth ("ranula") and, occasionally, the ventral aspect of the anterior tongue, and the cheeks are the sites of predilection; the upper lip and palate are rarely involved. The size may

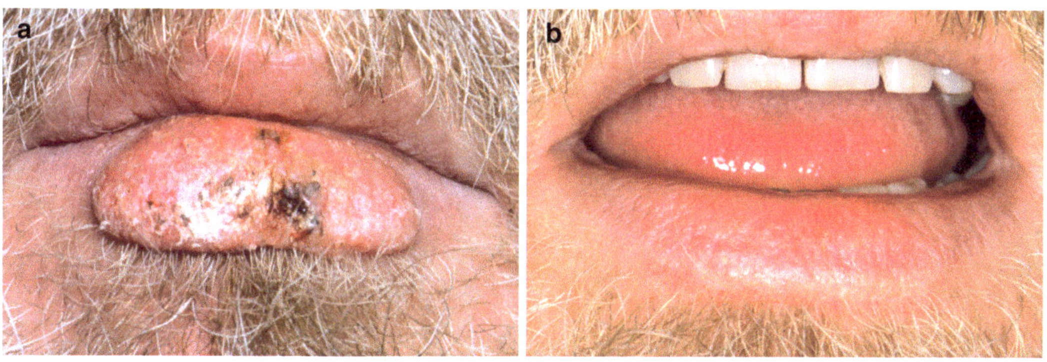

Fig. 3.16 (**a**) Giant keratoacanthoma of the lower lip. (**b**) Spontaneous healing within 6 months

vary from a few millimeters up to a centimeter (Fig. 3.17). The differential diagnosis of a mucocele on the lower lip mainly includes a phlebectasia ("varicosity"). In case of a mucocele-like swelling on the palate, a salivary gland neoplasm is the most likely diagnosis.

Histopathology

In the presence of an epithelial layer around the mucous material ("retention phenomenon"), some authors use the term "salivary duct cyst." In the extravasation type, the mucous material is surrounded by a layer of granulation tissue (Fig. 3.18).

Treatment

Enucleation, including part of the overlying epithelium in order to prevent early rupture of the "cyst." There is an ongoing debate whether it should be advised to remove also the surrounding minor salivary glands in order to prevent recurrence. However, recurrences after removal of mucoceles are very rare, irrespective of the extent of the removal.

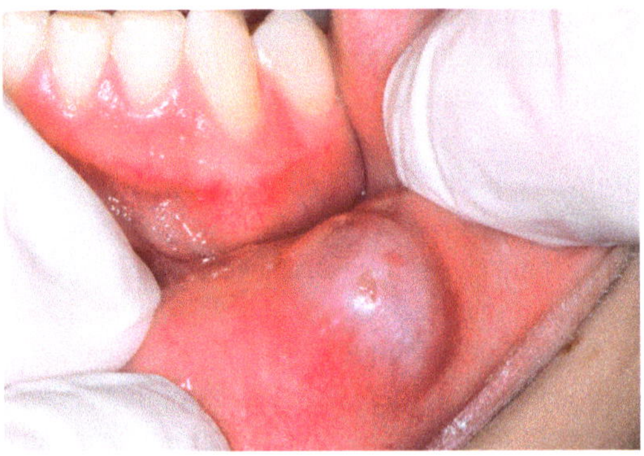

Fig. 3.17 Mucocele of the lower lip

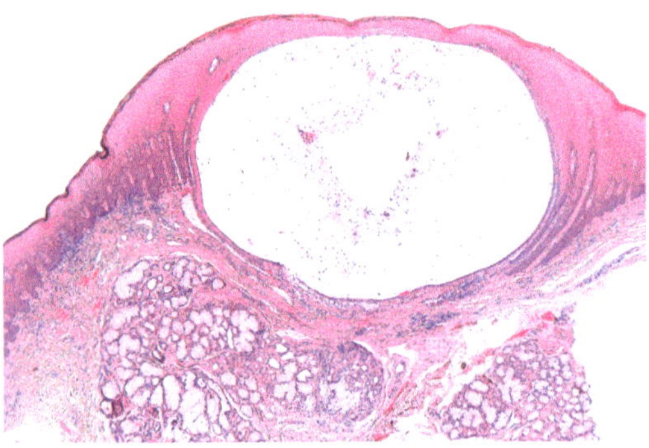

Fig. 3.18 Low-power view of a mucocele

3.8 Other Lesions Occurring on the Lips

3.8.1 Arteriovenous Malformation ("Hemangioma")

Some Characteristics

Arteriovenous malformations are usually present shortly after birth and may affect the upper and lower lip (Fig. 3.19); see also Chap. 2. Small vascular malformations may mimic a mucocele or a cystic salivary gland tumor. However, the diagnosis can almost always be made on the basis of the history.

3.8.2 Double Lip

Some Characteristics

Extremely rare phenomenon consisting of hyperplasia of the mucosal part of the lip, most likely representing a developmental anomaly. Usually, the upper lip is involved. Can be part of Ascher syndrome that includes recurrent edema of the upper eyelids and enlargement of the thyroid gland.

In severe cases, surgical correction may be indicated.

3.8.3 Granular Cell Tumor

Some Characteristics

Granular cell tumors may occur everywhere in the body, but mainly affect the oral cavity (see also

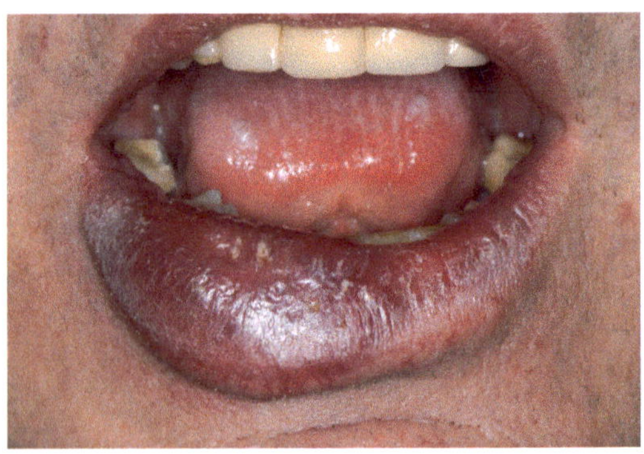

Fig. 3.19 Arteriovenous malformation of the lower lip

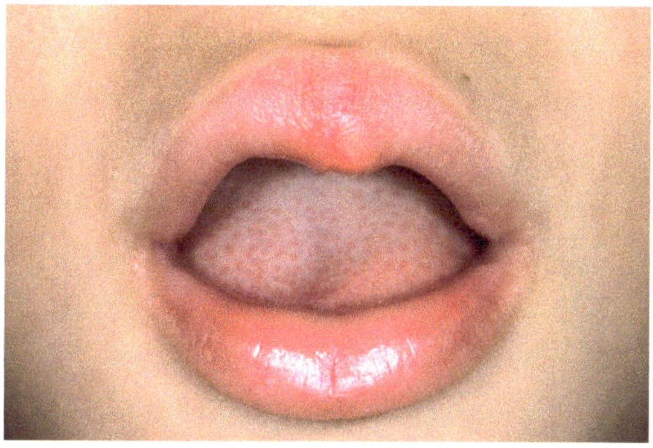

Fig. 3.20 Granular cell tumor on the upper lip in a 4-year-old child

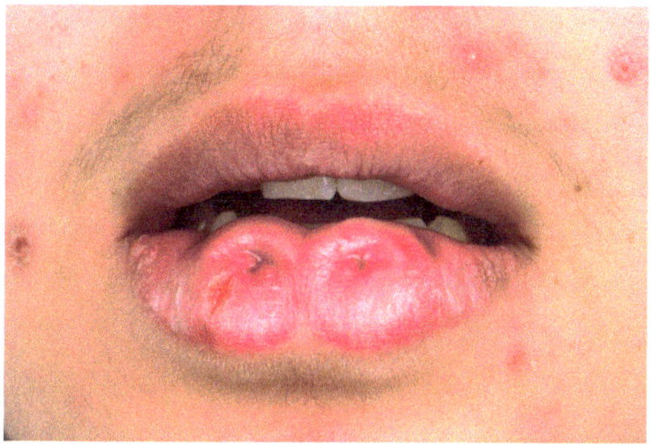

Fig. 3.21 Bilateral lip pits in patients affected by Van der Woude syndrome

Chap. 2). Most oral granular cell tumors are located on the tongue, either solitary or in a multiple fashion. Involvement of the lips is extremely rare (Fig. 3.20). Treatment consists of surgical removal.

3.8.4 Labial Pits

Some Characteristics
Labial pits are blind ducts or pits in the commissures or the lips (Fig. 3.21), present since birth. It is a rare event. Occasionally, there is excretion of mucous material.

Labial pits may be part of the Van der Woude syndrome (a genetic disorder characterized by the combination of lower lip pits, cleft lip with or without cleft palate; hypodontia, syndactyly of the hands, and ankyloglossia may be other features of this syndrome).

There is rarely a need for surgical correction.

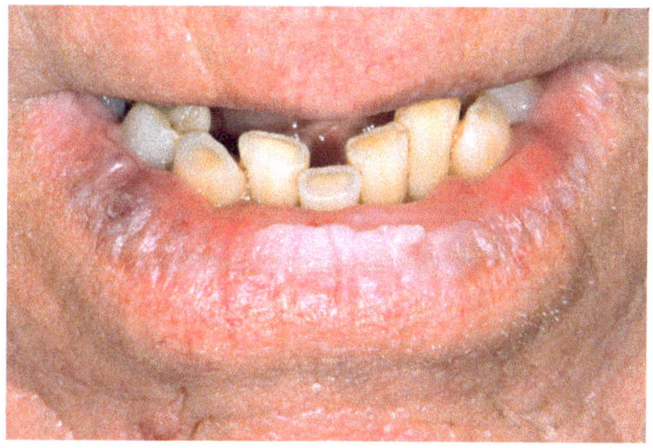

Fig. 3.22 Homogeneous leukoplakia of the lower lip

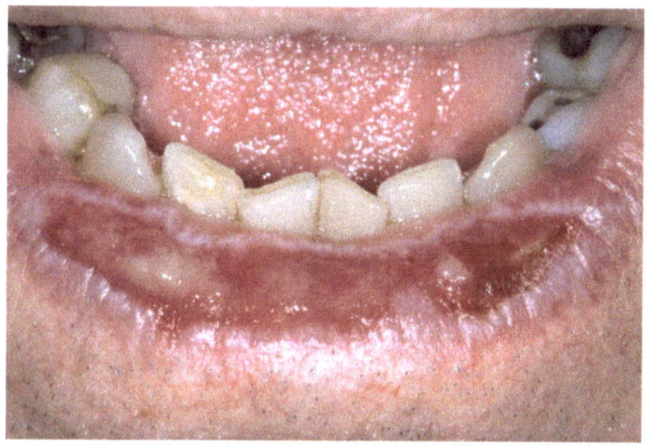

Fig. 3.23 Erosive lichen planus; also lichen planus manifestations elsewhere in the mouth

3.8.5 Leukoplakia and Erythroplakia

Some Characteristics
Leukoplakia and erythroplakia have been discussed in Chap. 2. Although the lower lip is one of the sites of predilection for squamous cell carcinoma, occurrence of leukoplakia or erythroplakia on the lips is rather rare (Fig. 3.22). The management of leukoplakia and erythroplakia has been discussed in Chap. 2.

3.8.6 Lichen Planus

Some Characteristics
Lichen planus has been discussed in Chap. 2. The lips, mainly the lower lip, is not a very common site for lichen planus (Fig. 3.23); in this event, there are always other expressions of oral lichen planus in the mouth. Furthermore, lichenoid

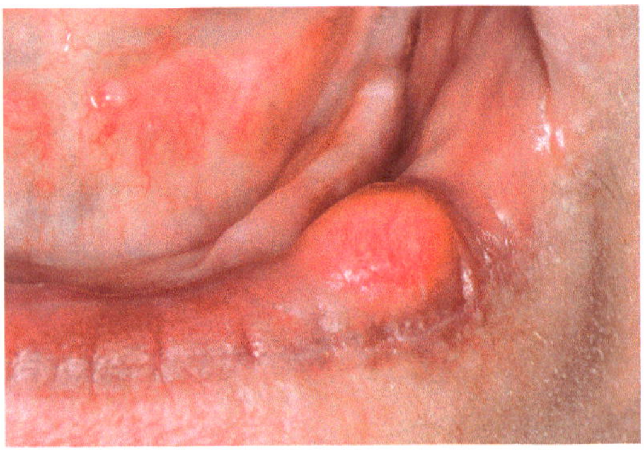

Fig. 3.24 Lipoma of the lower lip

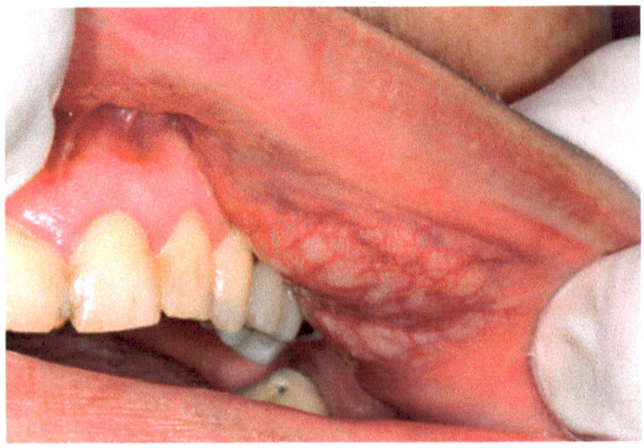

Fig. 3.25 Non-Hodgkin lymphoma as the first and only manifestation of the disease

lesions may occur on the lower lip in chronic graft-versus-host disease.

3.8.7 Lipoma

Some Characteristics
Lipomas rarely occur on the upper or lower lip (see also Chap. 2), usually above the age of 40 years. Often pedunculated, yellowish swelling, being asymptomatic otherwise (Fig. 3.24).

There are various histopathological subtypes, such as fibrolipoma, angiolipoma, and spindle cell lipoma. Malignancy, i.c. liposarcoma, is extremely rare.

Treatment consists of surgical removal.

3.8.8 Malignancies Other Than Squamous Cell Carcinomas

Some Characteristics
Malignancies other than squamous cell carcinomas, such as melanomas, sarcomas, and non-Hodgkin lymphomas, rarely affect the lips (Figs. 3.25 and 3.26). The presence in the lips of a metastasis derived from a malignancy located elsewhere in the body is almost nonexisting.

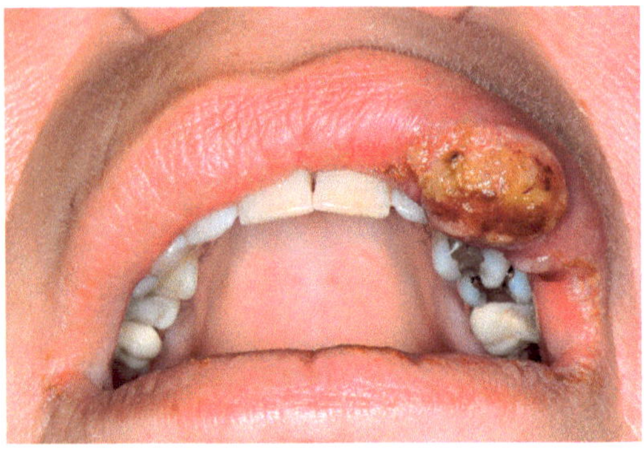

Fig. 3.26 Rhabdomyosarcoma of the upper lip

3.8.9 Pyogenic Granuloma ("Lobular Capillary Hemangioma")

Some Characteristics
Excessive tissue reaction to nonspecific local irritation (see also Chap. 2). Soft, pedunculated, and usually partly ulcerated swelling, usually asymptomatic otherwise. May occur at any site in the oral cavity, including the lips (Fig. 3.27).

At histopathologic examination, lobular vascular spaces are observed surrounded by clusters of endothelial cells ("lobular capillary hemangioma"); there may be secondary signs of inflammation.

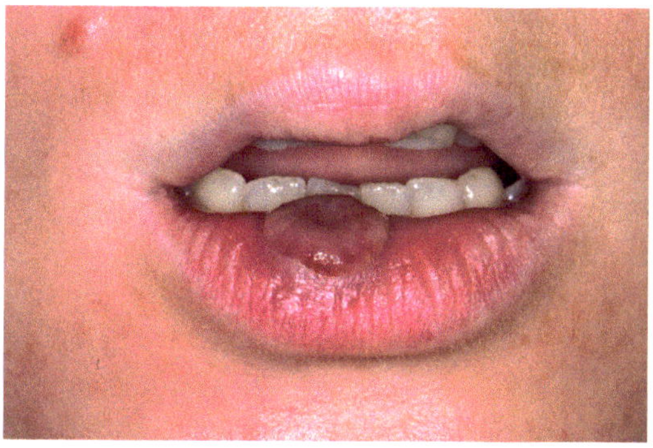

Fig. 3.27 Pyogenic granuloma of the lower lip

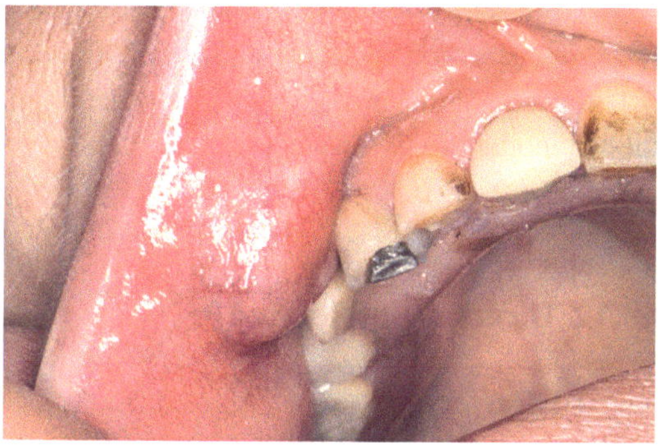

Fig. 3.28 Salivary gland tumor in the upper lip; could be benign or malignant

Treatment consists of conservative surgical excision; recurrences are rare.

3.8.10 Salivary Gland Tumors

Some Characteristics

Neoplasm arising from the salivary gland parenchyma (see also Chap. 2). Salivary gland tumors may occur in the upper lip (Fig. 3.28); involvement of the lower lip is extremely rare. There are no clinical characteristics to distinguish a benign intraoral salivary gland tumor from a malignant one.

There is a wide range of benign and malignant epithelial salivary gland tumors (see Chap. 2). Interestingly, the canalicular adenoma almost exclusively occurs in the upper lip, sometimes presenting as multiple small nodules.

Surgical removal is the treatment of choice. In selected cases, postoperative irradiation is indicated.

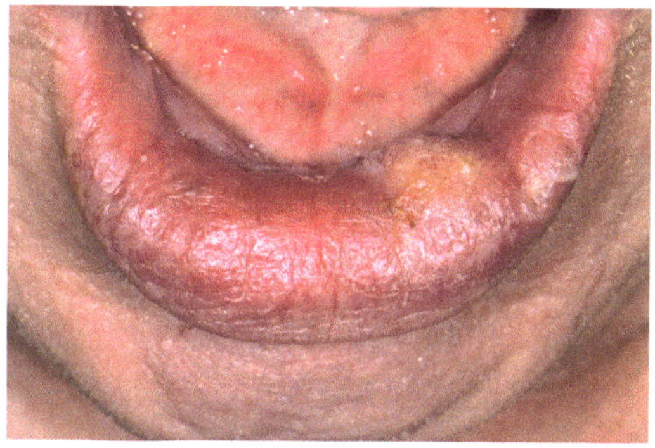

Fig. 3.29 Squamous cell carcinoma of the lower lip in an elderly man

3.8.11 Squamous Cell Carcinoma

Some Characteristics

The lower lip is one of the sites of predilection of an oral squamous cell carcinoma (Fig. 3.29). The upper lip is, indeed, rarely involved. A squamous cell carcinoma of the lower lip mainly occurs in men. Excessive exposure to sunlight is an important etiologic factor.

The clinical presentation is usually a slow-growing ulcerative swelling on the lower lip, sometimes mimicking actinic cheilitis. Also a keratoacanthoma may strongly resemble a squamous cell carcinoma, but this lesion is usually characterized by pain and rapid growth.

Lymph node metastases of squamous cell carcinomas of the lower lip are rather rare, but may develop late, sometimes even after a few years.

In most oncologic centers in the world, treatment consists of surgical excision. In small tumors, a wedge excision can be performed with primary

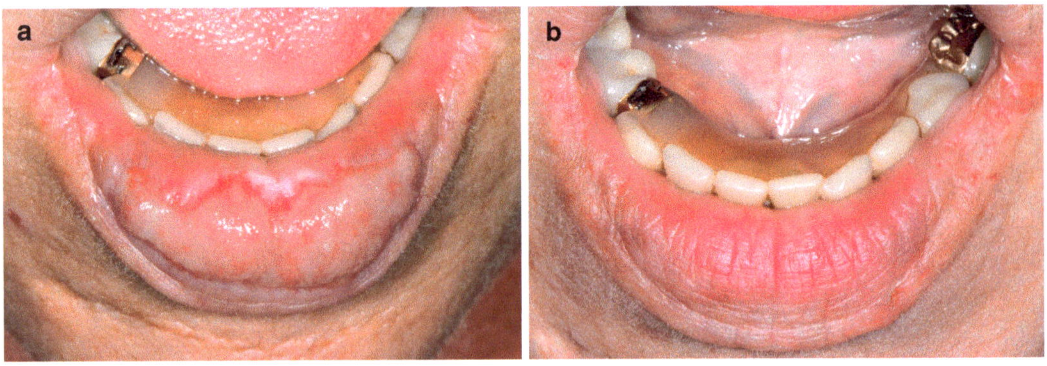

Fig. 3.30 (**a**) Ulcerative changes of the vermillion border due to the use of methotrexate for chronic rheumatoid disease. (**b**) Healing of the lip within a few weeks after withdrawal of the methotrexate

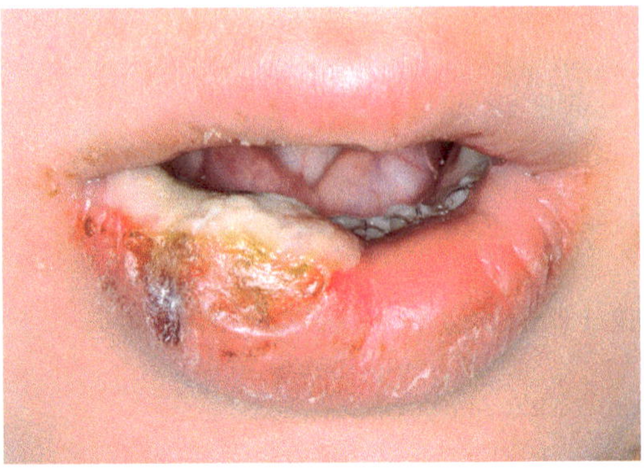

Fig. 3.31 Traumatic ulcer in a child after a mandibular block with local anesthetics

closure. If indicated, the wedge excision can be combined in continuity with a lip shave. In larger tumors, there is a need for immediate surgical reconstruction for which various flaps are available. Particularly in large tumors in elderly patients, there is a role for primary treatment by radiotherapy.

The 5-year survival rate of T1N0 squamous cell carcinoma of the lower lip is approximately 85–90 %.

3.8.12 Ulcers, Drug Related

Some Characteristics

Some drugs may result in stomatitis (drug stomatitis) or ulceration. Such ulceration is sometimes limited to the lips (Fig. 3.30a, b).

3.8.13 Ulcer, Traumatic

Some Characteristics

Traumatic ulcers of the lip are less common than one would expect (see also Chap. 2).

It may affect the lower lip in children after administration of a mandibular block in local anesthesia (Fig. 3.31).

4 Diseases of the Tongue

4.1 Introduction

Almost all lesions and diseases that may affect the oral mucosa may also occur on the tongue. On the other hand, there are some diseases that exclusively or almost exclusively affect the tongue. In this chapter, the emphasis is on the latter group of diseases.

4.2 Amyloidosis

Definition
Amyloidosis refers to the precipitation of certain proteins in various tissues of the body.

Classification

- Primary amyloidosis (AL type), in which the protein fibrils consist of monoclonal light chain immunoglobulins
- Secondary amyloidosis (AA type), in which there is an underlying disease; the proteins are derived from the acute phase of apolipoprotein precursors
- Hereditary amyloidosis
- Amyloidosis in chronic hemodialysis patients due to precipitation of β-2-microglobulins in the carpal ligaments

Etiology
The cause of the protein precipitation is unknown.

Epidemiology
Rather rare disease, mainly affecting people above the age of 60 years.

Clinical Aspects
Amyloidosis may present in the mouth as the first manifestation of the disease, most commonly by a slowly enlarging tongue. This may lead to difficulties with speech and swallowing (Fig. 4.1). In the majority of cases of oral amyloidosis, the patient is suffering from multiple myelomas (Kahler's disease).

The diagnosis of amyloidosis is based on histopathologic findings of a biopsy.

Histopathologic Examination
On histopathologic examination, amyloid presents as a hyaline-like, amorphous material.

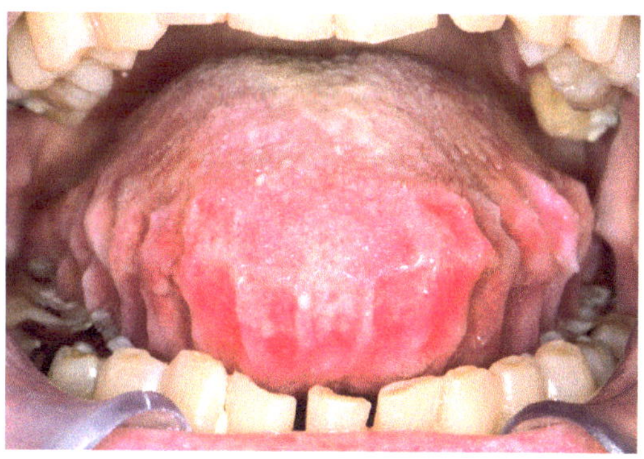

Fig. 4.1 Macroglossia due to amyloid deposition. Notice also the impressions from the teeth ("crenated tongue")

I. van der Waal, *Atlas of Oral Diseases: A Guide for Daily Practice*,
DOI 10.1007/978-3-662-48122-6_4

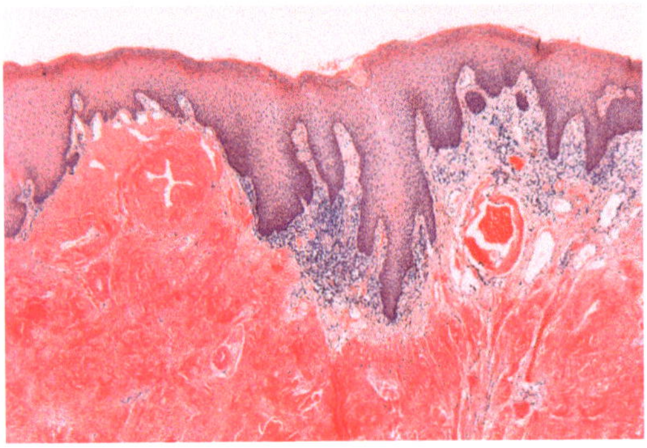

Fig. 4.2 Positive Congo red stain confirms the presence of amyloid deposition

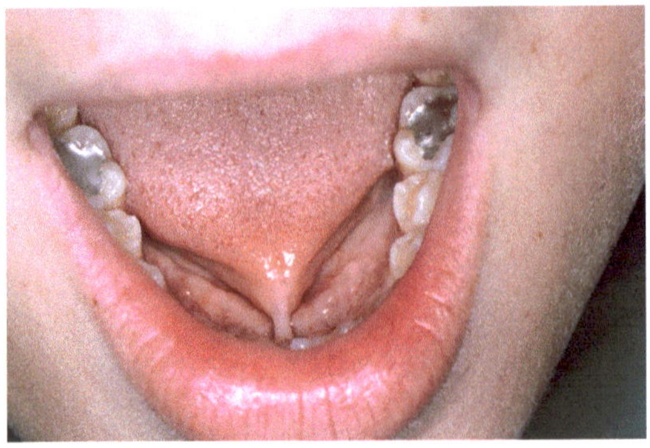

Fig. 4.3 Ankyloglossia ("tongue tie")

This amorphous material stains positive in a Congo red stain that shows a yellowish-greenish birefringence when using polarized light (Fig. 4.2).

Treatment

There is no effective treatment for primary amyloidosis. In secondary amyloidosis, the underlying disease should be treated, if feasible. In localized amyloid deposition, surgical excision may be considered.

4.3 Ankyloglossia ("Tongue Tie")

Definition

Developmental disorder in which the frenulum of the tongue is shortened, thereby limiting the mobility of the tongue (Fig. 4.3).

Epidemiology

Rather rare developmental phenomenon; there is no gender preference.

Clinical Aspects

Ankyloglossia rarely results in speech problems or eating problems.

Treatment

Surgical correction is rarely indicated and, if so, should in general not be performed before puberty. If performed, treatment consists of a Z-plasty; just cutting the frenulum is not effective and usually results in scar formation.

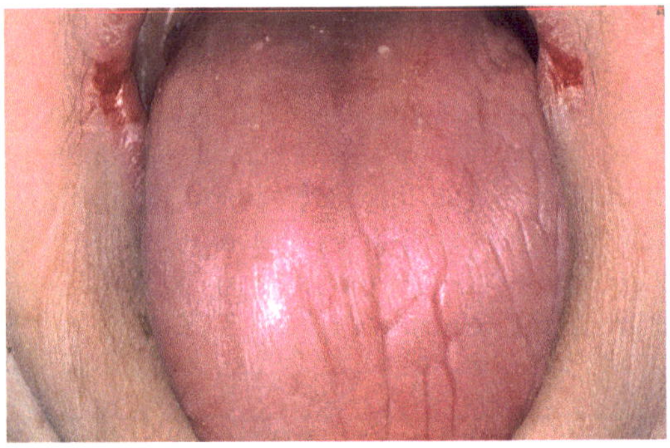

Fig. 4.4 Atrophy of the mucosal lining of the tongue. Notice also the presence of angular cheilitis in the corners of the mouth

4.4 Atrophy of the Mucosa of the Dorsum of the Tongue

Definition

Atrophy of the epithelium of the lingual mucosa of the dorsal surface of the tongue.

Etiology

Atrophy of the lingual mucosa of the dorsal surface of the tongue is probably more or less an aging phenomenon and is rarely caused by an underlying disease, such as pernicious anemia.

Clinical Aspects

The dorsal surface of the tongue may show a rather smooth, depapillated aspect (Figs. 4.4 and 4.5). The color of the mucosa may vary from pale to fiery red. The patient may or may not complain of a burning sensation.

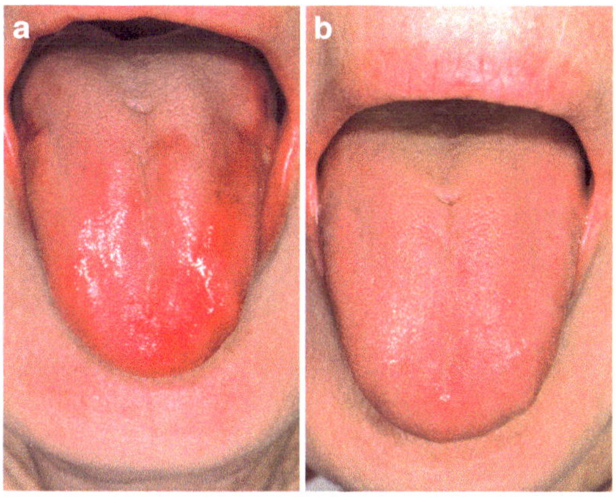

Fig. 4.5 Partly atrophic aspect of the lingual mucosa due to underlying pernicious anemia (**a**); normal aspect of the mucosa after vitamin B12 supplementation (**b**)

Treatment
In the absence of a treatable underlying disorder, there are no effective treatment modalities.

4.5 Ectomesenchymal Chondromyxoid Tumor

Definition
Rare, benign neoplasm that almost exclusively occurs on the dorsum of the tongue.

The exact origin of the neoplastic cells is unknown.

Clinical Aspects
Slow-growing swelling, usually on the anterior part of the dorsal surface, not characteristic otherwise (Fig. 4.6).

Histopathology
Well-circumscribed neoplasm consisting of myxoid tissue in which monomorphic clear cells are dispersed (Fig. 4.7); these cells may mimic salivary gland cells but may also have a somewhat (rhabdomyo)sarcomatous appearance.

Treatment
Surgical excision; because of the rarity of reported cases, limited information of possible recurrences is available.

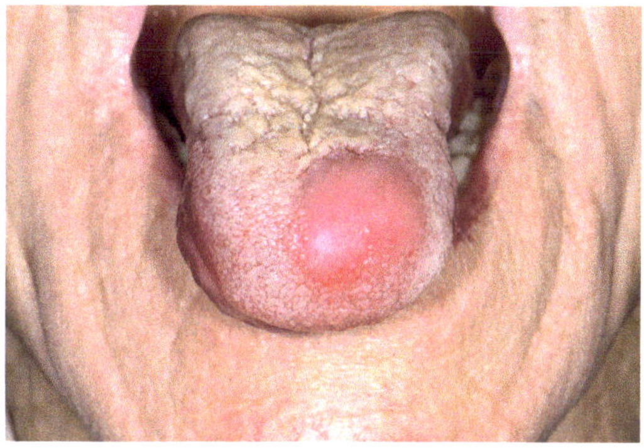

Fig. 4.6 Clinical nonspecific presentation of ectomesenchymal chondromyxoid tumor

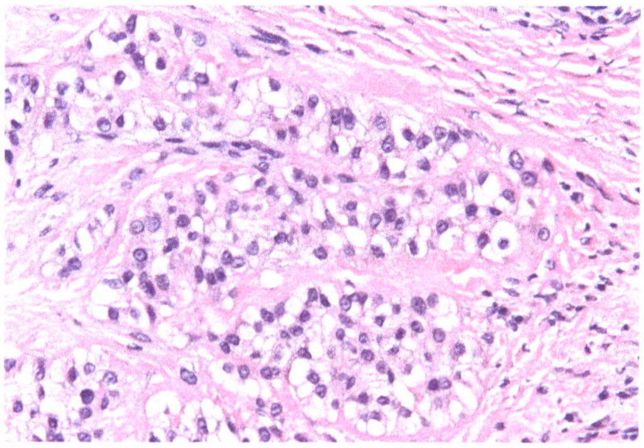

Fig. 4.7 Low-power view of ectomesenchymal chondromyxoid tumor

4.6 Fissured Tongue (Lingua Fissurata)

Definition
Presence of fissures in the dorsal surface of the tongue.

Etiology
Fissured tongue is to be regarded as a more or less anatomical variation and not as a disease.

Epidemiology
Common phenomenon; becomes usually not apparent before adulthood but may occasionally be encountered in children and adolescents.

Clinical Aspects
The pattern and the extent of the fissures may vary considerably (Fig. 4.8). Most patients are asymptomatic otherwise. May be associated with

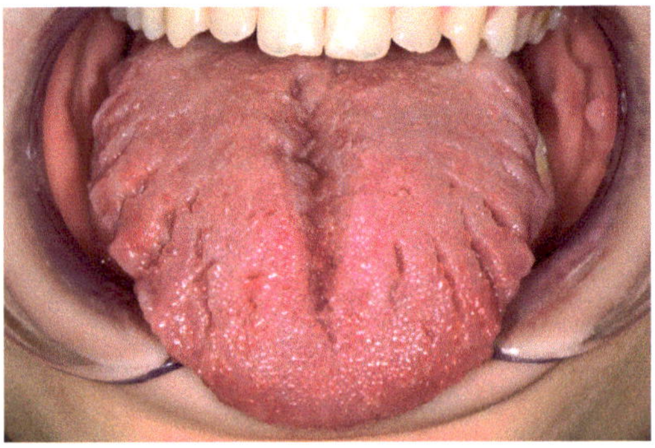

Fig. 4.8 Fissured tongue

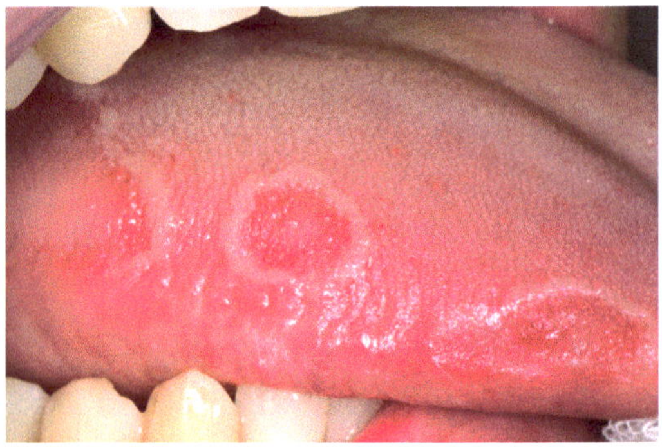

Fig. 4.9 Geographic tongue

geographic tongue. Fissured tongue may be part of Melkersson-Rosenthal syndrome, the other features being granulomatous cheilitis and transient facial nerve paralysis; this triad is not necessarily present at the same time.

Treatment

In case of symptoms, brushing the tongue twice a day may be helpful in some patients.

4.7 Geographic Tongue (Lingua Geographica; Migrating Glossitis)

Definition

Benign condition of the lingual mucosa characterized by migrating areas of smooth, reddish discolorations of the mucosal surface of the anterior tongue. The reddish areas are surrounded by a whitish border of desquamated epithelial cells.

Etiology

The etiology is unknown; stress has been mentioned as a possible predisposing factor. Due to the somewhat similar histopathologic aspects, a possible association with psoriasis has been suggested.

Epidemiology

The estimated prevalence is approximately 1 %. Geographic tongue may occur on all ages, even in young children.

Clinical Aspects

Smooth reddish changes on the dorsal surface of the tongue and sometimes also on the borders of the tongue, surrounded by a whitish slough (Figs. 4.9 and 4.10a, b). The reddish, depapillated areas will recover spontaneously in a matter of days, weeks, and sometimes months, showing up again at other sites of the tongue and, in rare instances, outside the tongue ("geographic stomatitis", "ectopic geographc tongue") (Fig. 4.11).

Geographic tongue may cause symptoms of burning when using spicy food or drinking juices and may be associated with fissured tongue.

The diagnosis of geographic tongue is usually a clinical one, and there is rarely a need for a biopsy.

Histopathology

The histopathologic appearance is characterized by numerous polymorphonuclear leukocytes that migrate through the epithelium, giving rise to the formation of spongiform pustules or small abscesses, called Munro abscesses, in the upper epithelial layers (Fig. 4.12). The stratum spinosum may be thickened and edematous. In the smooth, red areas, the papillae of the connective tissue may reach high up close to the surface, mimicking to some extent the histologic appearance of psoriasis.

Treatment

There are no means to treat geographic tongue effectively. The condition probably persists lifelong, although there may be remissions for a long period of time.

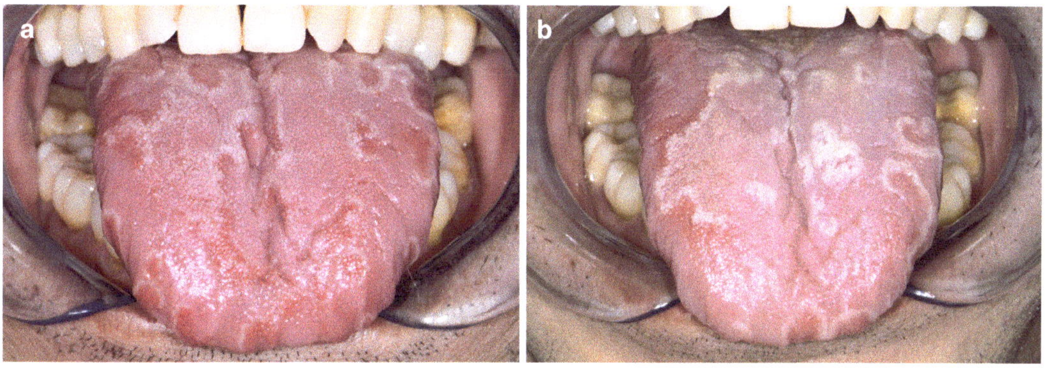

Fig. 4.10 (**a**) Geographic tongue. (**b**) Same patient 1 month later; notice the different pattern

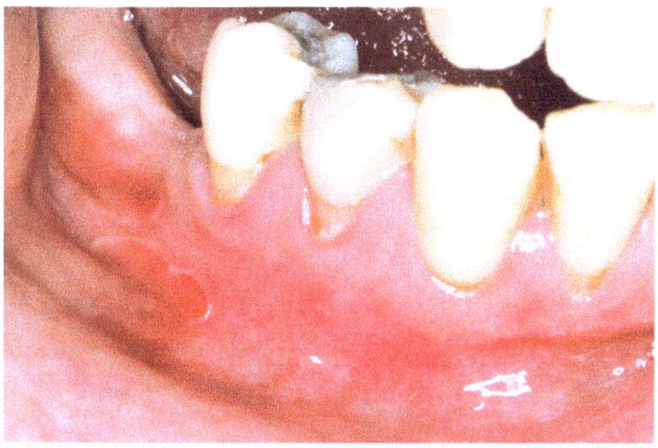

Fig. 4.11 Geographic stomatitis ("ectopic geographic tongue") affecting the lower mucobuccal fold

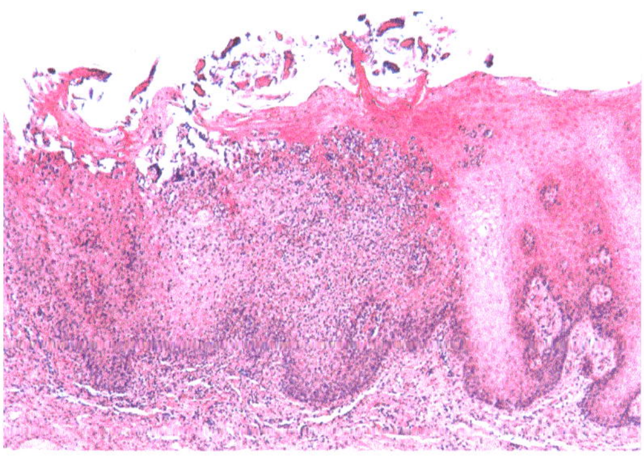

Fig. 4.12 Low-power view of geographic tongue

4.8 Glossodynia and Burning Mouth Syndrome

Definition

Bilateral painful or burning sensation of the tongue and/or other oral mucosas in the absence of clinically visible lesions. Dry mouth (xerostomia) and taste disturbances may be accompanying symptoms. When only the tongue is involved, without other symptoms, the term glossodynia or glossopyrosis may be used. In case of other involved subsites, the term burning mouth syndrome (BMS) is used.

In case of a burning sensation of only the palatal mucosa in a denture wearer, without clinically visible abnormalities, the term denture sore mouth (DSM) is used, not to be mixed up with denture stomatitis in which there is a fiery red appearance of the palatal mucosa.

Etiology

The etiology of BMS is unknown. Although a variety of causes have been mentioned in the literature, the most common one being an underlying psychiatric disorder, there is no proven causative etiological factor. Burning mouth is rarely, if ever, based on hormonal disturbances, vitamin deficiencies, or side effects of medication.

Epidemiology

The estimated prevalence is less than 0.01 %. BMS rarely occurs below the age of 40 years and is much more common among women than men.

Clinical Aspects

Normal aspect of the mucosa (Fig. 4.13). In patients complaining of dry mouth, there may be a sufficient amount of saliva as being observed during oral examination. However, xerostomia refers to the subjective feeling of dryness as experienced by the patient, while hyposalivation

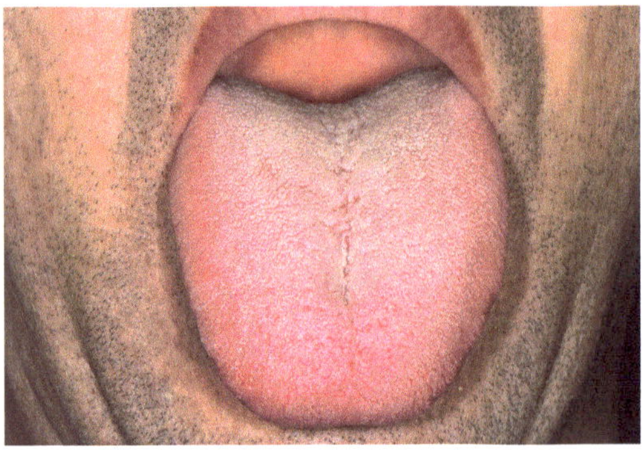

Fig. 4.13 Normal aspect of the tongue in patient with glossodynia

refers to an objectively measured decrease of the salivary flow.

Laboratory Studies
Laboratory studies of whatever type (e.g., vitamin levels, iron, etc.) rarely if ever contribute to the management of the symptoms. Nevertheless, such studies can be performed in case of unusual BMS, e.g., occurring in patients below the age of 30 years (Table 4.1).

Management
Always perform a thorough examination of the mouth, even when the symptoms are highly suggestive of BMS. Occasionally, the burning sensation is caused by mucosal lesions or disorders such as erosive lichen planus or erythroplakia.

Take time for the patient to explain the complexity of this syndrome and avoid giving the patient the impression of suffering from a psychiatric disorder, since there is no evidence for such suggestion. Reassure the patient that the symptoms are not caused by an underlying systemic disease, including malignancy.

In the majority of patients, the burning sensation will disappear in a matter of years. Some patients may need professional support to learn to cope with these symptoms. In severe cases, the prescription of antidepressive drugs may be indicated. This such suggestion is usually declined by the patient.

Do not perform any dental or surgical procedures that are not truly indicated. Do not refer the patient unless you know a qualified colleague who is more knowledgeable in this particular subject.

4.9 Granular Cell Tumor

Definition
Benign neoplasm probably derived from Schwann cells or from neuroendocrine cells.

Etiology
Unknown.

Epidemiology
Rare tumor that may occur already in children, more often in females than in males.

Clinical Aspects
A granular cell tumor may occur everywhere in the body but most often affects the tongue.

It is usually a solitary tumor but multiple tumors may occur as well. The clinical presentation is that of a yellowish nodule of the tongue or, occasionally, of other oral sites, being asymptomatic otherwise (Fig. 4.14a, b). In an exceptional case, simultaneous granular cell tumors may occur elsewhere in the body, e.g., in the lungs.

Histopathology
Somewhat circumscribed but not encapsulated tumor consisting of large polygonal cells with a granular cytoplasm. The granular cells are positive for S-100 immunohistochemically. In the overlying epithelium, pseudoepitheliomatous hyperplasia may be encountered; this phenomenon may be mistaken for a squamous cell carcinoma (Fig. 4.15a, b).

Treatment
Local excision usually suffices, although no true radicality may be obtained at the histopathologic level. Nevertheless, recurrences are rare.

Table 4.1 Management of patients with symptoms of burning mouth syndrome

- Patient < 30 years[a]
  - Laboratory studies[b]
    - Positive
      - Treatment accordingly
    - Negative → Patient information
- Patient > 30years
  - Bilateral symptoms → Patient information
  - Unilateral symptoms
    - Neurologic examination
      - Negative → Patient information
      - Positive
        - Treatment accordingly

Patient information
- The cause is unknown
- It is not a psychiatric illness
- It is rarely a side effect of medication
- The symptoms rarely are based on an allergic reaction
- The symptoms are no signs of an underlying disease of whatever type, including cancer elsewhere in the body
- In most patients the symptoms will disappear spontaneously, but this may take several months or even years
- There are no effective means to treat the symptoms
- There are no specific dietary guidelines
- Some patients benefit from the use of chewing gum
- In severe cases one may consider the use of antidepressants (not because of the presence of depression but because of the ineffectiveness of regular pain killers)

- Explanation not accepted
  - -Avoid any dental or surgical treatment that is not really indicated
  - -Offer psychological help, not because of the presence of a psychiatric illnes, but in order to get support in coping with the symptoms
  - -Only dedicated referral is justified (to a person who is knowledgable in this area); do not create high expectations of such referral
- Explanation accepted

[a]The cut-off point of 30 years is somewhat arbitrarily chosen and is not evidence based.

[b]The laboratory studies include:
- Complete blood count (CBC)
- Mean corpuscular volume (MCV)
- Mean corpuscular hemoglobin (MCH)
- White cell count
- Vitamin B_{12} (one may consider to include B_1, B_2, and B_6 as well)
- Folate (serum and red blood cells)
- Serum iron
- Total iron binding capacity (TIBC)
- Ferritin levels and % transferin saturation

Show your understanding

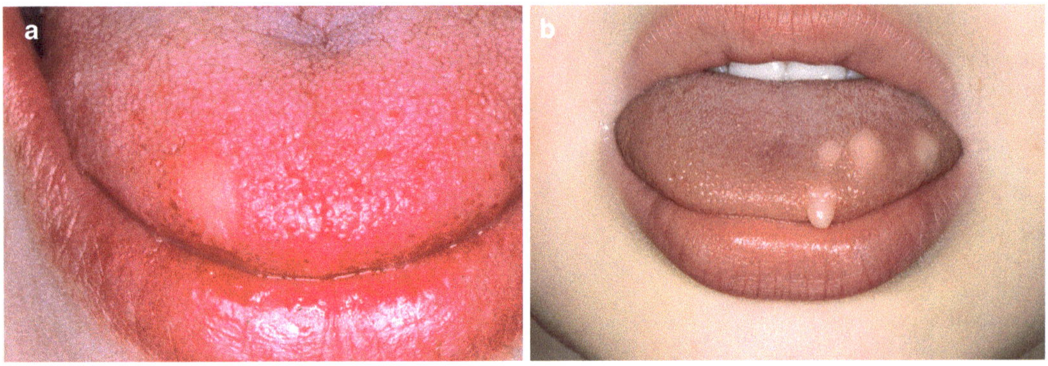

Fig. 4.14 (a) Rather characteristic aspect of a granular cell tumor. (b) Multiple granular cell tumors in a child

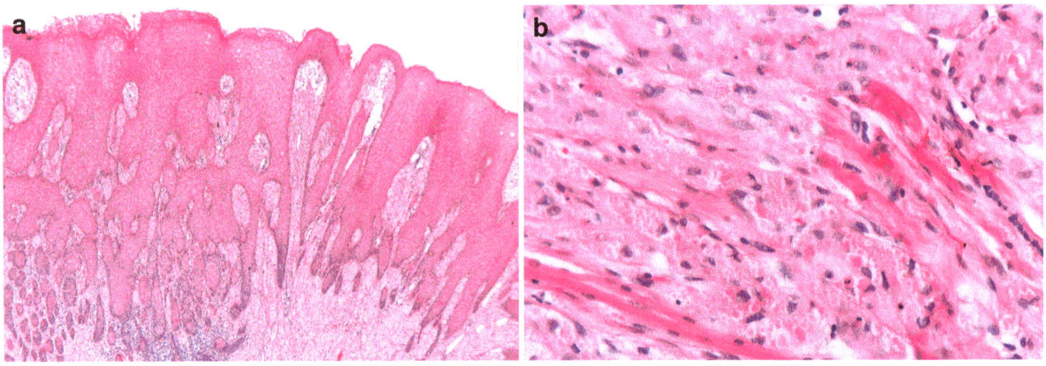

Fig. 4.15 (a) Pseudoepitheliomatous hyperplasia overlying a granular cell tumor. (b) Low-power view of granular cell tumor

4.10 Hairy Leukoplakia

Definition

Benign whitish change of the mucosa of the borders of the tongue in immunocompromised patients.

Note: The term "leukoplakia" for this condition is unfortunate since leukoplakia refers to a white lesion that cannot be identified as any other known white lesion. Hairy leukoplakia is a well-defined "known" lesion. Furthermore, "true" leukoplakia is premalignant, while hairy leukoplakia is not. In addition, the use of "hairy" may cause confusion with regard to hairy tongue and even with regard to the term hairy cell leukemia. Besides, the clinical aspect is not always "hairy."

Etiology

Hairy leukoplakia may be caused by immunodeficiency, e.g., by HIV infection or by the prolonged use of immunosuppressive drugs, e.g., after solid organ transplantation. In other words, hairy leukoplakia is not necessarily an expression of HIV infection.

Epidemiology

Apparently, in many parts of the world, hairy leukoplakia has become a rare disease among the HIV population, probably due to early detection and intervention of the infection.

Clinical Aspects

White, either flat or verrucous ("hairy"), non-wipeable mucosal changes on both borders of the tongue (Fig. 4.16a, b). Hairy leukoplakia is usually asymptomatic otherwise. The differential diagnosis of bilateral white lesions on the borders of the tongue includes:

- Candidiasis, pseudomembranous type
- Morsicatio (habitual biting or chewing on the tissues)

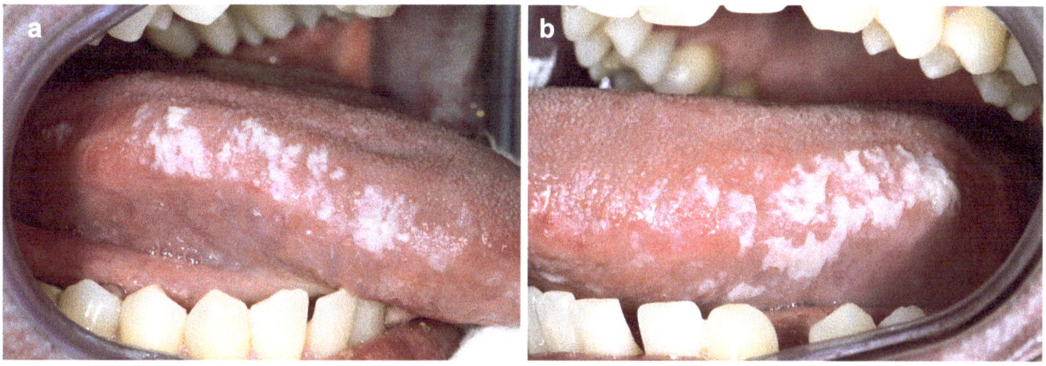

Fig. 4.16 (a) Hairy leukoplakia of the right border of the tongue. (b) Same patient; the other side. The diagnosis cannot be made on clinical grounds alone

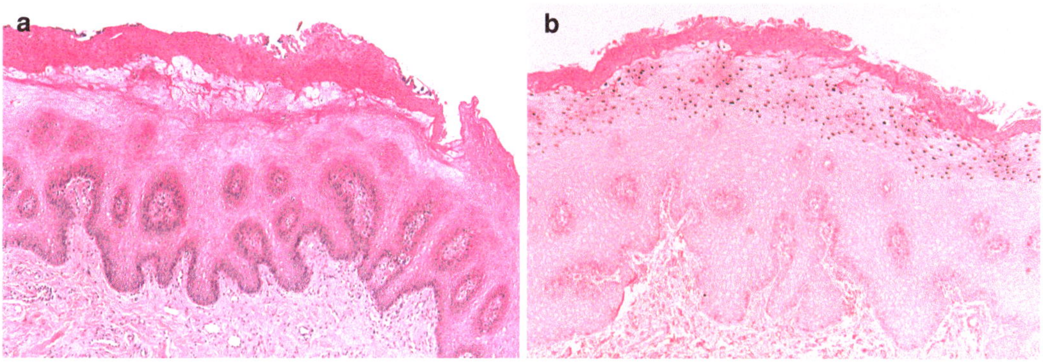

Fig. 4.17 (a) Low-power view of hairy leukoplakia. (b) Epstein-Barr virus positivity in the upper epithelial layer, being confirmative for a diagnosis of hairy leukoplakia

- Lichen planus, plaque type
- White sponge nevus
- Pachyonychia congenita
- Bilateral "true" leukoplakia

In an (HIV-)unidentified patient, it is not possible to diagnose the lesion on clinical grounds alone. In such event, one may either discuss with the patient the possibility of an HIV infection or another cause of immunosuppression or perform a biopsy.

Histopathology
In addition to a regular H-E stain, the immunohistochemical presence of Epstein-Barr virus should be demonstrated before allowing a firm diagnosis of "hairy leukoplakia" (Fig. 4.17a, b). As has been mentioned before, a firm diagnosis of "hairy leukoplakia" is no final proof of an underlying HIV infection but may also occur in patients who are immunosuppressed for other reasons. In some cases, there is secondary candidal involvement.

Treatment
Treatment with antiviral drugs usually results in disappearance of the lesion. After cessation of such treatment, the lesion will recur.

4.11 Hairy Tongue (Lingua Villosa; Coated Tongue)

Definition
Coated or hairy aspect of the dorsal surface of the tongue. Some authors use, somewhat arbitrarily, the term hairy tongue when the height of the papillae is more than 3 mm. In general, the terms coated and hairy tongue are used as synonyms.

Etiology

The etiology is actually unknown; the condition may perhaps be the result of an altered shedding pattern of the lingual papillae. Furthermore, *C. albicans* may play a role, as well as smoking.

Epidemiology

Hairy tongue may be seen in young adults and elderly persons; the prevalence is approximately 0.5 %.

Clinical Aspects

The coating of the dorsal surface may vary in color from yellowish-brown to black and sometimes even white ("black tongue," "white tongue") (Figs. 4.18 and 4.19a, b). Patients may complain of discomfort or a faulty taste.

Treatment

Since the cause is actually unknown, there are no effective means to treat this condition. Cessation of smoking habits may result in improvement. Some, but not all, patients benefit from cleaning the tongue twice a day with a toothbrush or a tongue scraper, with or without the use of a toothpaste.

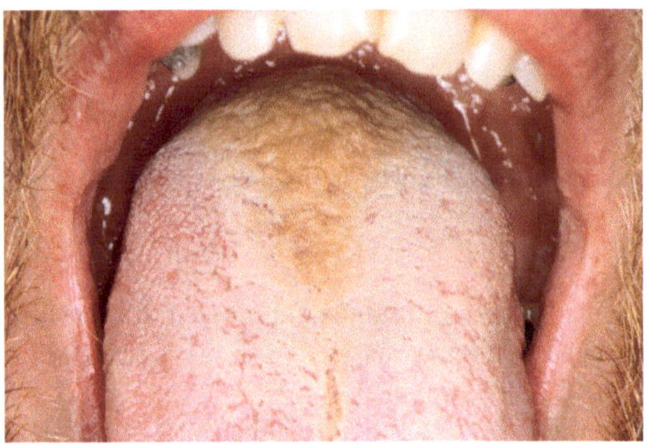

Fig. 4.18 Coated tongue

4.12 Lingual Thyroid

Definition

Developmental proliferation of thyroid tissue in the base of the tongue (Fig. 4.20).

Epidemiology

Rare phenomenon; occurs more often in women than in men. Usually becomes manifest during puberty.

Clinical Aspects

Firm elastic swelling, usually in the midline of the tongue at the junction of the mobile tongue and the base of the tongue (Fig. 4.21). May cause swallowing difficulties. Malignant transformation is extremely rare. The differential diagnosis includes:

- Salivary gland neoplasm
- Thyroglossal duct cyst
- Osteoma/osteochondroma

Laboratory Studies

Measurement of serum thyroid hormone. Scintigraphy of the thyroid gland may reveal that the lingual thyroid is the only functioning thyroid tissue present. One may also consider to perform

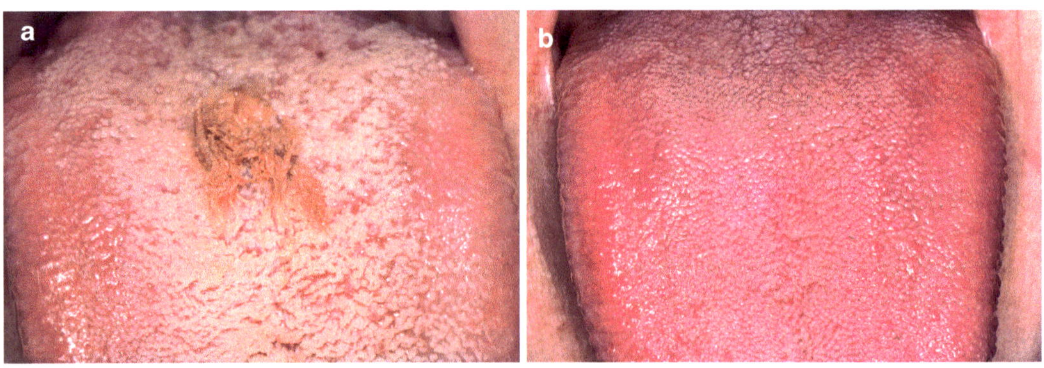

Fig. 4.19 (**a**) Hairy tongue; the patient was advised to brush the tongue twice a day. (**b**) Result after 2 weeks

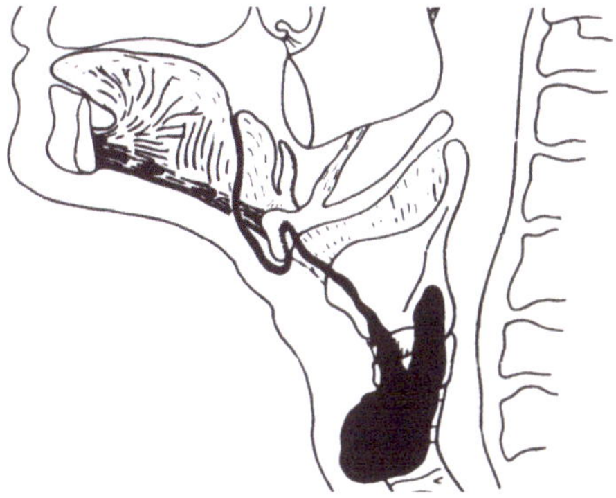

Fig. 4.20 Schematic drawing of thyroglossal tract

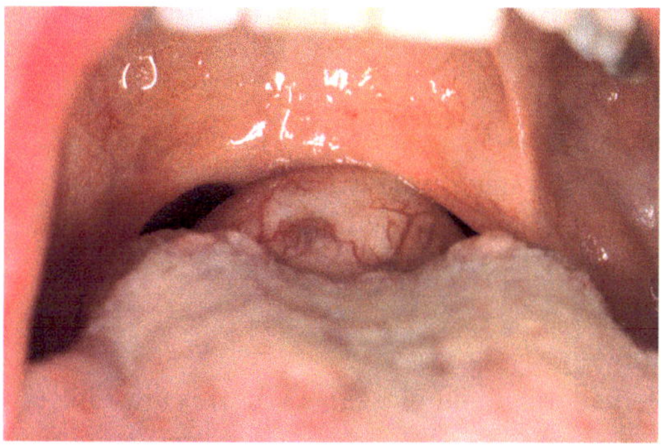

Fig. 4.21 Lingual thyroid in a 26-year-old woman

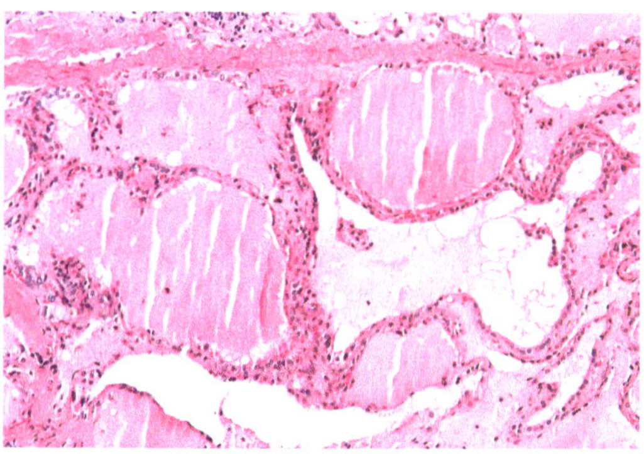

Fig. 4.22 The biopsy confirmed the clinical diagnosis of lingual thyroid in the patient shown in Fig. 4.21

aspiration cytology or to perform an incisional biopsy (Fig. 4.22).

Treatment

Substitutional therapy; there is rarely a need for surgical removal.

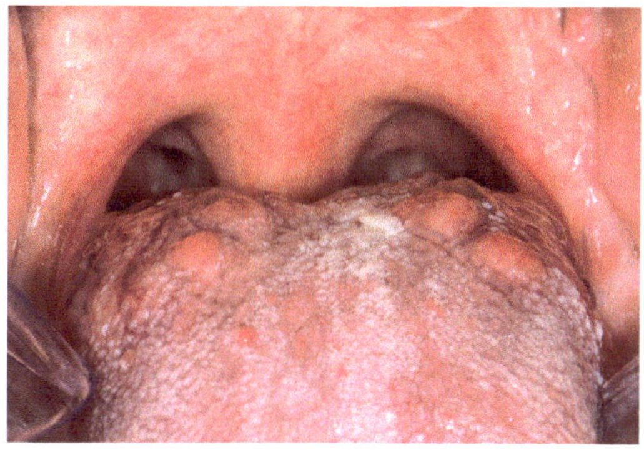

Fig. 4.23 Multiple tonsillar swellings on the base of the tongue

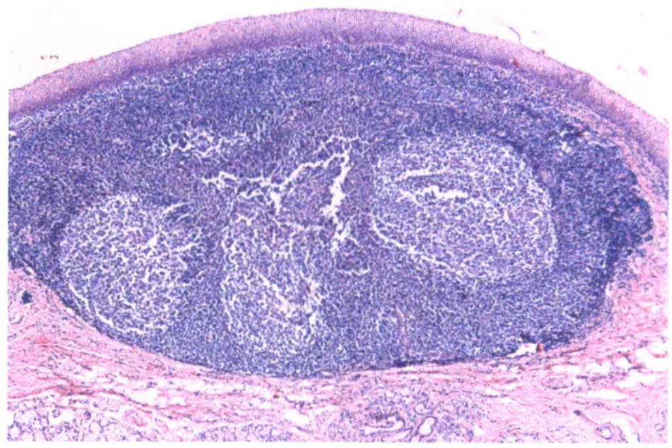

Fig. 4.24 Low-power view of lingual tonsillar tissue

4.13 Lingual Tonsils

Definition

Lymphoid tissue is normally present in the base of the tongue as part of Waldeyer's ring. These aggregates may be called lingual tonsils.

Clinical Aspects

Lingual tonsillar tissue may present as small nodules at the junction of the anterior part and the base of the tongue (Fig. 4.23). There is rarely a need for histopathologic confirmation.

Histopathology

Histopathologically, normal lymphoid tissue is observed (Fig. 4.24); in rare cases, pseudolymphoid hyperplasia may be encountered.

Treatment

No treatment indicated.

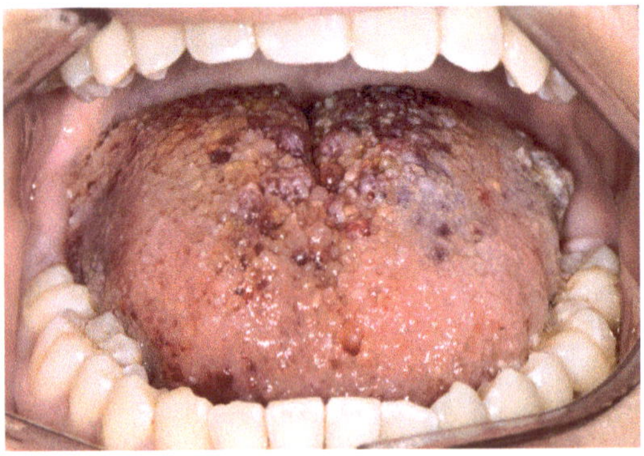

Fig. 4.25 Macroglossia caused by a lymphangioma

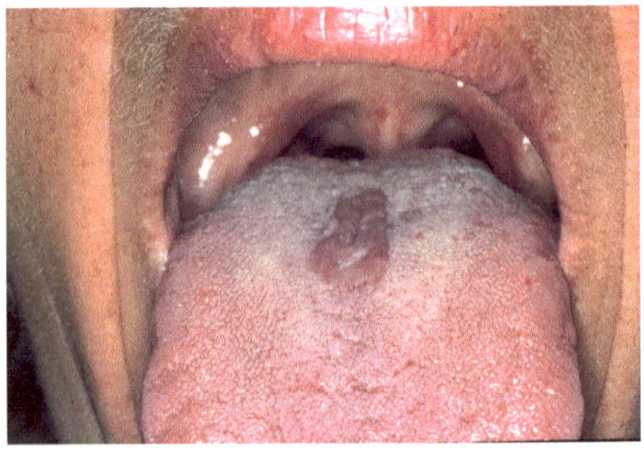

Fig. 4.26 Median rhomboid glossitis; asymptomatic

4.14 Macroglossia

Definition

Enlargement of the entire tongue. There are no objective means to define macroglossia. In general, the judgement of the size of the tongue is based on the patients' perception. Macroglossia can either be the result of a developmental disorder, such as a lymphangioma or syndromal disorders (e.g., Beckwith-Wiedemann syndrome, consisting of exomphalos, gigantism, and macroglossia, or Down syndrome), or being acquired, e.g., by cyst formation (e.g., a large dermoid cyst), a benign or malignant neoplasm, acromegaly, or the precipitation of amyloid.

Clinical Aspects

As mentioned above, lymphangiomas may cause macroglossia (Fig. 4.25). Particularly in case of malignant neoplasms, but also in case of amyloid deposition (see Fig. 4.1), the mobility of the tongue may be seriously limited. In case of a rapid enlargement of the tongue, impressions may arise at the borders of the tongue due to pressure from the teeth. This results in a "crenated" tongue (see Fig. 4.1).

Treatment

Treatment of macroglossia depends on the underlying cause.

4.15 Median Rhomboid Glossitis

Definition

Inflammatory-like lesion of the mucosa in the midline of the tongue, usually near the foramen cecum. There is often a rhomboid configuration, indeed, but other shapes may be encountered as well.

Etiology

Median rhomboid glossitis (MRG) is most likely caused by *C. albicans* infection, representing the erythematous form of candidiasis. May occur in patients using corticosteroids containing inhalers. Probably, also smoking plays a role in the etiology of MRG.

Epidemiology

MRG is rather common in adults and is, indeed, rarely observed in children or adolescents.

Clinical Aspects

The lesion may be either flat or granular and sometimes elevated and lobular (Fig. 4.26). MRG may occur not only in the foramen cecum area but also on the anterior part of the tongue in or close to the midline. MRG may cause local irritation. Quite often, there is involvement of the opposite palatal mucosal surface ("Kissing lesion") (Fig. 4.27a, b).

In the majority of cases, the diagnosis of MRG can be made based on clinical grounds alone, partly

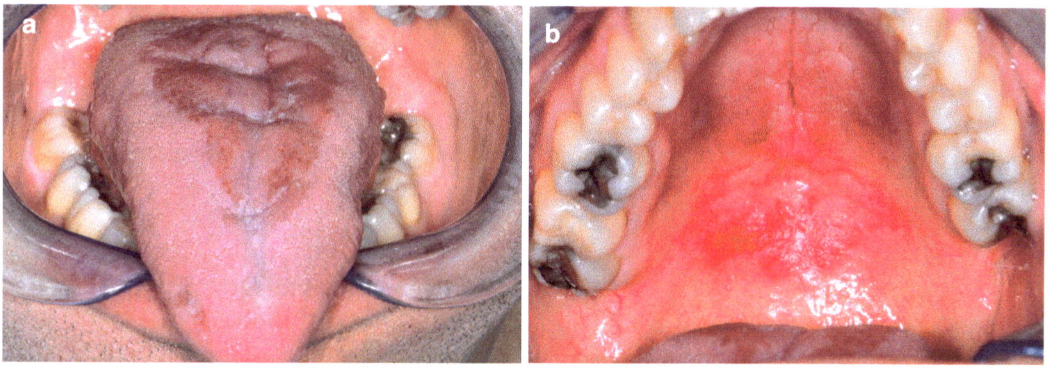

Fig. 4.27 (**a**) Median rhomboid glossitis in a patient using inhalers. (**b**) Palatal aspect in the same patient ("kissing lesion")

because of the fact that a squamous cell carcinoma rarely arises at the dorsal surface of the tongue. In case of doubt, a biopsy should be taken. In rare instances, a Kaposi sarcoma may be located on the tongue and may, indeed, somewhat mimic median rhomboid glossitis (see elsewhere in this chapter).

Histopathology

In case of a biopsy, one may observe epithelial hyperplasia and the presence of candidal hyphae in the superficial layers of the epithelium (see also Chap. 2). In case of a superficial biopsy, the pathologist may have difficulties in excluding the possibility of a squamous cell carcinoma.

Treatment

In the absence of symptoms, there is no need for antifungal treatment, either topically or systematically. The patient should be advised to quit smoking, if applicable. In case of the use of an inhaler, the patient should be advised to thoroughly rinse the mouth after its use.

4.16 Osteoma; Osteochondroma

Definition

Developmental disorder characterized by the formation of bone or cartilage in the soft tissues. In fact, this disorder is an example of a choristoma, being defined as the presence of tissue at an abnormal site in the body

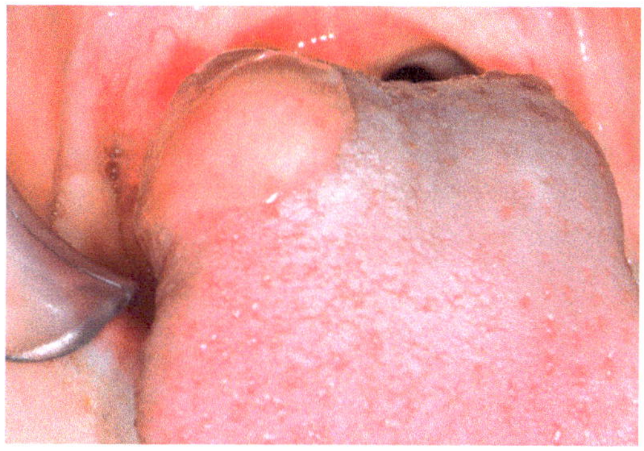

Fig. 4.28 Osteoma at the dorsum of the tongue; asymptomatic

Epidemiology

Rare phenomenon.

Clinical Aspects

Usually occurs on the dorsal surface of the tongue (Fig. 4.28). Occurs in adolescents and young adults. Is asymptomatic otherwise.

Treatment

Although treatment is not necessary, removal is usually advised for histopathologic confirmation of the diagnosis (Fig. 4.29).

4.17 Papillae Foliatae and Foliate Papillitis

Definition

In human beings, foliate papillae at the posterior lateral borders of the tongue are somewhat rudimentary; in rare instances, they may become inflamed ("foliate papillitis").

Etiology

The cause of secondary inflammation of these papillae is unknown; perhaps smoking plays a role.

Clinical Aspects

The papillae may become enlarged and may have a fiery red appearance. There is often a bilateral presentation (Fig. 4.30a, b). There is no induration on palpation. May cause a localized burning sensation. In case of doubt about the diagnosis, a biopsy should be taken.

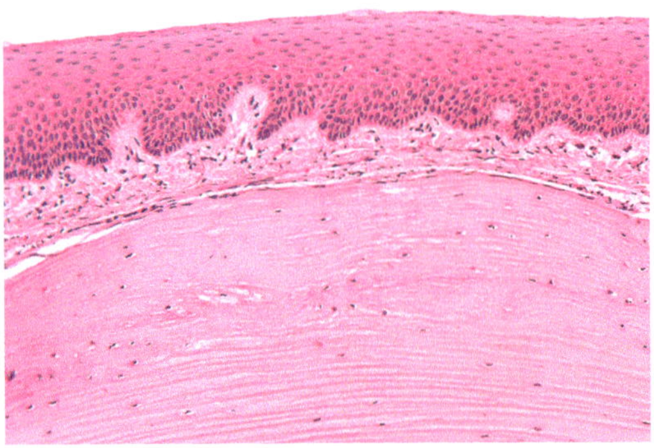

Fig. 4.29 Low-power view of osteoma of the tongue

Histopathology

Nonspecific chronic inflammatory changes.

Treatment

Not required; the symptoms usually disappear in a matter of a few months.

4.18 Thyroglossal Duct Cyst

Definition

Developmental cyst derived from epithelial remnants of the thyroglossal tract (Fig. 4.20).

Epidemiology

Rare cyst; usually becomes manifest during childhood.

Clinical Aspects

Cystic swelling that may occur at any site of the thyroglossal tract, either extraorally in the midline of the neck or intraorally in the foramen cecum area of the dorsum of the tongue (Fig. 4.31). The differential diagnosis includes a lingual thyroid and a salivary gland tumor.

Histopathology

At histopathologic examination, thyroid tissue is encountered in the cyst wall; malignant transformation is extremely rare.

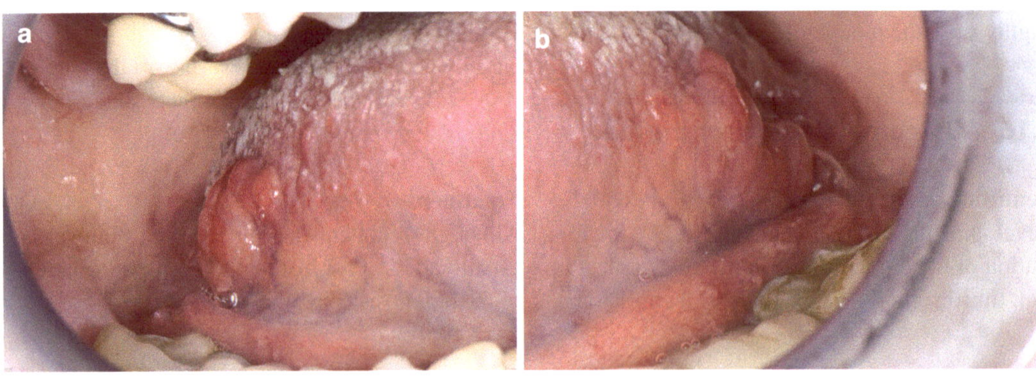

Fig. 4.30 (**a**) Papillae foliatae on the right side. (**b**) Same patient; at the other side, the papillae foliatae are less prominent

Treatment

Enucleation; it may be necessary to include a small portion of the hyoid bone ("Sistrunk procedure") in order to prevent a recurrence since the cyst may extend into the hyoid bone (Fig. 4.32).

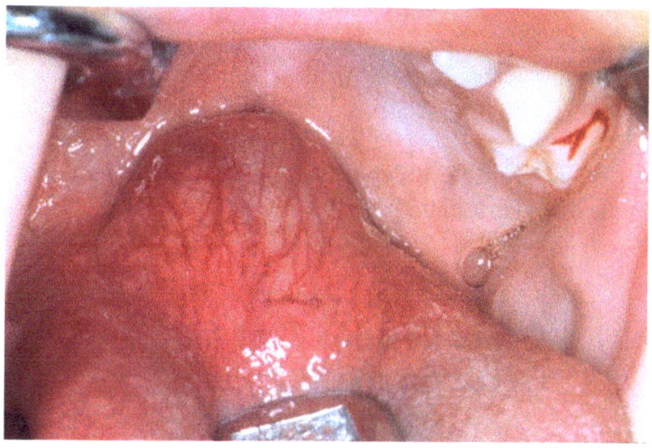

Fig. 4.31 Thyroglossal duct cyst in a child

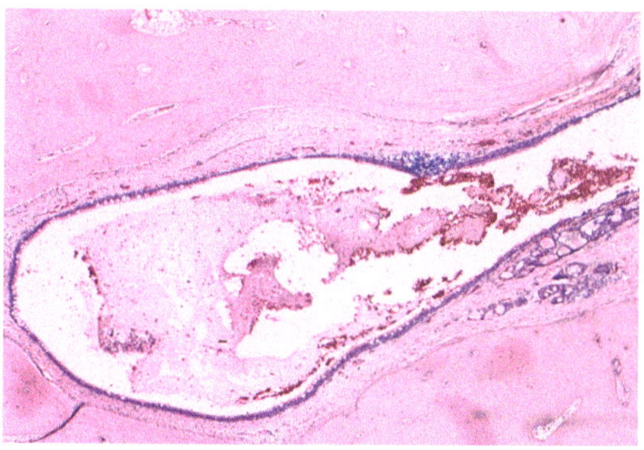

Fig. 4.32 Extension of thyroglossal duct cyst into the hyoid bone

4.19 Traumatic Eosinophilic Granuloma (Traumatic Ulcerative Granuloma with Stromal Eosinophilia (TUGSE))

Definition

Inflammatory disease characterized by the presence of numerous eosinophilic granulocytes.

Etiology

In spite of the terminology, the role of trauma is uncertain.

Clinical Aspects

Non-indurated and usually non-painful ulcer with a sharp border, most often occurring on the tongue (Fig. 4.33a, b). The ulcer may be present for several weeks without showing a tendency to heal and may mimic an ulcerative squamous cell carcinoma.

The ulcer in the ventral aspect of the tip of the tongue in Riga-Fede disease, due to the eruption of deciduous lower incisors, is regarded to be a variant of traumatic eosinophilic granuloma (see Chap. 2).

Histopathology

On histopathologic examination, a chronic inflammatory infiltrate will be encountered including the presence of various amounts of eosinophilic granulocytes (Fig. 4.34). The lymphocytic cells may be misdiagnosed as being part

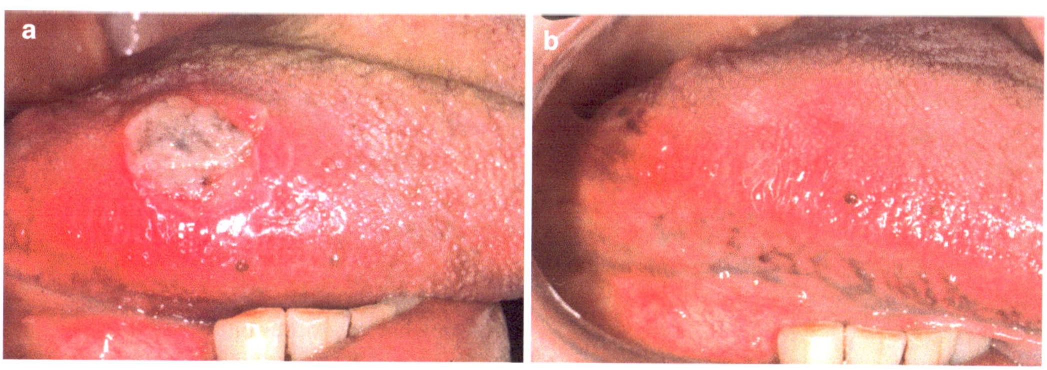

Fig. 4.33 (**a**) Non-characteristic presentation of eosinophilic granuloma, mimicking a squamous cell carcinoma. (**b**) Spontaneous healing in 2 weeks after a small incisional biopsy

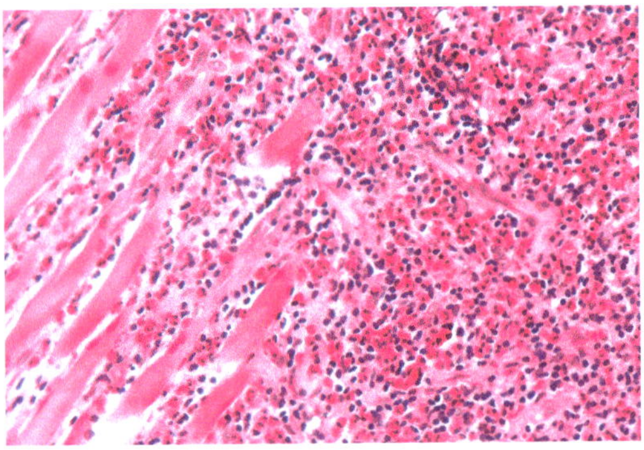

Fig. 4.34 Numerous eosinophils in a biopsy from traumatic eosinophilic granuloma

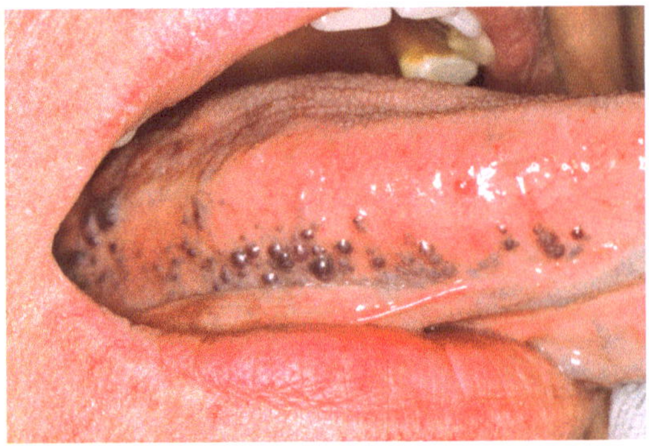

Fig. 4.35 Multiple phlebectasias on the border of the tongue ("caviar tongue")

of the spectrum of a non-Hodgkin lymphoma since there may be positivity for the tumor marker CD30.

Treatment
After the taking of an incisional biopsy, the lesion usually heals within a week.

4.20 Varices and Phlebectasias

Definition
Dilatation of part of a small blood vessel ("varix") or just a local dilatation of a blood vessel ("phlebectasia"); both terms are often used as synonyms (see also Chap. 2).

Etiology
Is regarded as an aging phenomenon and is not a sign of a compromised cardiovascular condition.

Clinical Aspects
May occur in a solitary or multiple fashion everywhere on the lips or the oral mucosa, but often involve the tongue. In the latter case, the term "caviar tongue" is sometimes used (Fig. 4.35). Varices and phlebectasias rarely cause symptoms. The diagnosis can usually be made on clinical grounds alone.

Treatment
No treatment or follow-up is required.

4.21 Other Lesions That May Occur on the Tongue

4.21.1 Aspirin Burn

Some Characteristics
The buccal mucosa and the borders of the tongue are the sites of predilection of an aspirin burn (Fig. 4.36a, b). Prolonged local application of paracetamol tablets may cause similar defects (see also Chap. 2).

4.21.2 Cowden's Syndrome (Multiple Hamartoma Syndrome)

Some Characteristics
In Cowden syndrome, also referred to as multiple hamartoma syndrome, multiple papules may involve the oral mucosa, including the tongue (Fig. 4.37). Recognition of this hereditary disorder is important because of the risk of developing benign and malignant neoplasms, such as of the thyroid and the breast.

4.21.3 Erythroplakia

Some Characteristics
Erythroplakia may occur on the tongue, both on the borders and the dorsal surface (Fig. 4.38). Usually, erythroplakias cause a local burning or

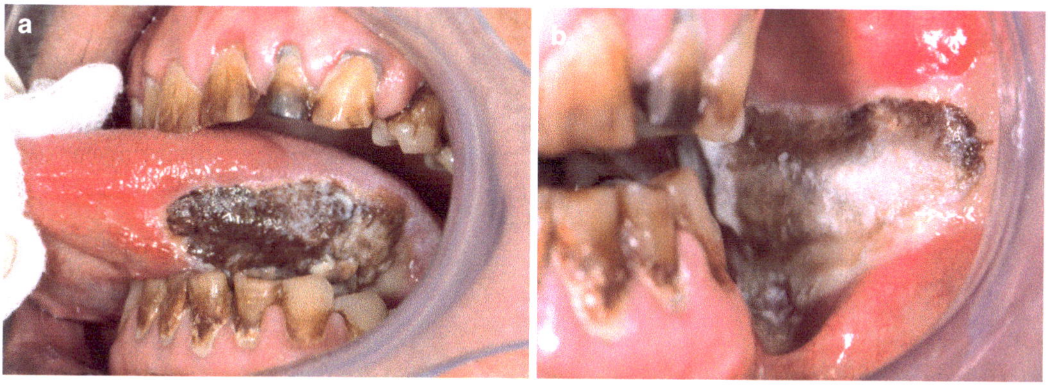

Fig. 4.36 (**a**) Ulcerative lesion caused by prolonged local application of paracetamol tablets for a toothache in a heavy smoker. (**b**) Same patient; in the buccal mucosa, the commonly whitish aspect of aspirin burns is preserved

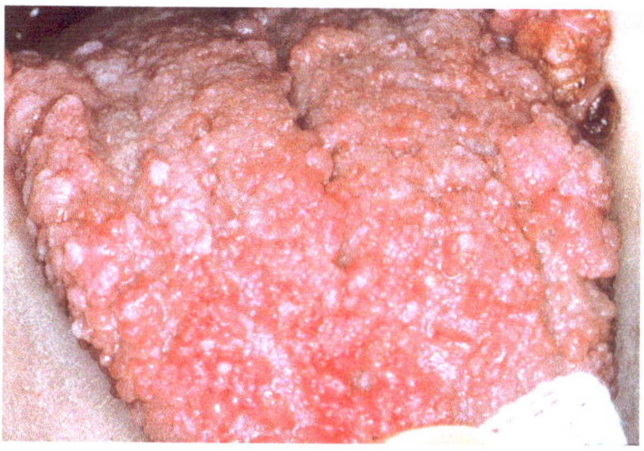

Fig. 4.37 Papillomatous aspect of the tongue in a patient with Cowden's syndrome

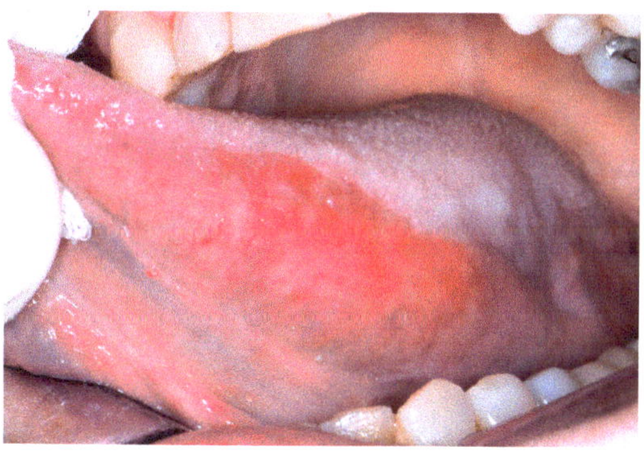

Fig. 4.38 Unilateral erythroplakia of the tongue

itching sensation (see also Chap. 2). As a rule, erythroplakias should always be biopsied for the assessment of epithelial dysplasia or even a squamous cell carcinoma.

4.21.4 Fibroma

Some Characteristics

Fibromas quite commonly occur on the tongue, particularly at the anterior part of the tongue (Fig. 4.39) (see also Chap. 2). In the majority of cases, the diagnosis can be made on clinical grounds alone; in case of doubt, an excisional biopsy should be taken.

4.21.5 Kaposi Sarcoma

Some Characteristics

Oral Kaposi sarcomas almost exclusively occur in HIV-infected patients. The palate, the gingiva, and the tongue are the sites of predilection (see Chap. 2). When the tongue is involved, it usually concerns the dorsum of the tongue (Fig. 4.40).

4.21.6 Leukoplakia

Some Characteristics

Most common potentially malignant disorder of the oral mucosa. May occur everywhere in the oral mucosa, including the tongue (Fig. 4.41) (see also Chap. 2). Leukoplakia of the tongue is relatively common among nonsmokers compared to smokers and carries a higher risk of malignant

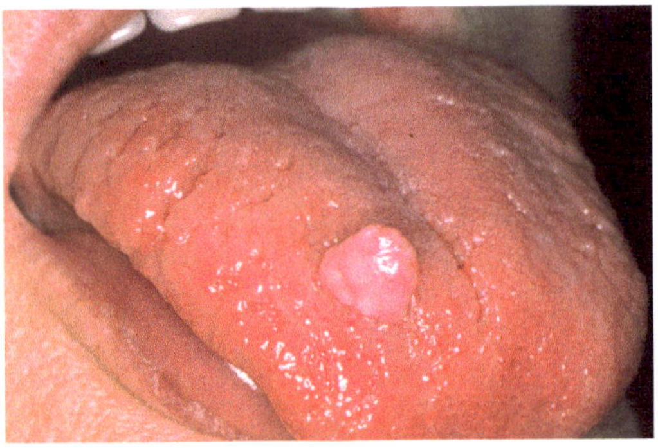

Fig. 4.39 Fibroma on the dorsum of the tongue

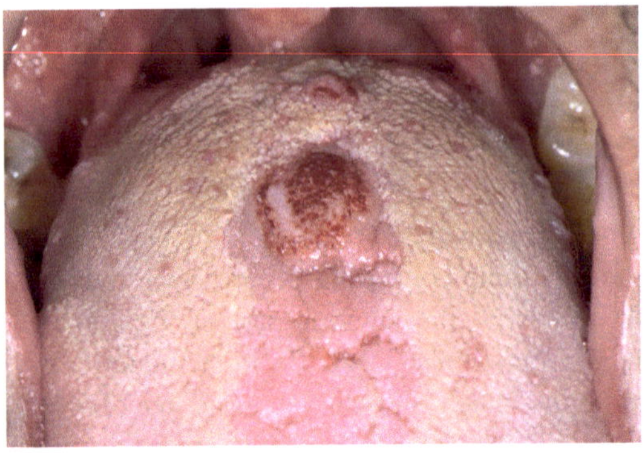

Fig. 4.40 Median rhomboid glossitis-like aspect of a Kaposi sarcoma; notice also the more posteriorly located lesion

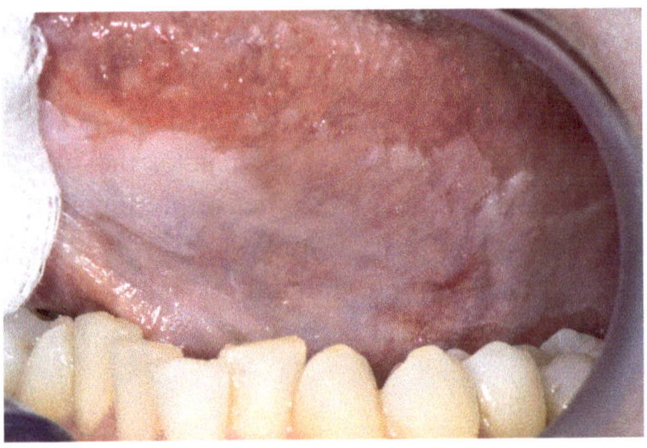

Fig. 4.41 Homogeneous leukoplakia

transformation than leukoplakias elsewhere in the mouth. Symptoms such as local burning or itching may be indicative of the presence of epithelial dysplasia or even a squamous cell carcinoma. Therefore, in case of symptoms, a biopsy is indicated.

4.21.7 Lichen Planus

Some Characteristics

Lichen planus has been discussed in Chap. 2. The buccal mucosa, the gingiva, and the tongue are the sites of predilection (Fig. 4.42). Sometimes it may be difficult to distinguish plaque-type lichen planus from leukoplakia. In such cases, a biopsy may be helpful, but there remain cases where no firm diagnosis can be established.

4.21.8 Lymphoepithelial Cyst

Some Characteristics

Lymphoepithelial cysts of the oral mucosa mainly occur in the floor of the mouth and in the tongue (Fig. 4.43). In case of doubt about the diagnosis, a biopsy is required (see also Chap. 2).

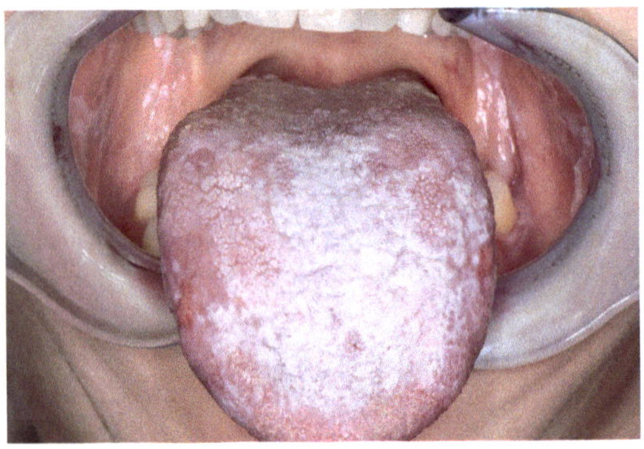

Fig. 4.42 Lichen planus of the dorsal surface

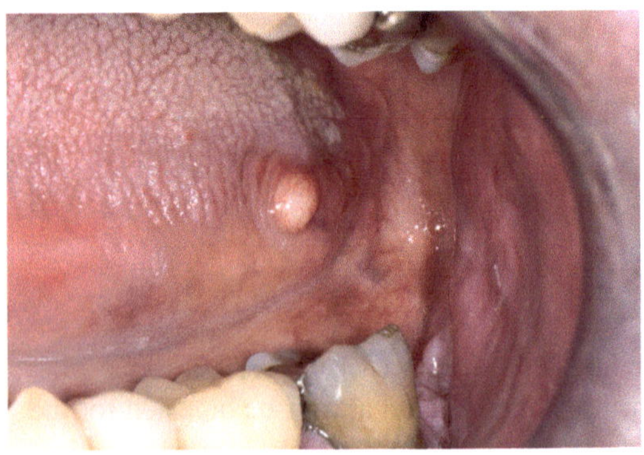

Fig. 4.43 Lymphoepithelial cyst on the border of the tongue

4.21.9 Morsicatio

Some Characteristics

Morsicatio may involve the lateral borders of the tongue. There is usually a bilateral distribution (Fig. 4.44a, b) (see also Chap. 2). Morsicatio may mimic clinically a number of other lesions, such as hyperplastic candidiasis, leukoplakia, lichen planus, hairy leukoplakia, and pachyonychia congenita. In case of doubt, a biopsy should be taken.

4.21.10 Mucous Cyst

Some Characteristics

Mucous cysts are most common on the lower lip and the floor of the mouth but may occur on the tongue as well, particularly at the ventral aspect of the tip of the tongue (Fig. 4.45) (see also Chaps. 2 and 3). In this particular location, there is a high risk of recurrence after conservative removal. Therefore, it is recommended to include all surrounding salivary gland tissue during the removal of the cyst.

4.21.11 Multifocal Epithelial Hyperplasia

Some Characteristics

Multifocal epithelial hyperplasia may occur everywhere on the lips or the oral mucosa, including the tongue, particularly at its borders (Fig. 4.46) (see also Chap. 2). The clinical picture is usually diagnostic. In case of a biopsy, a rather characteristic histopathologic picture is encountered (see Chap. 2). Treatment is not required. The lesions usually resolve spontaneously in a matter of months and sometimes years.

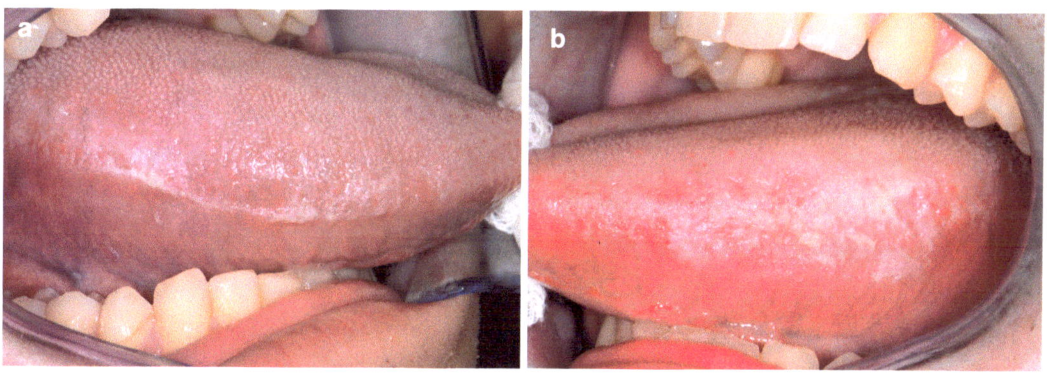

Fig. 4.44 (**a**) Morsicatio of the border of the tongue. (**b**) Same patient; left border

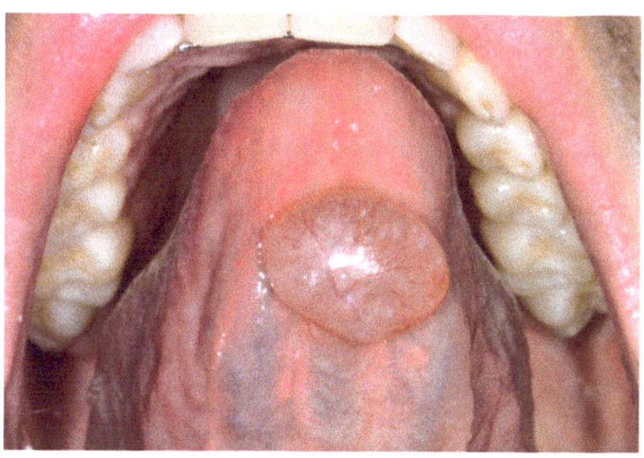

Fig. 4.45 Mucous cyst at the ventral aspect of the tongue

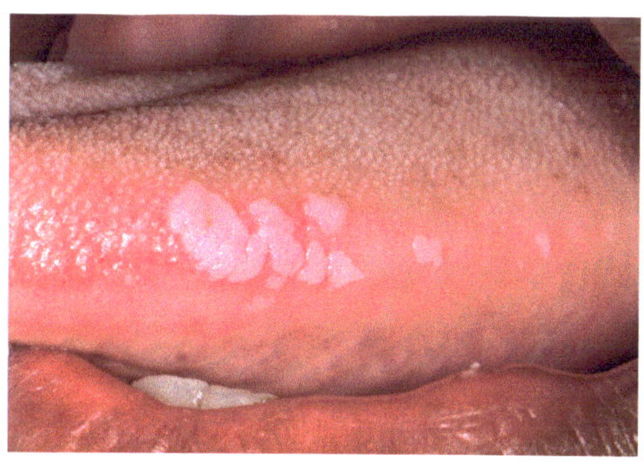

Fig. 4.46 Multifocal epithelial hyperplasia

4.21.12 Papilloma

Some Characteristics

Papillomas, either solitary or multiple, may occur everywhere in the oral mucosa, including the tongue (Fig. 4.47) (see also Chap. 2). May occur already during childhood.

Papillomas may somewhat resemble multifocal epithelial hyperplasia. Another differential diagnostic entity is condyloma acuminatum (see Chap. 2).

Recurrences after surgical removal are rare.

4.21.13 Pyogenic Granuloma

Some Characteristics

Excessive tissue proliferation after minor trauma, also referred to as lobular capillary hemangioma (see also Chap. 2). Pyogenic granulomas may occur everywhere in the mouth, including the tongue. The clinical presentation is a somewhat pedunculated, fibroma-like swelling with an ulcerative surface and may mimic a squamous cell carcinoma (Fig. 4.48). Treatment consists of surgical removal. Recurrences are rare.

4.21.14 Recurrent Aphthous Ulcers

Some Characteristics

Aphthous ulcers may occur on the tongue. The most common type is the minor type, often presenting in a multiple fashion. Major aphthous ulcers are relatively rare. When they present as a solitary lesion, there may strongly resemble a squamous cell carcinoma (Fig. 4.49a, b); see also Chap. 2.

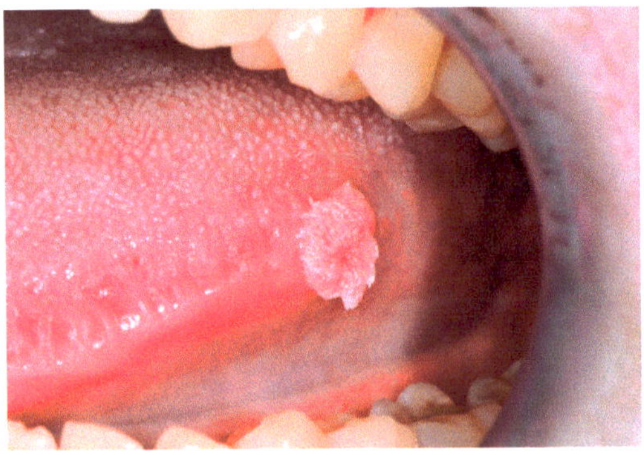

Fig. 4.47 Papilloma at the border of the tongue

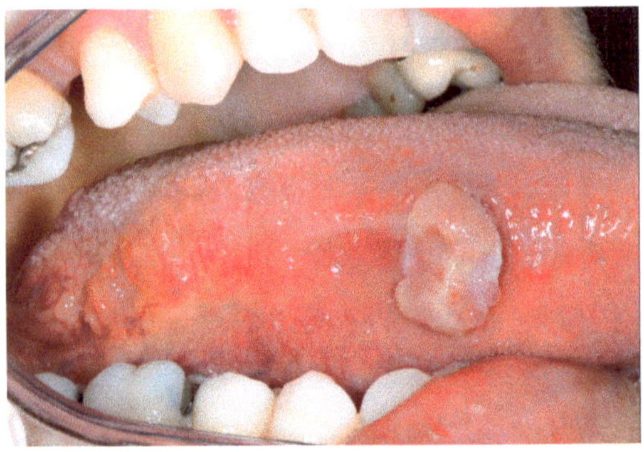

Fig. 4.48 Pyogenic granuloma

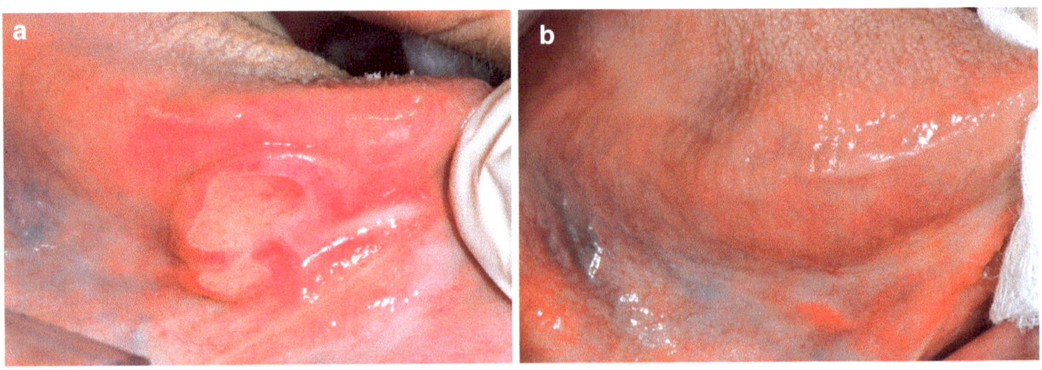

Fig. 4.49 (**a**) Patient with a history of major aphthous ulcers; the lesion very much mimics a squamous cell carcinoma. (**b**) Same patient 3 weeks later; spontaneous healing

4.21.15 Salivary Gland Tumors

Some Characteristics

Salivary gland neoplasms, either benign or malignant, rarely occur on the anterior two-thirds of the tongue (Fig. 4.50). The clinical presentation is an aspecific, slowly enlarging swelling of the soft tissues, often being asymptomatic otherwise.

4.21.16 Squamous Cell Carcinoma

Some Characteristics

The tongue is one of the sites of predilection of an oral squamous cell carcinoma. This neoplasm most often arises at the borders of the tongue and rarely on the dorsum (Fig. 4.51) (see also Chap. 2). The clinical presentation is usually an indurated, painful ulcer. There is a considerable risk of lymphatic spread to the neck nodes.

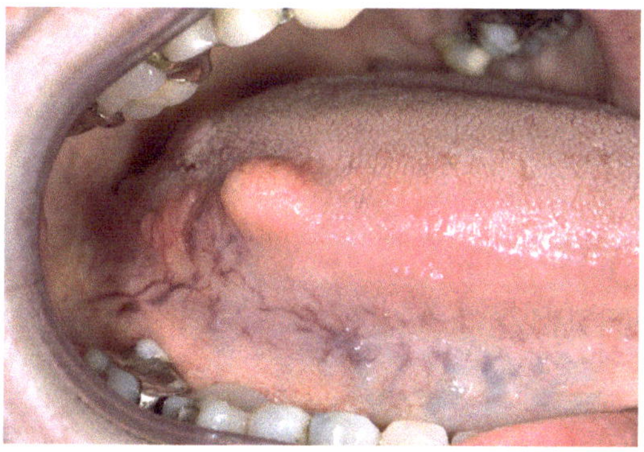

Fig. 4.50 Fibroma-like swelling based on a mucoepidermoid carcinoma

Small tongue cancers are primarily treated by surgery, while advanced cancers may be treated by surgery followed by radiotherapy or chemoradiation.

4.21.17 Syphilis

Some Characteristics

Primary syphilis may affect the tongue; this also applies to the second stage of this venereal disease (see also Chap. 2). The clinical presentation of a primary affect is an ulcer, usually on the dorsum of the tongue. In the second stage, the presentation may be that of "plaques muqueuses," lichenoid changes of the mucosa or red patches on the tongue or other parts of the mouth (Fig. 4.52).

4.21.18 Tongue Piercing

Some Characteristics

Tongue piercings have become quite common nowadays (Fig. 4.53). Although such piercings occasionally give rise to mucosal infections or injuries to the teeth, there are no strong reasons to discourage their application.

4.21.19 Vascular Malformations

Some Characteristics

Vascular malformations may affect almost all oral subsites, including the tongue. Occasionally,

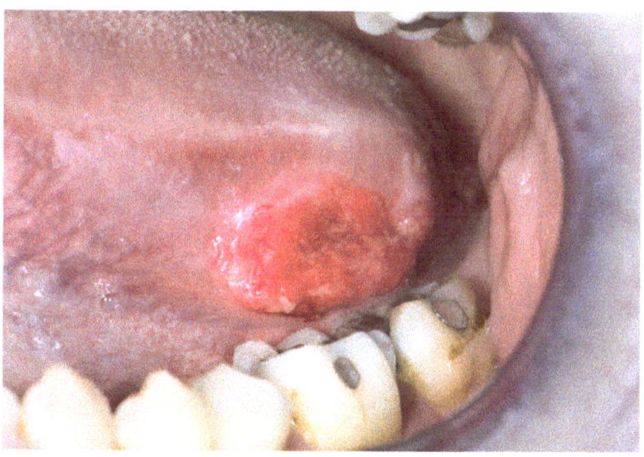

Fig. 4.51 Squamous cell carcinoma of the tongue

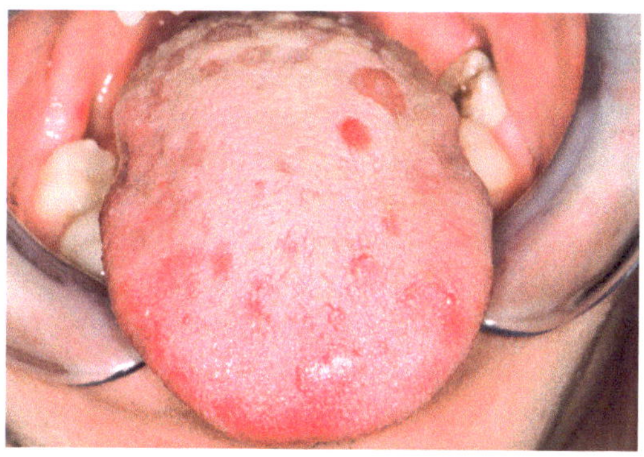

Fig. 4.52 Syphilis, second stage

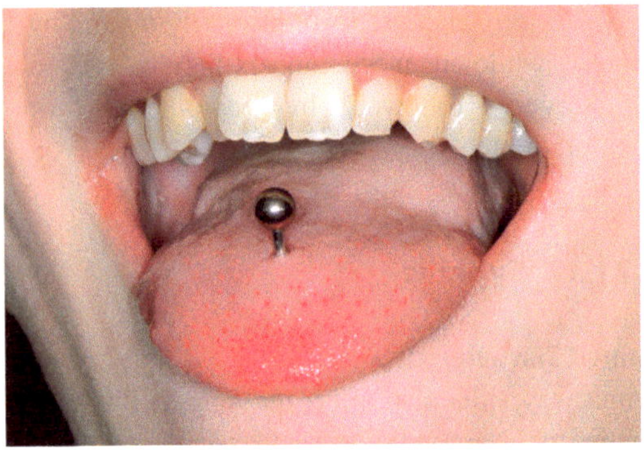

Fig. 4.53 Tongue piercing

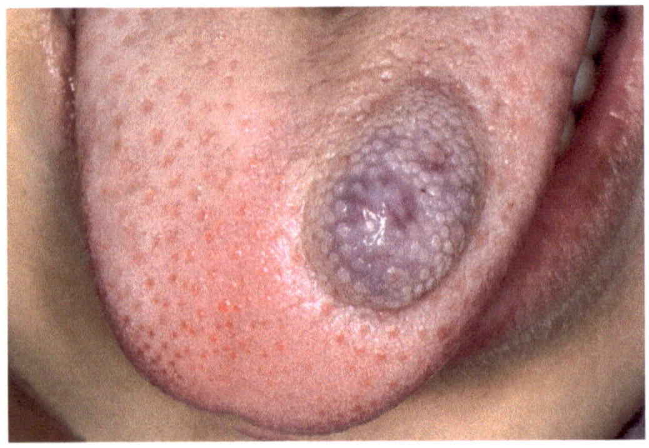

Fig. 4.54 Venous malformation in an 11-year-old child

such malformations, particularly in case of a lymphangioma, may interfere with swallowing, eating, or speech. Sometimes a patient asks for treatment because of esthetic reasons, particularly in case of location on the anterior part of the tongue (Fig. 4.54) (see also Chap. 2).

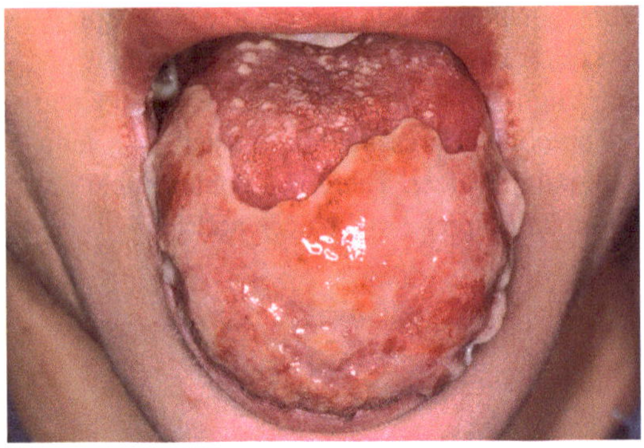

Fig. 4.55 Extensive involvement of the tongue in pemphigus vulgaris

4.21.20 Vesiculobullous Diseases

Some Characteristics

Vesiculobullous diseases, such as pemphigus vulgaris and mucous membrane pemphigoid, may occur everywhere in the oral cavity (see also Chap. 2). Sometimes large part of the dorsal surface of the tongue becomes affected (Fig. 4.55). Treatment usually consists of local application of corticosteroids. Systemic treatment with corticosteroids is only indicated in severe cases.

5 Diseases of the Gingiva and the Alveolar Mucosa

5.1 Introduction

The majority of diseases of the oral mucosa may also affect the gingiva and the mucosa of the alveolar ridges in edentulous part of the jaws. Some mucosal diseases rarely involve the gingiva, e.g., aphthous ulcers. On the other hand, there are diseases that only occur on the gingiva. In this chapter, examples of both categories of diseases will be discussed.

5.2 Cysts

5.2.1 Eruption Cyst

Definition
Odontogenic developmental cyst that can be regarded as a dentigerous or follicular cyst of an erupting tooth, usually a deciduous tooth. Some prefer to call this cyst an "eruption hematoma," suggesting that the lesion is caused by trauma during eruption resulting in a hematoma.

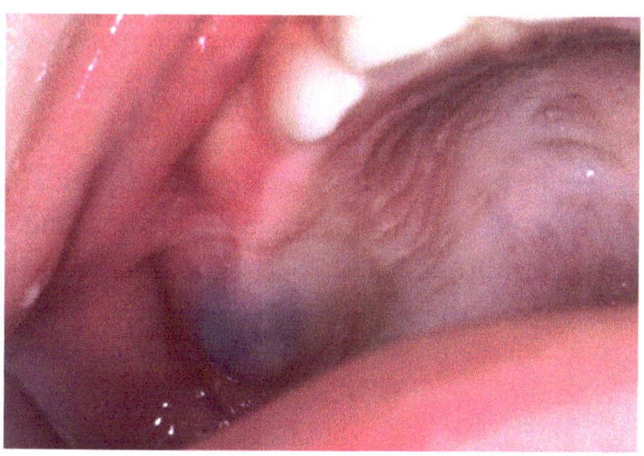

Fig. 5.1 Eruption cyst of 54

Epidemiology
Not very common phenomenon; no gender preference.

Clinical Aspects
Bluish, cystic lesion on the alveolar ridge at the site of an erupting tooth, usually a deciduous molar in the upper jaw (Fig. 5.1). It is questionable whether an eruption cyst is painful. The general belief is that it is not. The diagnosis can usually be made on clinical grounds alone without the need for a radiograph to demonstrate the presence of an underlying erupting tooth. A biopsy is only indicated in case of doubt.

Treatment
Treatment is not required. The underlying tooth will erupt in a normal way. Sometimes the parents insist on having the overlying operculum excised.

5.2.2 Gingival Cyst of the Adult

Definition
Odontogenic developmental cyst in the gingiva of an adult is to be regarded as the extraosseous counterpart of the intraosseous lateral periodontal cyst.

I. van der Waal, *Atlas of Oral Diseases: A Guide for Daily Practice*,
DOI 10.1007/978-3-662-48122-6_5

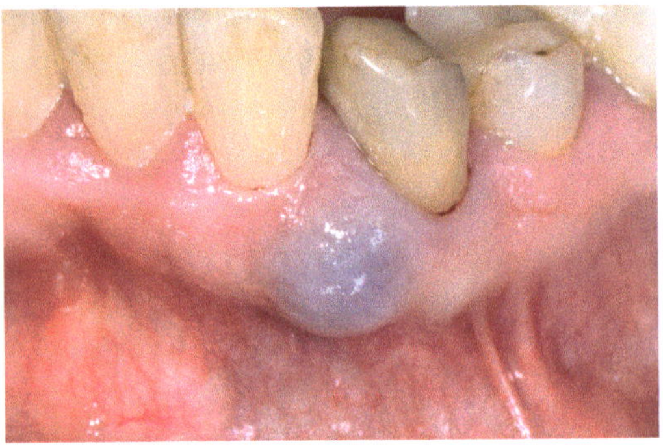

Fig. 5.2 Gingival cyst in an adult

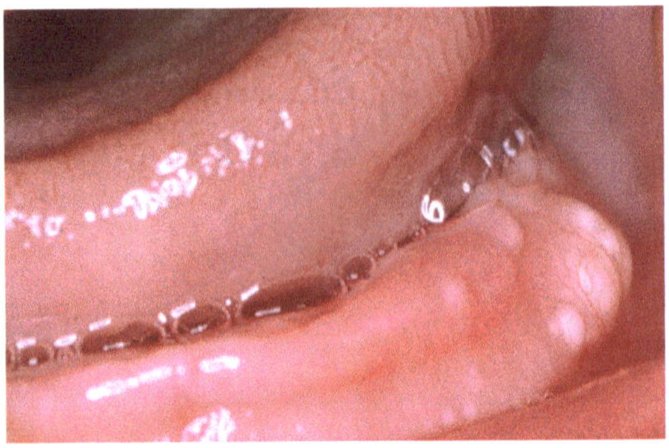

Fig. 5.3 Multiple gingival cysts in a newborn ("dental lamina cyst"); no treatment indicated

Epidemiology
Rather rare cyst; no gender preference.

Clinical Aspects
Cystic, often bluish lesion of the alveolar mucosa on the buccal aspect of a tooth, usually in the anterior region of the mandible or maxilla (Fig. 5.2). The gingival cyst is asymptomatic otherwise. Usually, a radiograph (periapical film) is taken to exclude the presence on an underlying intraosseous lesion.

Histopathology
Thin epithelial lining that may show features of a lateral periodontal cyst, such as formation of epithelial "plaques."

Treatment
Treatment consists of conservative excision; the cyst rarely recurs.

5.2.3 Gingival Cyst of the Newborn ("Dental Lamina Cyst of the Newborn")

Definition
Odontogenic developmental cyst on the alveolar ridge of a newborn.

Epidemiology
Probably quite common cyst.

Clinical Aspects
Solitary or multiple whitish-grayish nodules on the upper or lower alveolar ridge (Fig. 5.3). The diagnosis is a clinical one; only in rare instances, the taking of a biopsy may be considered.

Treatment
The cyst(s) will disappear spontaneously in a matter of weeks or a few months.

5.3 Epulis

Definition
Epulis is a clinical term for a localized swelling of the gingiva. It is, therefore, not a final diagnosis. Various diseases may present as a localized swelling of the gingiva. The "epulis of the newborn," consisting of granular cells resembling somewhat a granular cell tumor, will be discussed separately.

Epulis fissuratum, also referred to as "denture fibrous hyperplasia," has been dealt with in the paragraph on fibroma (see Chap. 2).

Etiology
The majority of epulides are caused by local irritation, e.g., by the presence of calculus, and consist of fibrous tissue such as is observed in fibrous hyperplasia. A fibrous epulis may occur during pregnancy, being referred to as pregnancy tumor. Epulis-like swellings of the gingiva may also be a side effect of some drugs, e.g., amlodipine.

Epidemiology
Rather common gingival swelling that may occur at all ages.

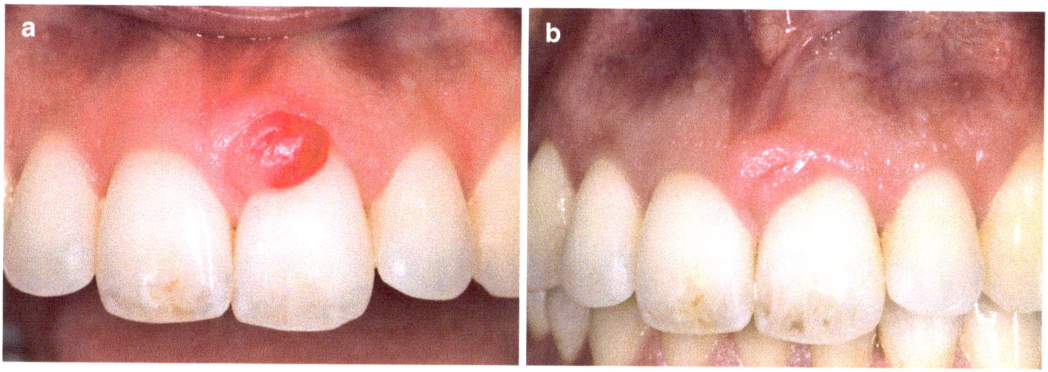

Fig. 5.4 (**a**) Local swelling of the gingiva ("epulis"). (**b**) Clinical aspect 3 months after excision

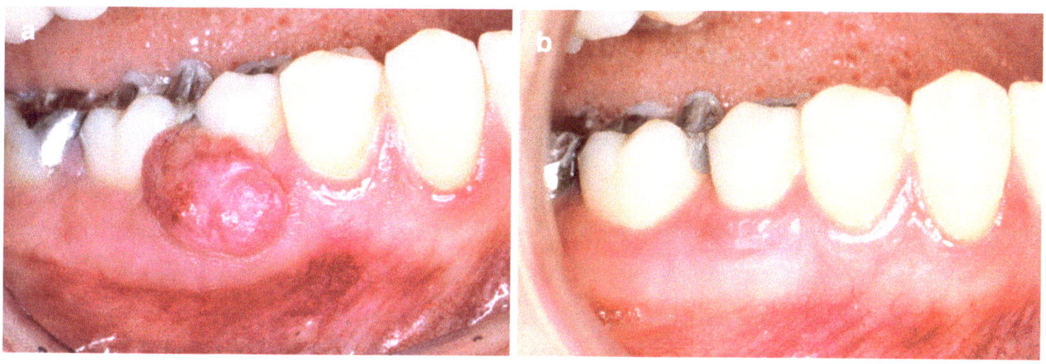

Fig. 5.5 (**a**) Pregnancy tumor in the mandible. (**b**) Spontaneous regression within a few months after the delivery

Clinical Aspects

Usually somewhat pedunculated swelling between two or more teeth, often only at the buccal side but sometimes also extending to the palatal side (Figs. 5.4a, b and 5.5a, b). The size may vary from a few millimeters to a few centimeters. The color may vary from that of the normal gingiva to a more bluish color in case of a peripheral giant cell lesion. There are usually no symptoms. The taking of a periapical film is recommended to exclude the presence of an underlying expanding intraosseous lesion. The differential diagnosis of an epulis includes:

- Metastasis of a malignancy located elsewhere in the body (Fig. 5.6)
- Non-Hodgkin lymphoma (Figs. 5.7 and 5.8)
- Peripheral giant cell lesion (Fig. 5.9a, b)
- Squamous cell carcinoma (Fig. 5.10)
- Sarcoma (Fig. 5.11)

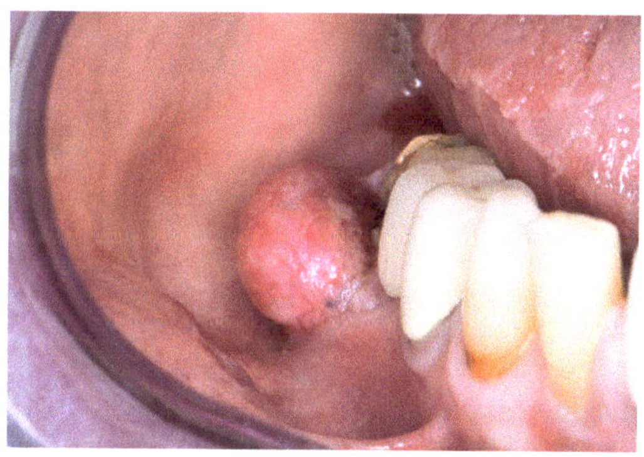

Fig. 5.6 Epulis caused by a metastasis of a cancer of the kidney

Histopathology

The majority of epulides will show fibrous hyperplastic tissue with or without signs of inflammation. In case of the presence of bone formation, the term "peripheral ossifying fibroma" is applied (Fig. 5.12). This lesion is not considered to be the

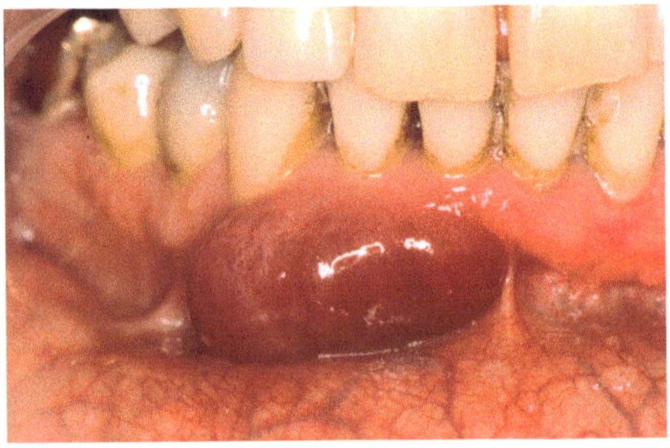

Fig. 5.7 Non-Hodgkin lymphoma of the gingiva and alveolar mucosa

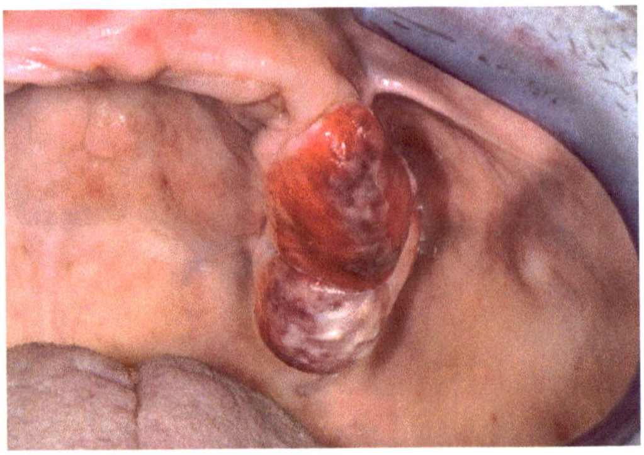

Fig. 5.8 Non-Hodgkin lymphoma of the alveolar mucosa

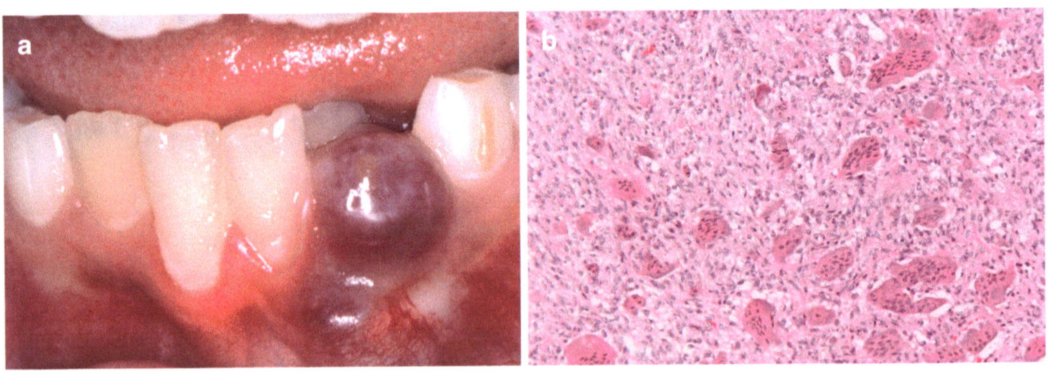

Fig. 5.9 (**a**) Peripheral giant cell lesion. (**b**) Low-power view of peripheral giant cell lesion

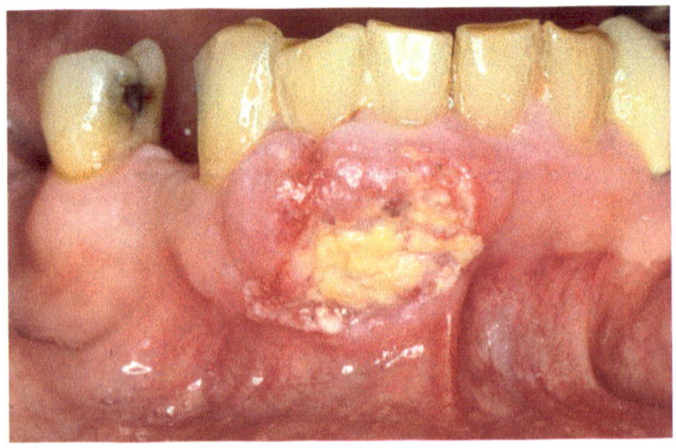

Fig. 5.10 Squamous cell carcinoma of the gingiva and alveolar mucosa

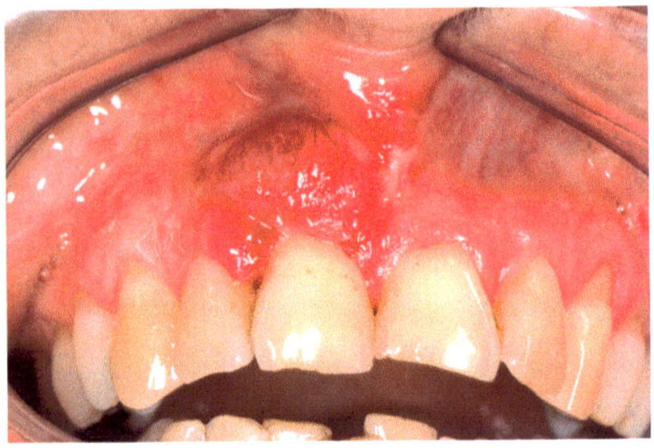

Fig. 5.11 Fibrosarcoma of the gingiva and alveolar mucosa

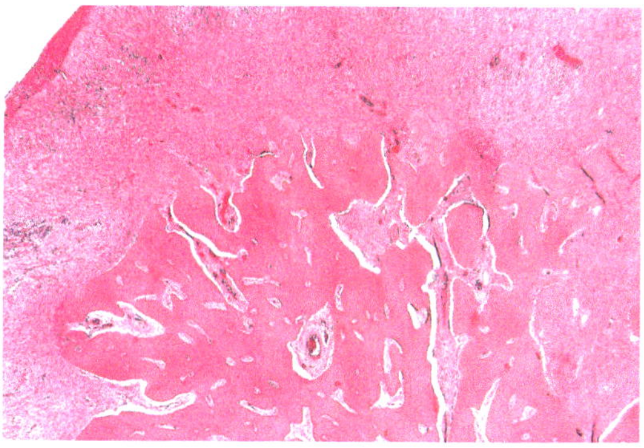

Fig. 5.12 Low-power view of peripheral ossifying fibroma

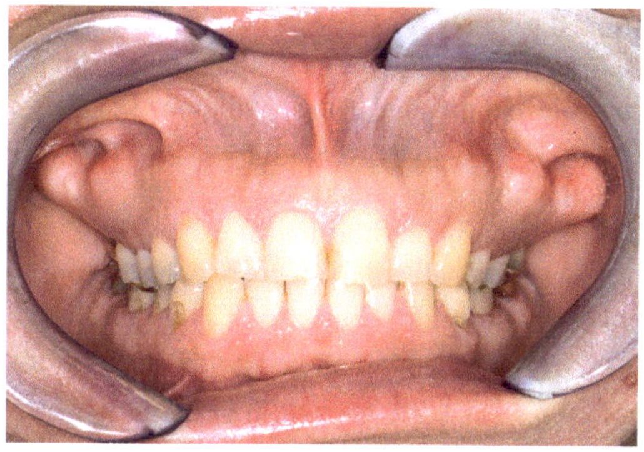

Fig. 5.13 Multiple exostoses at the buccal aspect of the maxilla

extraosseus counterpart of the central ossifying fibroma. In the presence of odontogenic epithelium, the term "peripheral odontogenic fibroma" is applied, being the extraosseous counterpart of the rare intraosseous odontogenic fibroma. In the presence of multinucleated giant cell, the term peripheral giant cell lesion is applied.

Treatment
Treatment of an epulis consists of excision. The underlying periosteum should be thoroughly curetted in order to minimize the risk of recurrence. Possible present calculus should be removed as well. Sometimes, an epulis behaves in a rather aggressive way by repeated recurrences after removal.

5.4 Exostoses

Definition
Exostoses are bony excrescencies that may occur on the buccal aspect of the maxillary or mandibular gingiva.

Etiology
Multiple exostoses of the gingiva are supposedly caused by chronic periodontal irritation.

However, when this hypothesis is true, one would expect to see these exostoses much more often.

Epidemiology
Occur exclusively in elderly people.

Clinical Aspects
Multiple bony, hard, localized swellings at the buccal aspect of the gingiva in the maxilla or mandible, being asymptomatic otherwise (Fig. 5.13).

Treatment
Surgical correction is only indicated in case of interference with the wearing of a denture.

5.5 Fibromatosis of the Gingiva

Definition
Generalized fibrous swelling of the gingiva.

Etiology
May be a side effect of certain drugs, e.g., phenytoine and cyclosporine. In the absence of a causative factor, the term idiopathic fibromatosis is used.

Clinical Aspects

Multiple fibrous swellings of the gingiva in the mandible and maxilla, being asymptomatic otherwise (Fig. 5.14). May cause eruption disturbances when occurring in children (Fig. 5.15a, b). In rare instances, a fibroma-like swelling of the gingiva or alveolar mucosa is based on a leukemic infiltrate (Fig. 5.16). Furthermore, there is a rare autosomal dominant syndrome consisting of fibromatosis of the gingiva and hypertrichosis on the face, the midback, and the extremities ("gingival fibromatosis-hypertrichosis syndrome").

Treatment

Adjustment of medication, if applicable. Surgical correction followed by a strict oral hygiene program.

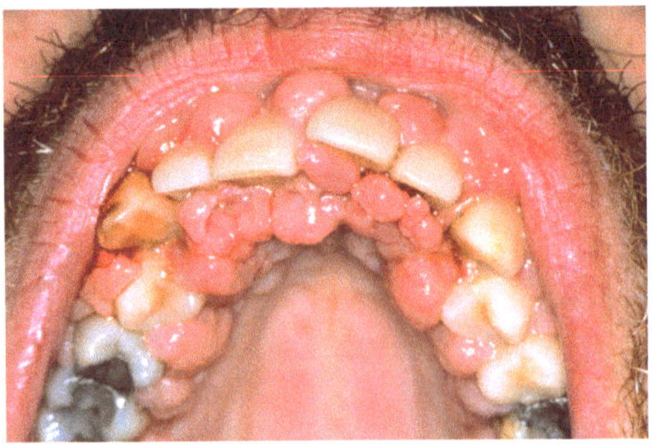

Fig. 5.14 Drug-induced fibromatosis of the gingiva

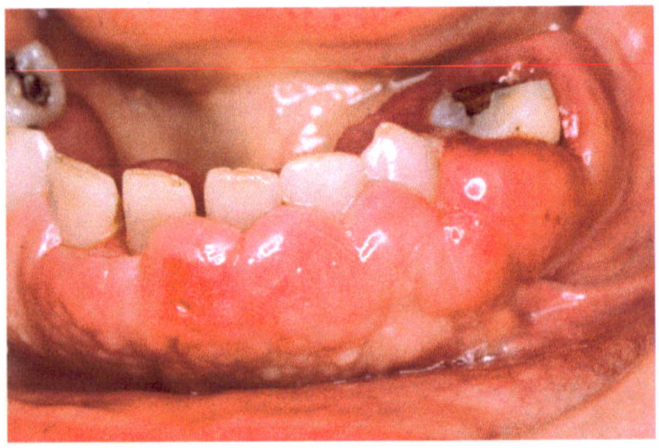

Fig. 5.16 Leukemic infiltrate of the mandibular gingiva

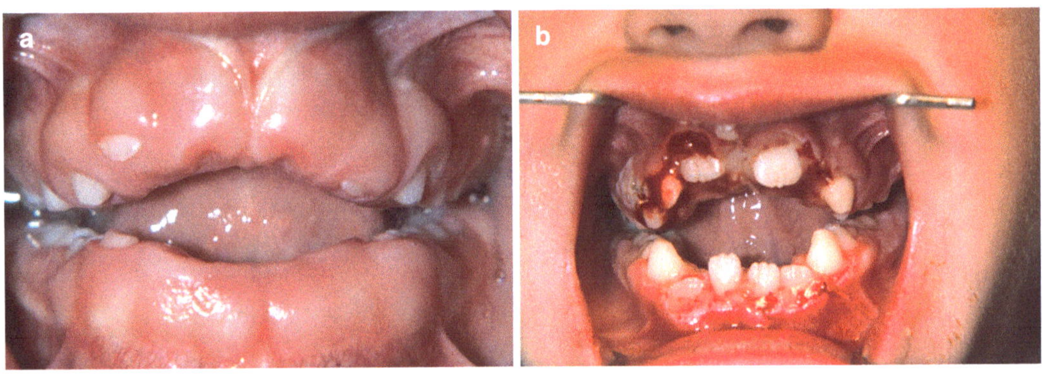

Fig. 5.15 (**a**) Fibromatosis of the gingiva in a child, due to the use of anticonvulsant drugs. (**b**) Clinical aspect immediate after surgical exposure of the teeth

5.6 Gingivitis and Periodontitis

Definition
Inflammation of the gingiva (gingivitis); when the inflammatory process has caused loss of alveolar bone, the term periodontitis is applied. A separate entity is necrotizing and ulcerative gingivitis/periodontitis (NUG and NUP).

Etiology
Poor oral hygiene with or without resulting calculus formation on the dental surfaces.

Smoking is an important contributory factor in the etiology of periodontal diseases. In NUG and NUP, there may be an underlying systemic disease, e.g., HIV infection. Apparently, diabetes mellitus may be a contributing cause of periodontal disease as well.

In the literature, the entity of plasma cell gingivitis is mentioned. Supposedly, this lesion is due to allergy for cinnamon, e.g., as being present in chewing gum.

Epidemiology
May occur already during childhood (prepuberal periodontitis) and adolescence, but mainly becomes manifest in adults.

Clinical Aspects
Usually fiery red appearance of the gingiva, with or without swelling of the gingiva and (pseudo) pocket formation (Fig. 5.17). Calculus formation may or may not be present (Fig. 5.18a, b). Gingivitis and periodontitis may be localized, but are often generalized, and are usually not painful. In some patients, bleeding at brushing the teeth may occur.

In necrotizing and ulcerative gingivitis/periodontitis, loss of interdental papillae occurs (Figs. 5.19 and 5.20). In this type of gingivitis, the gingiva is extremely painful; the patient is febrile and there is a strong foetor ex ore ("halitosis").

In case of severe periodontal bone loss, the teeth become mobile (Fig. 5.21).

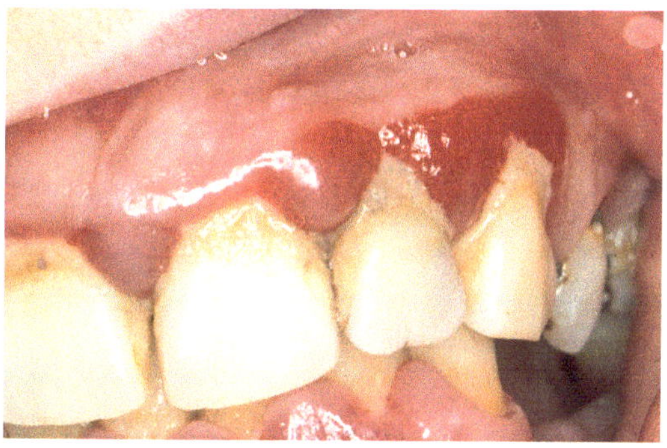

Fig. 5.17 Gingivitis due to poor oral hygiene

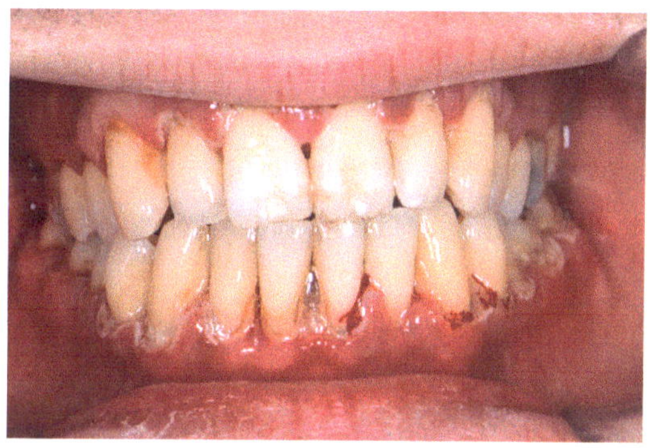

Fig. 5.19 Necrotizing and ulcerative gingivitis

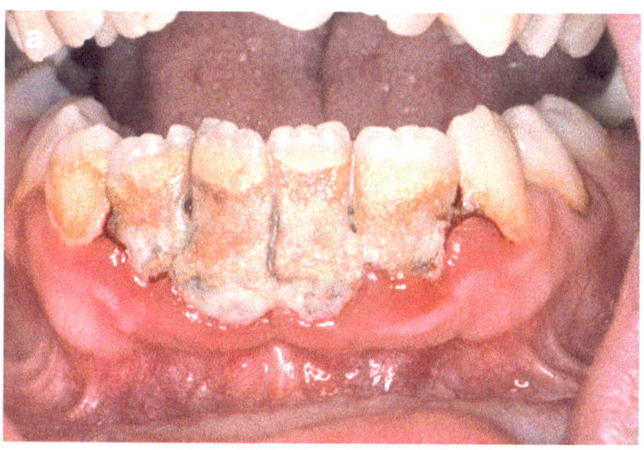

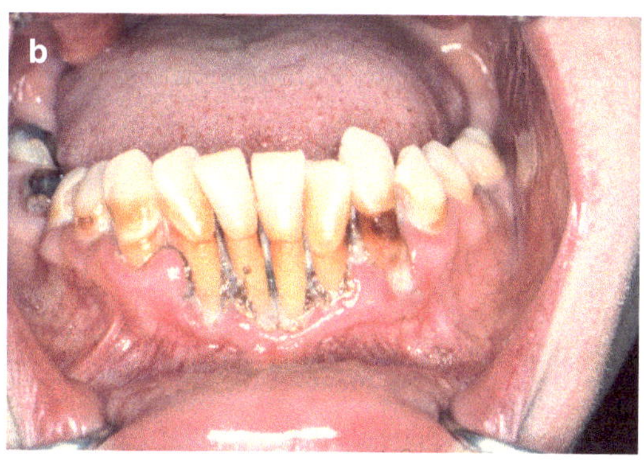

Fig. 5.18 (**a**) Chronic gingivitis and periodontitis with massive calculus formation. (**b**) Same patient after removal of the calculus

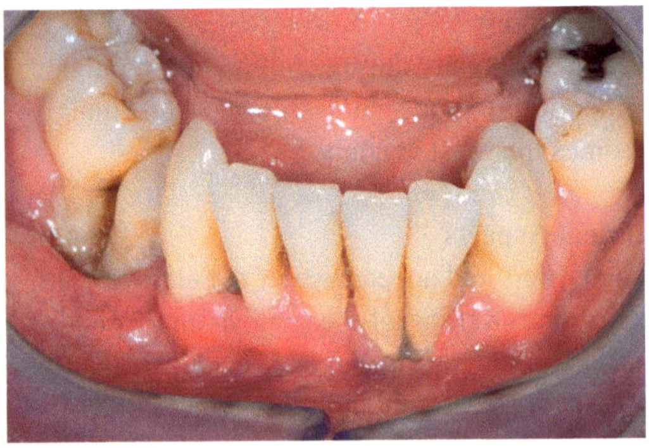

Fig. 5.20 Necrotizing and ulcerative periodontitis in an HIV-infected patient

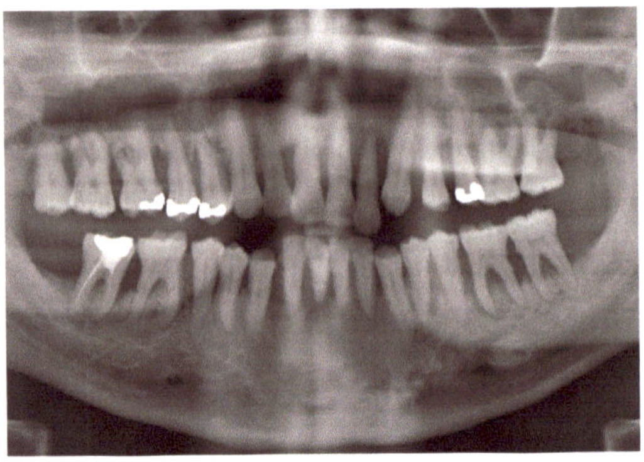

Fig. 5.21 Extensive periodontal bone loss in the mandible and maxilla

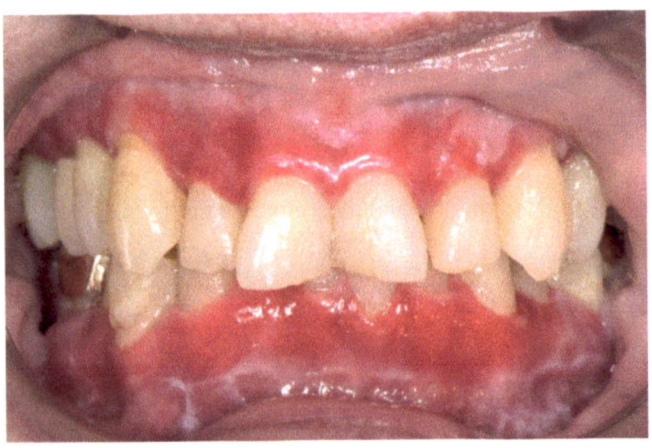

Fig. 5.22 Erosive lichen planus of the gingiva

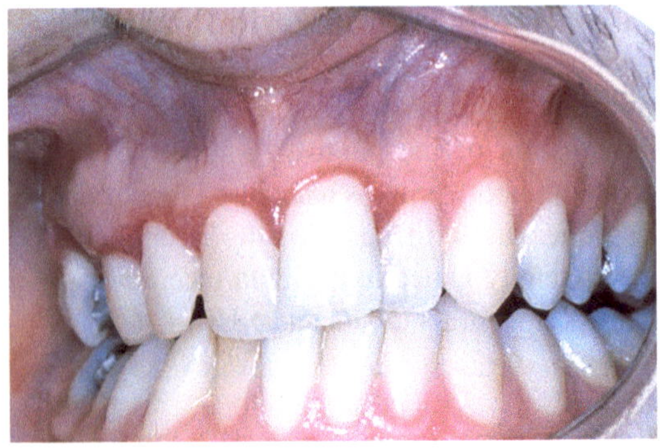

Fig. 5.23 Gingivitis-like aspect, caused by an intraosseous arteriovenous malformation

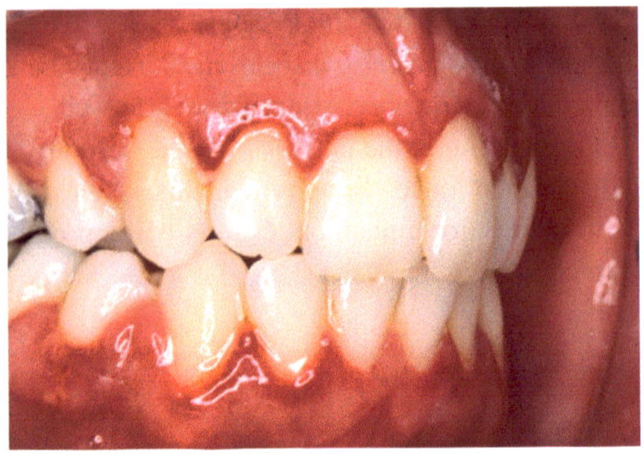

Fig. 5.24 Herpetiform gingivostomatitis

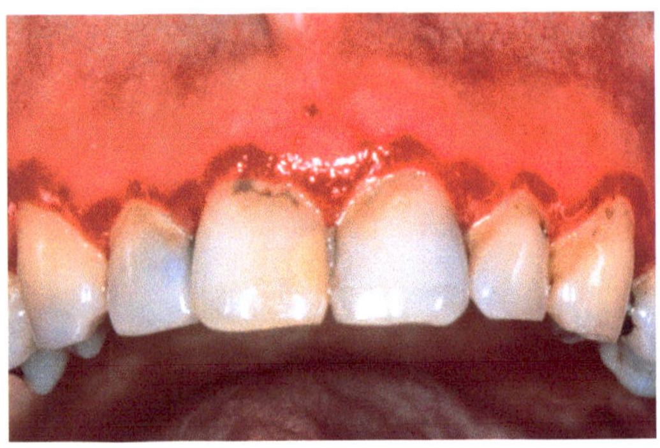

Fig. 5.25 Linear gingiva erythema in HIV-infected patient

The differential diagnosis of gingivitis includes:

- Erythematous lichen planus (see also Chap. 2) (Fig. 5.22)
- Arteriovenous malformation in the underlying bone (see also Chaps. 2 and 7) (Fig. 5.23)
- Herpetiform gingivostomatitis (see also Chap. 2) (Fig. 5.24)
- HIV-related inflammation, e.g., linear gingival erythema (Fig. 5.25)
- Langerhans cell histiocytosis (see also Chap. 7) (Fig. 5.26)

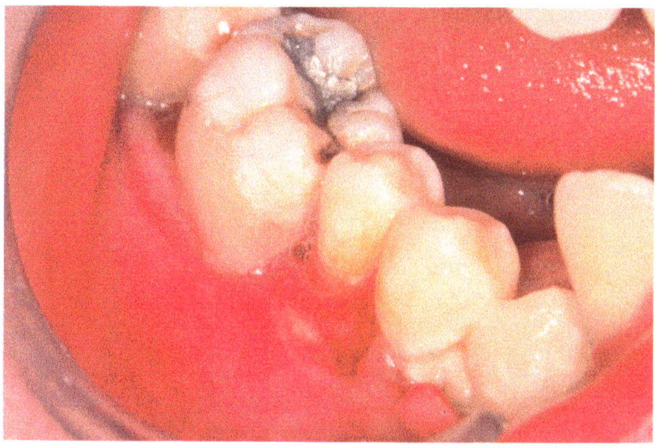

Fig. 5.26 Gingivitis-like aspect in Langerhans cell histiocytosis

- Acute leukemia (Fig. 5.27)
- Linear IgA disease
- Mucous membrane pemphigoid (see also Chap. 2) (Fig. 5.28a, b)
- Traumatic lesion due to vigorous toothbrushing (Fig. 5.29)

Diagnostic Aids

Radiographs are required to assess possible periodontal bone loss. Culturing may be indicated in patients who are resistant to normal dental

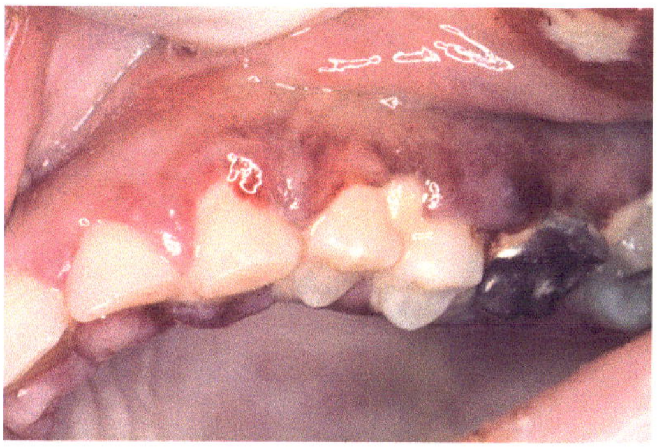

Fig. 5.27 Gingivitis-like aspect in patient suffering from acute leukemia

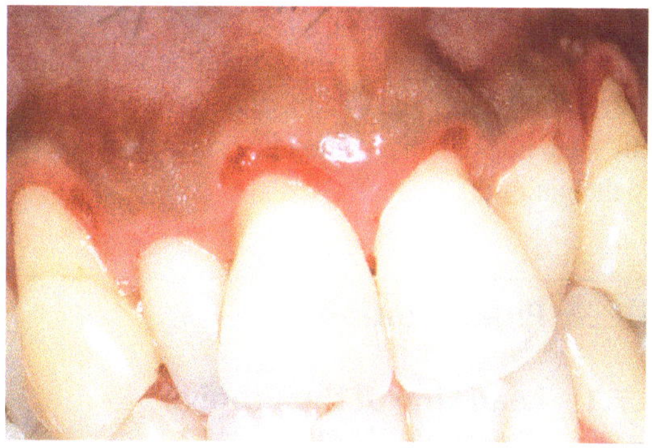

Fig. 5.29 Traumatic changes of the gingiva due to vigorous toothbrushing

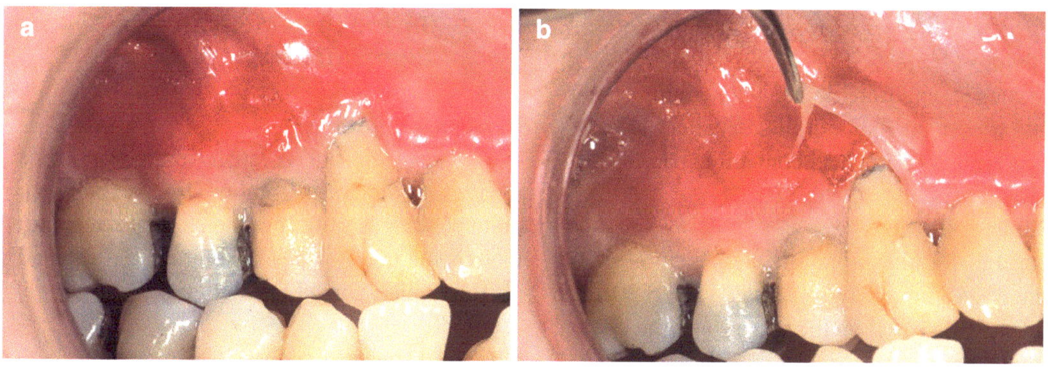

Fig. 5.28 (**a**) Mucous membrane pemphigoid of the gingiva. (**b**) The mucosa can be easily lifted up

hygiene programs. This also applies to the indication for a biopsy. When an underlying disease is suspected, e.g., HIV infection, testing may be considered but only after careful counseling. Blood examination is only indicated when the possibility of leukemia is considered.

Treatment

Instructions about proper dental and oral hygiene, if needed supported by professional cleaning of the teeth. In acute stages of NUG or NUP, the temporary use of mouthrinses with chlorhexidine 0.12 % is indicated. The use of antibiotics may be indicated in selected cases but should not routinely be prescribed.

In periodontitis, there may be, quite rarely, an indication for surgical treatment in order to eliminate deep pockets that cannot be properly cleaned by the patient.

5.7 Pigmentations

5.7.1 Lead Line of the Gingiva (Burton's Line)

Definition

Generalized bluish-grayish pigmentation of the gingiva due to deposition of lead particles.

Etiology

Prolonged exposure to lead-containing chemicals, e.g., in patients working in battery factories, or in painters using lead-containing paint.

Clinical Aspects

Generalized bluish-grayish pigmentation of the gingiva, asymptomatic otherwise (Fig. 5.30). The diagnosis is based on the history and the clinical presentation.

Laboratory Examination

In case of suspected lead poisoning, tests for lead intoxication should be performed.

Treatment

There are no means to remove the lead pigmentation.

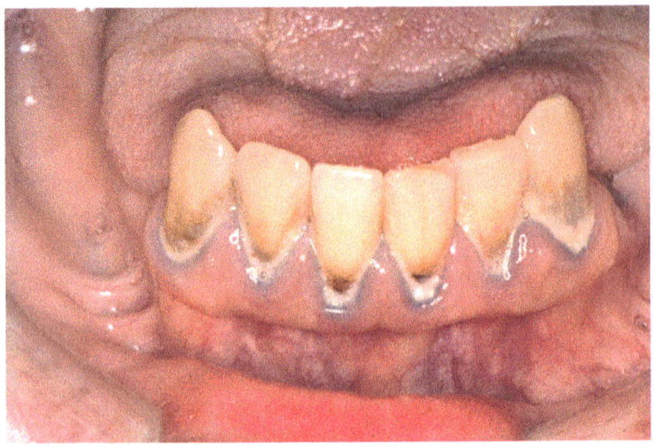

Fig. 5.30 Lead deposition in the gingiva ("Burton's line") in a patient with lead poisoning

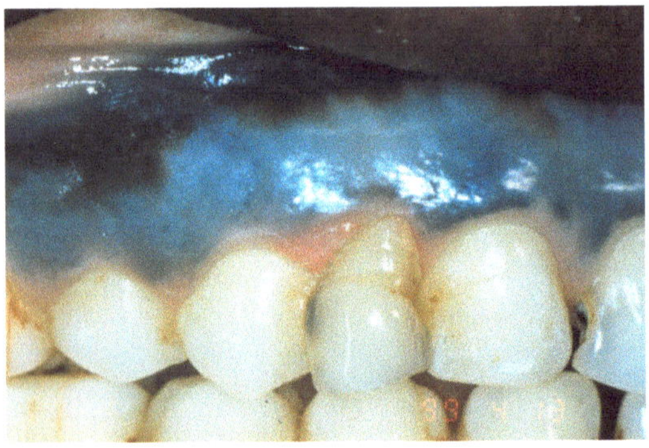

Fig. 5.31 Traditional tattooing of the alveolar mucosa in a woman from Sudan

5.7.2 Tattoos and Melanin Pigmentations

Definition

Tattooing of the skin is rather common practice today. Tattooing of the oral mucosa is becoming quite popular as well. In some parts of the world, there is the tradition of tattooing the gingiva and alveolar mucosa in adolescent girls.

Clinical Aspects

In traditional tattooing, there is a brownish or bluish discoloration of the gingiva and the alveolar mucosa (Fig. 5.31). Tattoos are often applied on the inner side of the lower lip. The differential diagnosis of pigmented gingival lesions includes:

- Racial pigmentation (see Chap. 2) (Fig. 5.32)
- Smokers melanosis (see Chap. 2)

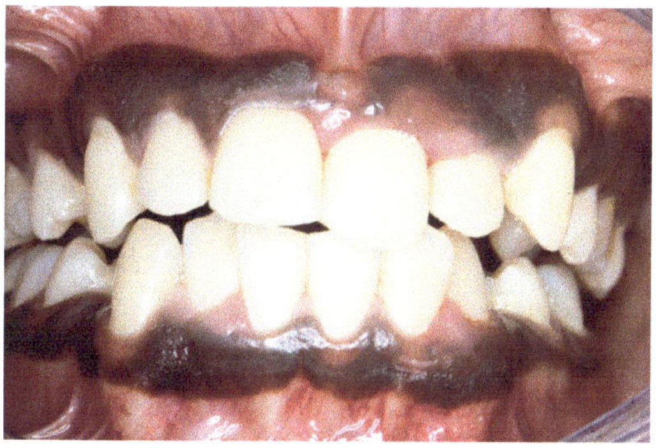

Fig. 5.32 Racial pigmentation of the gingiva and the alveolar mucosa

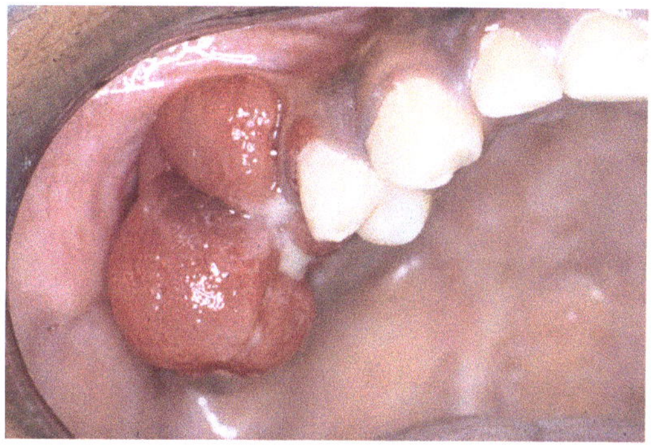

Fig. 5.34 Prolapse of antral lining due to a chronic oroantral communication after tooth extraction

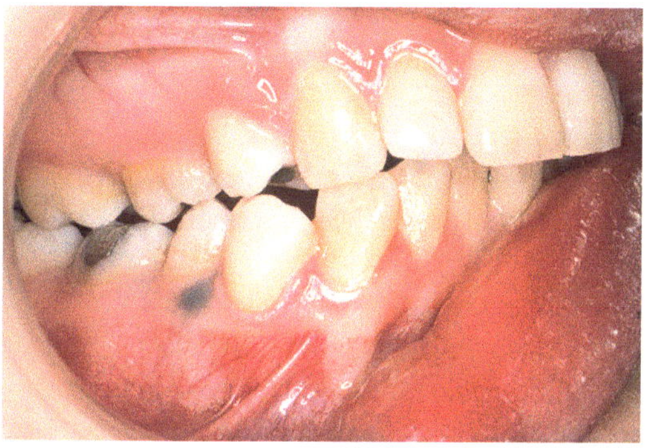

Fig. 5.33 Amalgam tattoo in the gingiva

- Melanoma (see Chap. 2 and also the present chapter)
- Amalgam tattoo (see Chap. 2) (Fig. 5.33)

Treatment

Tattoos can sometimes effectively be removed by CO_2 laser evaporation. In case of melanin pigmentation, a biopsy is often required, particularly when melanoma is suspected.

5.8 Lesions Arising from the Maxillary Sinus That May Extend into the Mouth

5.8.1 Chronic Oroantral Communication

In a chronic oroantral communication after a tooth extraction, hyperplastic mucosa of the antrum may protrude into the mouth (Fig. 5.34). Treatment consists of removal of the hyperplastic tissue and closure of the oroantral communication. It may be necessary to clean the entire antrum from polypoid tissue that may have obliterated the antrum.

5.8.2 Surgical Ciliated Cyst (Postoperative Maxillary Cyst)

Cyst formation after a previous surgical exposure of the maxillary sinus whereby antral epithelium has been entrapped. Therefore, some authors use the term "postoperative maxillary cyst." The clinical presentation is usually a swelling in the upper mucobuccal fold (Fig. 5.35a–c). May or may not be shown on a radiograph. On histopathologic examination, a cyst lining of ciliated epithelium is encountered. Treatment consists of enucleation.

5.8.3 Malignant Neoplasms Arising from the Maxillary Sinus That May Protrude into the Mouth

Malignant neoplasms arising in the maxillary sinus may protrude into the mouth. Occasionally, this protrusion is the first manifestation of the tumor. Complaints may consist of a nonhealing ulcer along the border of a denture or an ill-fitting upper denture (Fig. 5.36).

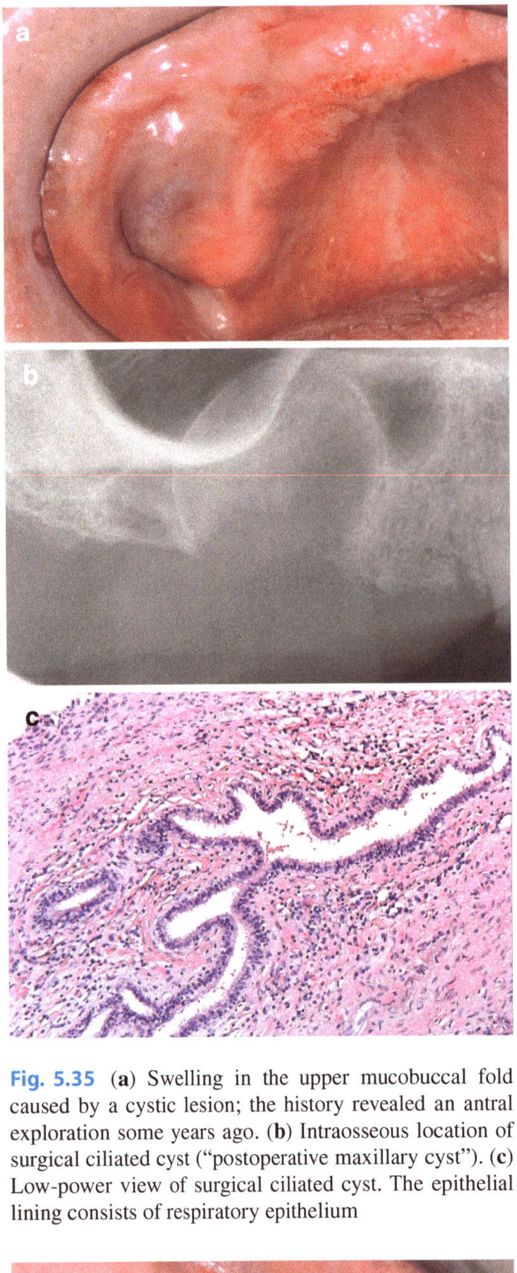

Fig. 5.35 (**a**) Swelling in the upper mucobuccal fold caused by a cystic lesion; the history revealed an antral exploration some years ago. (**b**) Intraosseous location of surgical ciliated cyst ("postoperative maxillary cyst"). (**c**) Low-power view of surgical ciliated cyst. The epithelial lining consists of respiratory epithelium

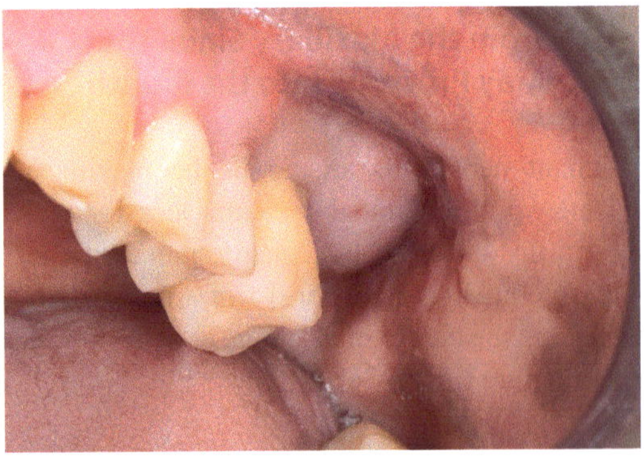

Fig. 5.36 Epulis-like swelling as the first manifestation of a malignant tumor in the maxillary sinus

5.9 Some Other Lesions of the Gingiva and the Alveolar Ridges

5.9.1 Epulis of the Newborn

Some Characteristics

Benign, developmental lesion of the mucosa in the anterior part of the upper and sometimes of the lower alveolar ridge in a newborn (Fig. 5.37a, b). Tends to regress spontaneously in a matter of several months. If excised, histopathological examination will show the characteristics that somewhat resemble those of a granular cell tumor (see Chap. 4), but with immunohistochemically negative staining for the S-100 protein.

5.9.2 Leukoplakia and Leukoplakia Lesions and Erythroplakia

Some Characteristics

Whitish changes of the gingiva seem often to be the result of mechanical irritation due to vigorous toothbrushing habits ("frictional lesion") (Fig. 5.38a, b). Some authors suggest to exclude these white changes from the category of (premalignant) leukoplakia and refer to these lesions as "benign frictional keratosis" (see also Chap. 2). A similar suggestion has been made in the literature for white changes of the mucosa of an edentulous part of the alveolar ridges ("alveolar ridge keratosis") (Fig. 5.39). A misleading clinical aspect can be a skin graft used during a vestibuloplasty, being performed many years ago (Fig. 5.40).

In spite of the previous considerations, one should try to eliminate possible etiologic factors, including smoking habits, and in case of persistence of the lesion, the taking of a biopsy should be considered. In all instances, annual follow-up is recommended.

Erythroplakias rarely affect the gingiva but may occasionally be located in the mucosa of an edentulous part of the mandible or maxilla (see Chap. 2).

5.9.3 Lichen Planus

Some Characteristics

Lichen planus often affects the gingiva, sometimes without involvement of other oral subsites.

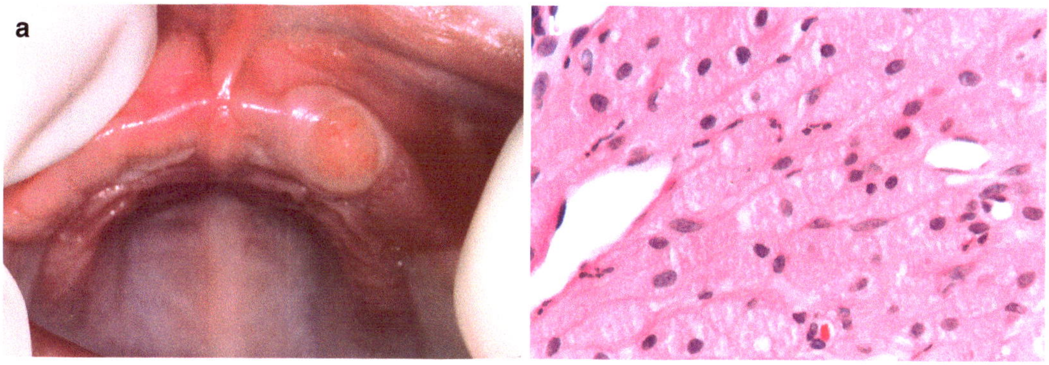

Fig. 5.37 (**a**) Epulis of the newborn. (**b**) Granular cells in epulis of the newborn

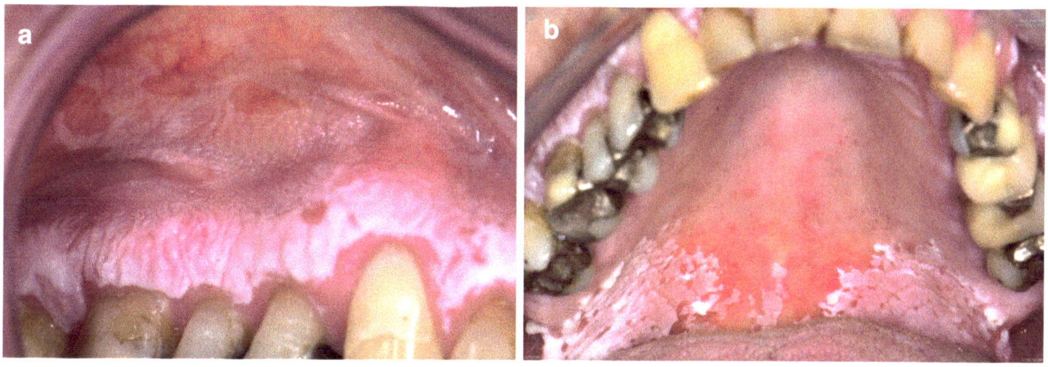

Fig. 5.38 (**a**) Extensive white changes of the gingiva and alveolar mucosa. (**b**) Palatal leukoplakia in the same patient. It does not seem logical to consider the changes shown in (**a**) as (benign) frictional lesions and the palatal changes in (**b**) as (potentially malignant) leukoplakia

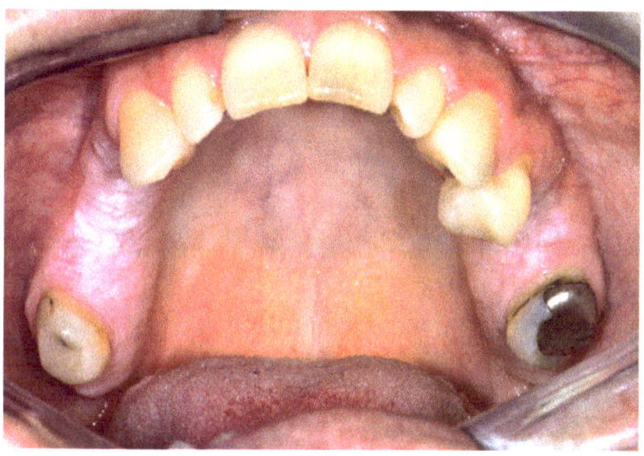

Fig. 5.39 Leukoplakia or "alveolar ridge keratosis." The patient has not been wearing a (partial) denture. Management according to the leukoplakia guidelines is recommended (see Chap. 2)

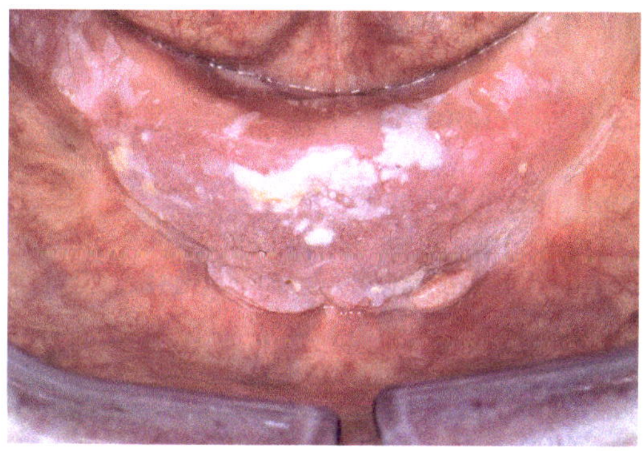

Fig. 5.40 Leukoplakia-like aspect of skin graft applied during a vestibuloplasty

Women may suffer from the vulvovaginal-gingiva syndrome (see also Chap. 2).

In gingival involvement, the majority of patients suffer from the erosive type (Fig. 5.41), while the reticular type is quite rare, indeed (Fig. 5.42). Gingival lichen planus can be quite painful and often causes bleeding on brushing the teeth. Some patients complain about the unpleasant esthetic aspect. Proper dental hygiene is important in order to prevent secondary gingivitis.

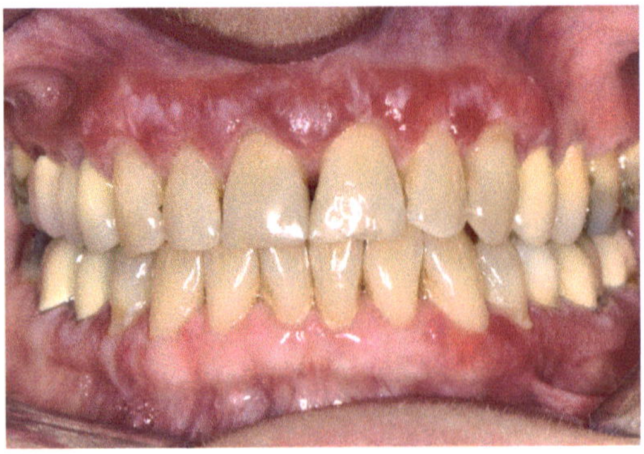

Fig. 5.41 Erosive or erythematous lichen planus

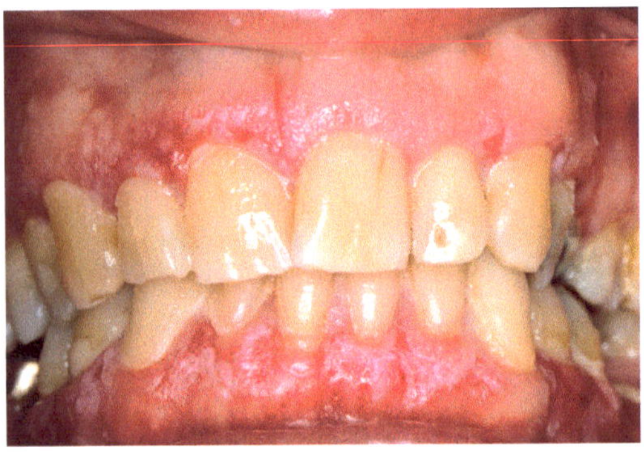

Fig. 5.42 Lichen planus, partly reticular, of the gingiva

In severe cases, an acrylic splint can be made to facilitate the local application of corticosteroids.

5.9.4 Melanoma

Some Characteristics

Oral melanomas are rare. Sites of preference are the palate and the upper and lower gingiva (Fig. 5.43). The usual presentation is a localized or more widespread brown or black pigmented flat or elevated mucosal or gingival lesion, often being asymptomatic otherwise.

Treatment consists of radical surgery. The 5-year prognosis is rather poor due to local recurrences and regional and distant metastases (see also Chap. 2).

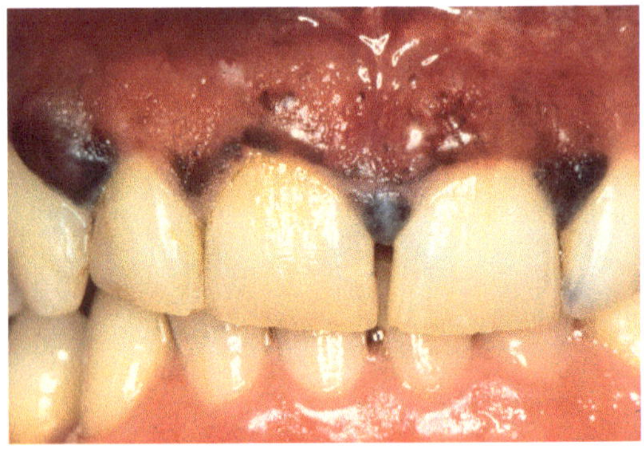

Fig. 5.43 Melanoma of the gingiva

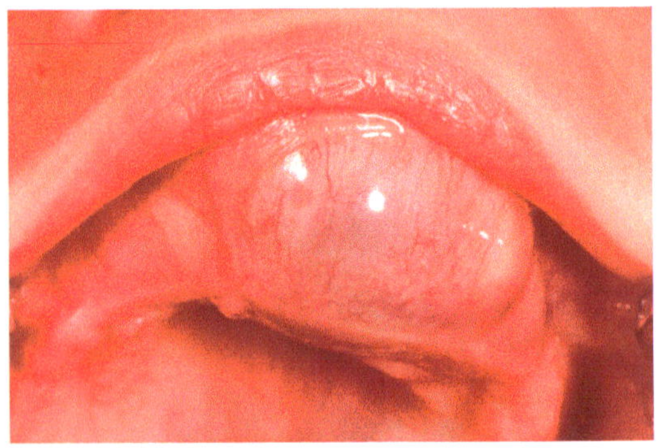

Fig. 5.44 Melanotic neuroectodermal tumor of infancy; the underlying bone is intact

5.9.5 Melanotic Neuroectodermal Tumor of Infancy

Some Characteristics

Extremely rare, usually benign neoplasm derived from neural crest cells. Usually presents in the first year of life. Mainly occurs in the anterior part of the maxilla (Fig. 5.44). May cause destruction of the underlying bone. Rarely metastasizes. High concentrations of vanillylmandelic acid may be found in the urine.

Treatment consists of surgical removal. Recurrences are uncommon.

5.9.6 Peripheral Giant Cell Lesion of the Edentulous Alveolar Ridge

Some Characteristics

A peripheral giant cell lesion arising in the mucosa of an edentulous part of the alveolar ridge is quite uncommon (Fig. 5.45). The cause is unknown. A radiograph should be taken to exclude a possible underlying intraosseous lesion. The histopathology is similar as in intraosseous giant cell lesions, including the resemblance to lesions caused by hyperparathyroidism.

5.9.7 Recurrent Aphthous Stomatitis

Some Characteristics

Recurrent aphthous stomatitis has been discussed in Chap. 2. Involvement of the gingiva is extremely rare, in contrast to occurrence in the alveolar mucosa (Fig. 5.46).

5.9.8 Squamous Cell Carcinoma

Some Characteristics

A squamous cell carcinoma (SCC) arising from the gingiva is a rather rare phenomenon (Figs. 5.47 and 5.48). However, an SCC

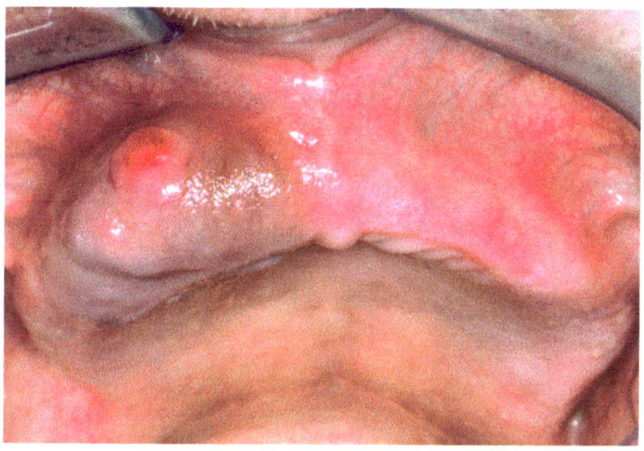

Fig. 5.45 Peripheral giant cell lesion; no bone involvement

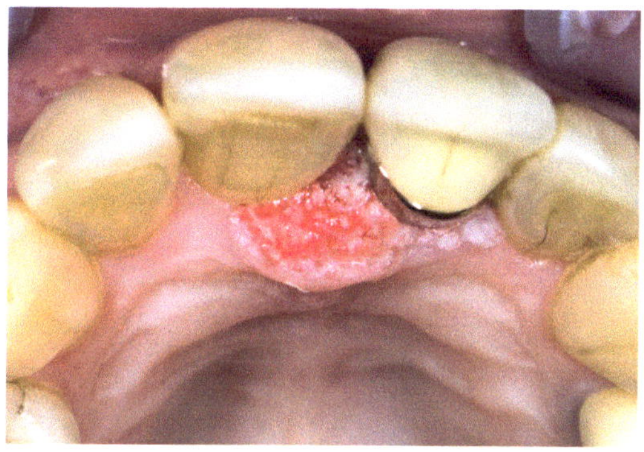

Fig. 5.47 Rare presentation of squamous cell carcinoma of the palatal gingiva

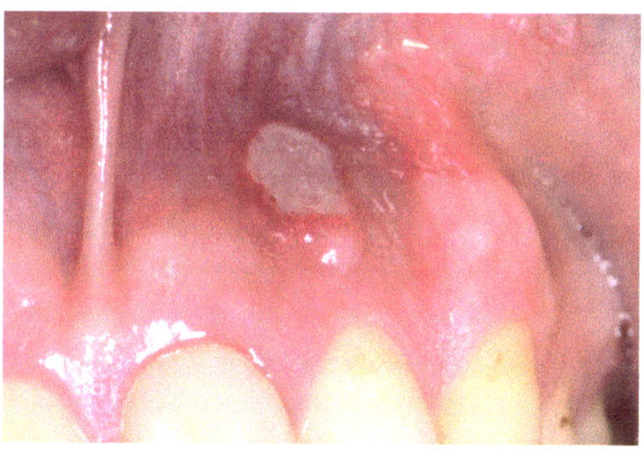

Fig. 5.46 Recurrent aphthous ulcer affecting the alveolar mucosa

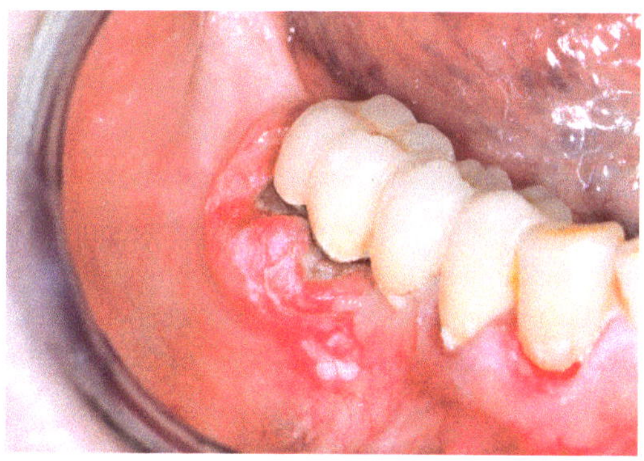

Fig. 5.48 Squamous cell carcinoma of the gingiva

is not a rare phenomenon on an edentulous part of the alveolar ridge, particularly in the mandible (see also Chap. 2). Treatment may consist of surgery or combined treatment such as surgery followed by radiotherapy or by chemoradiation.

5.10 Some Syndromes with Gingival Involvement

5.10.1 Cowden Syndrome

Some Characteristics

Cowden syndrome (the hereditary multiple hamartoma syndrome) may be associated with numerous tiny papules of the oral mucosa, including the alveolar mucosa (Fig. 5.49) (see also Chap. 4).

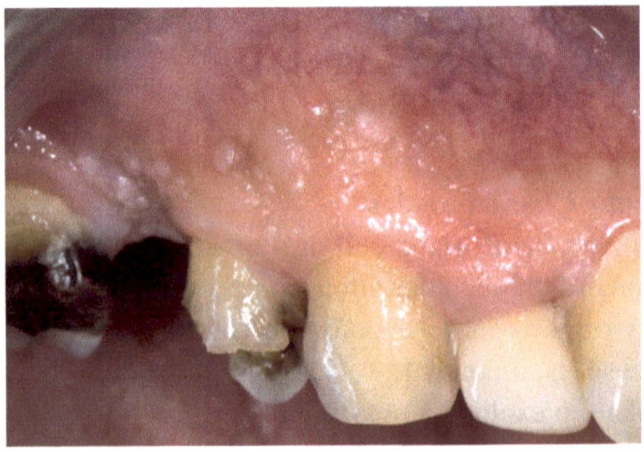

Fig. 5.49 Discrete papules of the alveolar mucosa in a patient with the hereditary Cowden syndrome

5.10.2 Neurofibromatosis

Some Characteristics

In patients suffering from neurofibromatosis type I, numerous neurofibromas may occur throughout the body. When the oral cavity is involved, neurofibromas may occur on the tongue, the palate, and the gingiva (Fig. 5.50). There is effective treatment (see also Chap. 2).

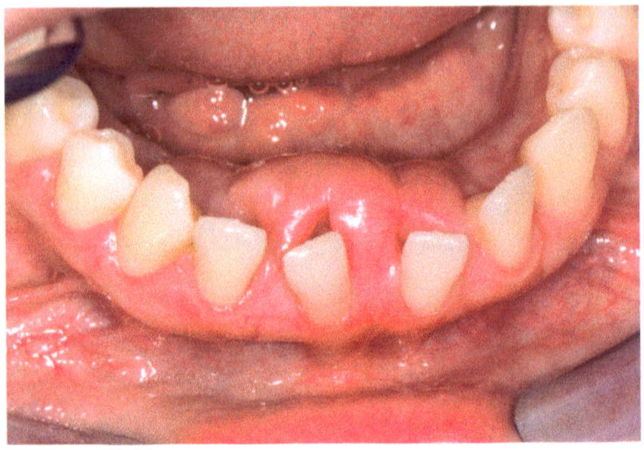

Fig. 5.50 Gingival involvement in patient suffering from neurofibromatosis

5.10.3 Tuberous Sclerosis

Some Characteristics

In tuberous sclerosis, a (sometimes hereditary) syndrome in which a variety of abnormalities may occur, oral involvement consists a.o. of fibrous hyperplasia of the gingiva (Fig. 5.51) (see also Chap. 2).

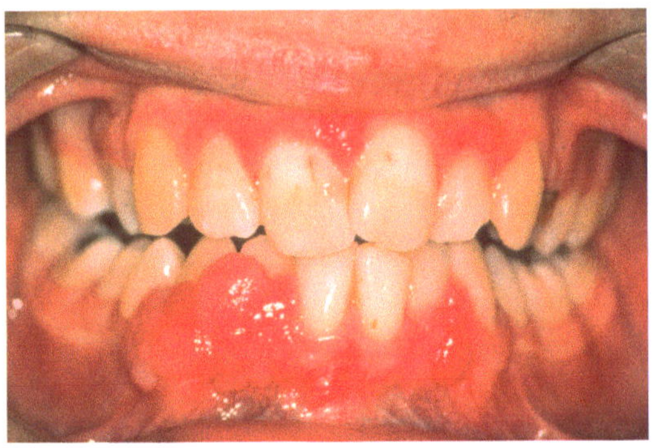

Fig. 5.51 Fibrous hyperplasia of the gingiva in a patient suffering from tuberous sclerosis

Diseases of the Palate 6

6.1 Introduction

The palate may be the site of various diseases of the oral mucosa and the underlying minor salivary glands. With regard to palatal lesions, it is somewhat artificial to make a distinction between hard and soft palate. Nevertheless, in this chapter, the focus is on lesions of the hard palate.

A limited number of lesions are more or less limited to the palate such as nicotinic stomatitis and angina bullosa hemorrhagica. Also non-Hodgkin lymphoma is one of the diseases that has a predilection for occurrence on the palate.

6.2 Angina Hemorrhagica Bullosa (Blood Blister)

Definition

Angina bullosa hemorrhagica is the Latin term for a blood blister. Some authors refer to this lesion as epidermolysis bullosa acquisita (see also Chap. 2).

Etiology

The etiology is unknown, although trauma is suggested to be the most likely cause.

Epidemiology

Rather rare phenomenon. Occurs more often in women than in men, usually at an older age.

Clinical Aspects

Sudden development of a solitary blood blister accompanied by a painful sensation.

The palate is the site of predilection (Fig. 6.1); other affected sites may be the buccal mucosa and the lateral borders of the tongue. The blister ruptures in a matter of hours, leaving a superficial ulcer behind.

Treatment

Because of the spontaneous rupture of the blister, there is no need for treatment. Some patients will experience recurrences; there are no means to prevent such events.

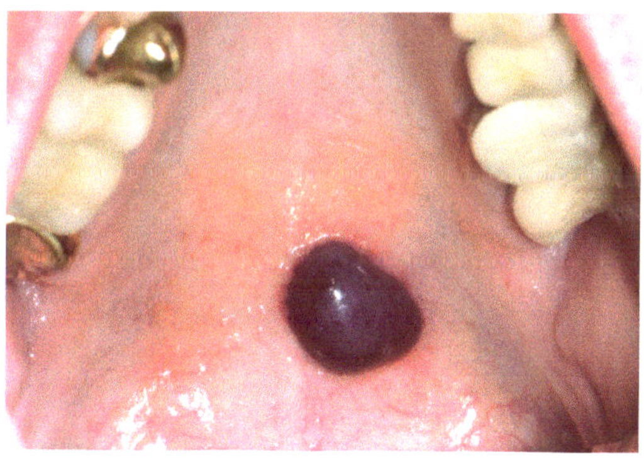

Fig. 6.1 Suddenly arising blood blister ("angina hemorrhagica bullosa") on the palate

I. van der Waal, *Atlas of Oral Diseases: A Guide for Daily Practice*,
DOI 10.1007/978-3-662-48122-6_6

6.3 Midline Granuloma

Definition
Descriptive, somewhat obsolete, term for an ulcerative lesion in the midline of the hard palate after having excluded any etiologic factor.

Etiology
A midline granuloma is often caused by a natural killer T-cell lymphoma. There are several lesions and conditions that may cause palatal ulceration or even perforation, including malignancies other than lymphomas, Wegener's granulomatosis, traumatic ulcers due to an ill-fitting denture, third stage of syphilis, and cocaine abuse.

Epidemiology
Rare event.

Clinical Aspects
Ulcerative, destructive changes of the palatal mucosa sometimes resulting in palatal perforation (Fig. 6.2). The differential diagnoses includes Wegener's granulomatosis (Fig. 6.3), squamous cell carcinoma, non-Hodgkin lymphoma, and a defect due to the use of cocaine.

Treatment
Depends on the final diagnosis.

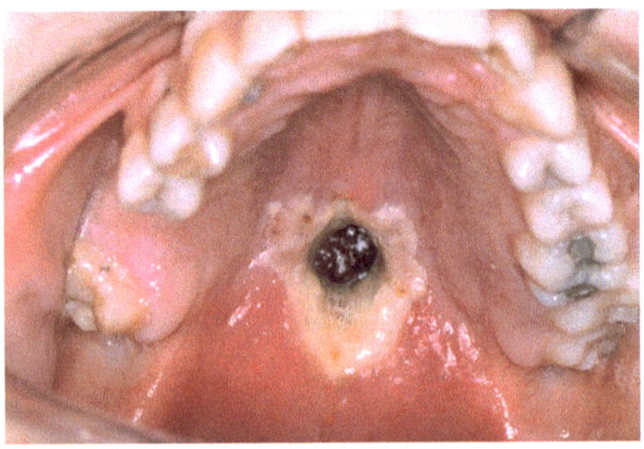

Fig. 6.2 Midline granuloma after having excluded all other diagnoses, including non-Hodgkin lymphoma

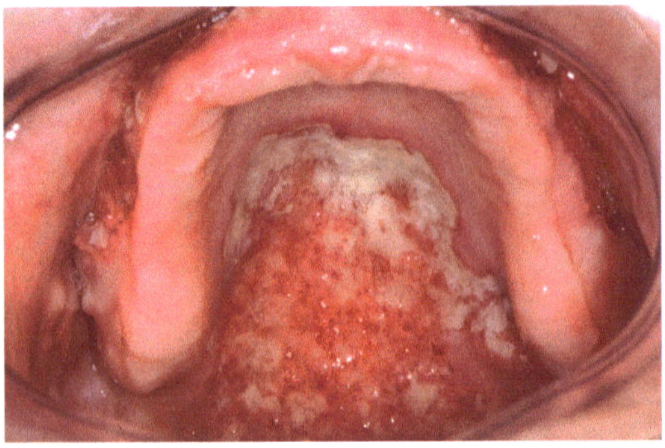

Fig. 6.3 Granulomatous aspect of the palatal mucosa, compatible with a diagnosis of Wegener's granulomatosis

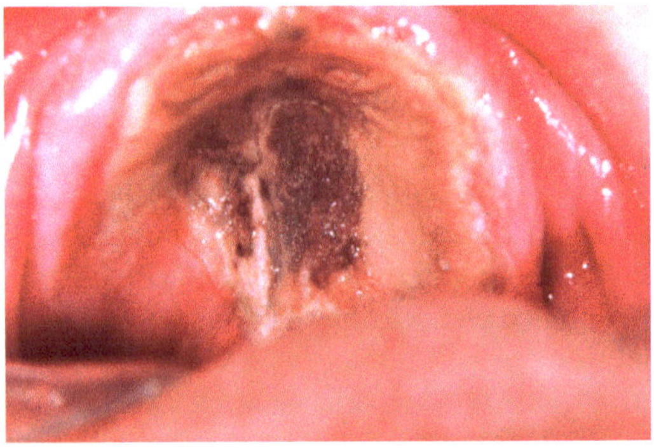

Fig. 6.4 Rather typical presentation of mucormycosis of the palate

6.4 Mucormycosis

Definition
Opportunistic mycotic infection.

Etiology
Predisposing factors are dysregulated diabetes mellitus, chronic renal failure, and immunodeficiency.

Clinical Aspects
The typical oral presentation is a dehiscence of the palatal bone that becomes necrotic, acquiring a brown-black appearance (Fig. 6.4).

Laboratory Examination
Cytologic smears may be used for the demonstration of the fungus (Fig. 6.5).

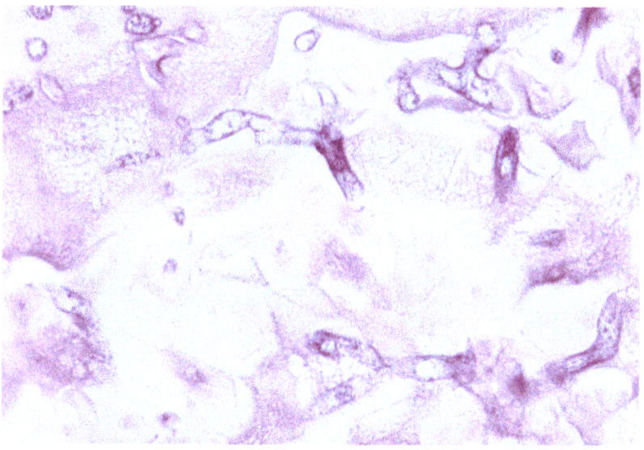

Fig. 6.5 Cytologic aspect of mucormycosis; notice the branching of the fungi

Treatment
Treatment of the underlying cause, if possible. Removal of the necrotic bone. Antifungal treatment, e.g., with high-dose amphotericin B.

6.5 Nasopalatine Duct Cyst

Definition
Developmental non-odontogenic cyst derived from epithelial rests of the nasopalatine duct.

Epidemiology
Rather uncommon cyst that usually does not appear before the age of 30–40 years.

Clinical Aspects
A nasopalatine duct cyst occasionally causes a swelling at the palatal aspect of the upper front teeth, typically located in the midline (Fig. 6.6); the teeth remain vital. In the rare event of occurrence in a child, the typical presentation is just a small, slightly elevated bluish lesion behind the upper incisors (Fig. 6.7). In rare instances, the cyst formation occurs in the papilla incisiva, outside the bone. A nasopalatine duct cyst may also arise in an edentulous part of the alveolar ridge.

Radiographic Aspects
A nasopalatine duct cyst presents as a round or oval, well-defined radiolucency in or close to the midline, sometimes mimicking a periapical radiolucency (Fig. 6.8). When the teeth are vital, the diagnosis of nasopalatine duct cyst may be made based on the radiograph only, although the differential diagnosis theoretically includes a variety of odontogenic and non-odontogenic cysts and tumors.

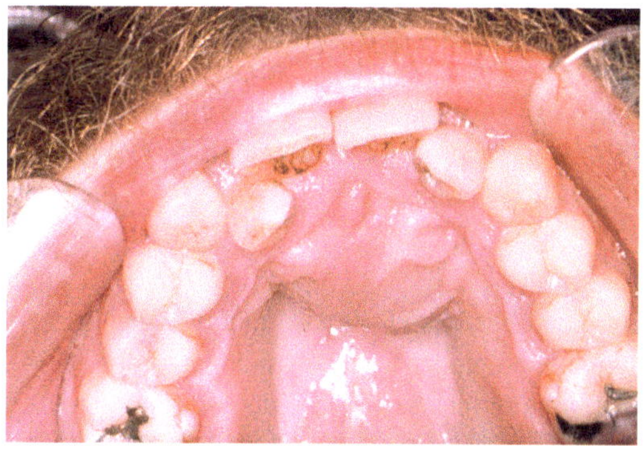

Fig. 6.6 Palatal swelling caused by a nasopalatine duct cyst

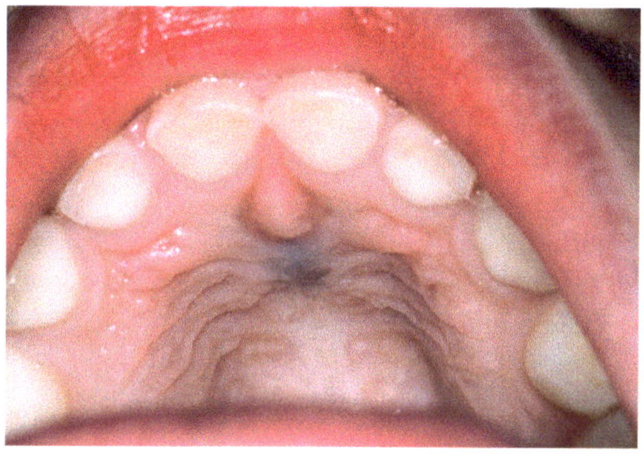

Fig. 6.7 Typical presentation of a nasopalatine duct cyst in a child

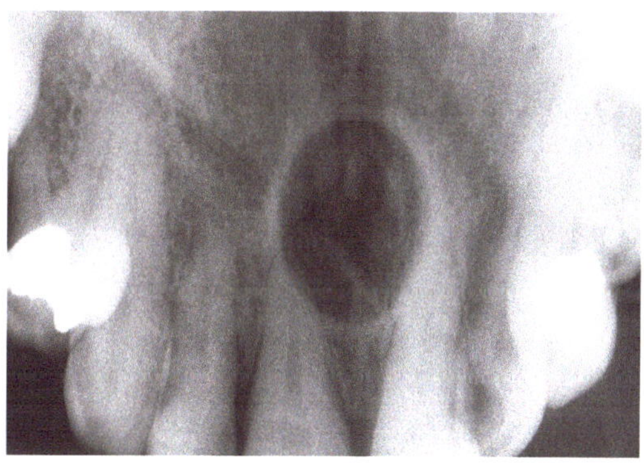

Fig. 6.8 The radiograph shows a well-defined radiolucency in the midline; almost diagnostic of nasopalatine duct cyst

Histopathology
The cyst lining consists of stratified squamous epithelium and sometimes cuboidal or ciliated epithelium. In contrast to odontogenic cysts, the cyst wall may contain nerves.

Treatment
An asymptomatic well-defined radiolucency in the midline of the upper front is a rather common incidental finding on a radiograph and does not necessarily require treatment. In the absence of a swelling or symptoms, there is no need for treatment or follow-up. In case of symptoms, enucleation or marsupialization is indicated. Recurrences are rare.

6.6 Palatal Ulcer Due to the Use of Local Anesthetics

Definition
Ulcer of the palatal mucosa due to local injection of an anesthetic solution (see also Chap. 2).

Etiology
A palatal ulcer may be caused by infiltration with a local anesthetic containing epinephrine. This may result a few days later in an ischemic ulcer.

Clinical Aspects
Clinically, a nonspecific, usually painful ulcer near the midline of the palate will be observed (Fig. 6.9a, b). The underlying bone will remain intact. When in doubt about the nature of the ulcer, a biopsy should be taken.

Histopathology
A biopsy will show necrotic changes of the parenchyma of the palatal salivary glands. The salivary ducts usually persist and may show squamous metaplasia ("necrotizing sialometaplasia"). These changes may mimic a squamous cell carcinoma or a mucoepidermoid carcinoma (Fig. 6.10).

Treatment
Treatment is not required. Healing takes place in several weeks.

6.7 Papillomatosis of the Palate

Definition
Papillary hyperplasia of the palatal mucosa.

Etiology
Papillomatosis of the palate is mainly observed in denture wearers and is probably caused by wearing the denture day and night. Probably, *C. albicans* plays a role in the etiology.

Clinical Aspects
Papillary, reddish aspect of the palatal mucosa (Fig. 6.11). There may be symptoms of a burning sensation.

Histopathology
Papillary epithelial hyperplasia often associated with candidal hyphae.

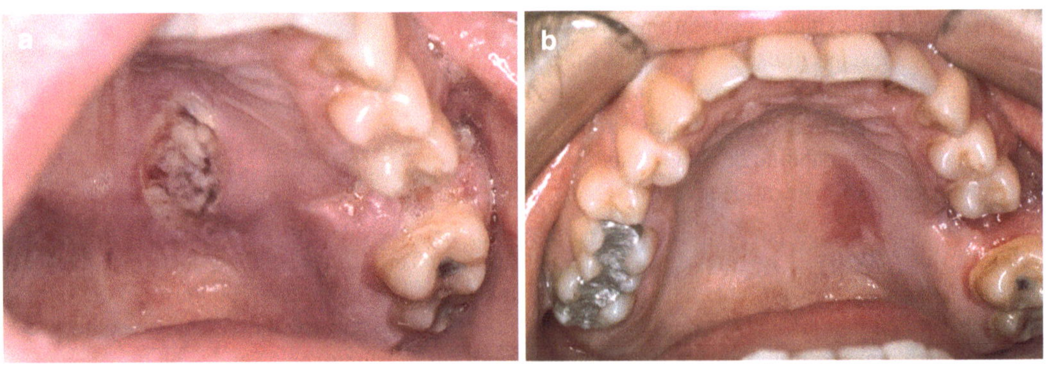

Fig. 6.9 (**a**) Ulcer caused by an injection with local anesthetics for the removal of 26 a few days before. (**b**) Spontaneous healing within a month

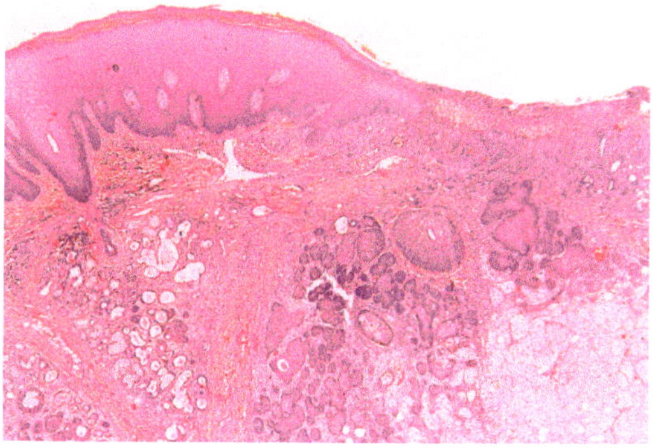

Fig. 6.10 Low-power view of ulcer shown in Fig. 6.9, showing necrotizing sialometaplasia

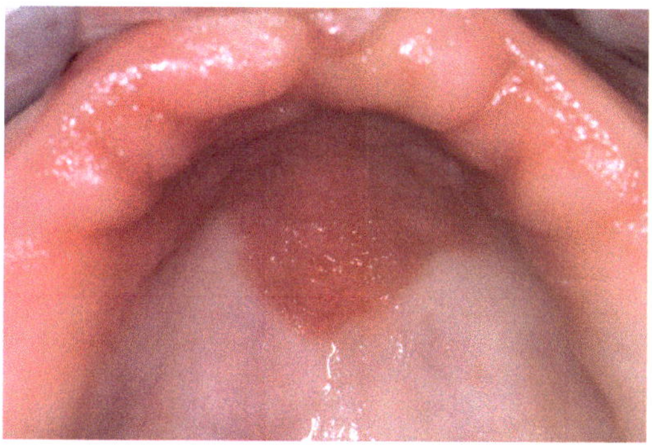

Fig. 6.11 Papillomatosis of the palate; clinical diagnosis

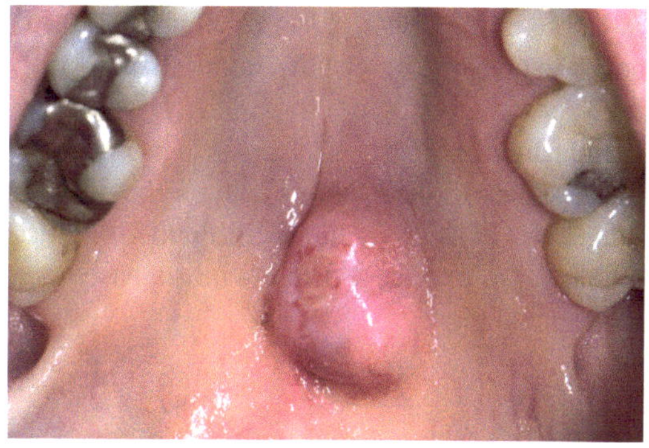

Fig. 6.12 Fibromalike swelling; the biopsy showed the presence of a benign salivary gland tumor

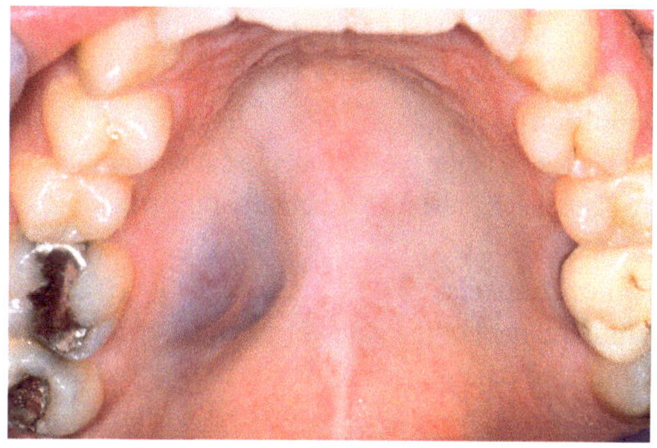

Fig. 6.13 Bluish, cystic, and otherwise asymptomatic swelling of a few years duration; mucoepidermoid carcinoma

Treatment

Improvement of the oral hygiene; if insufficient, the denture should be relined and may even have to be renewed.

6.8 Salivary Gland Tumors

Definition

Neoplasm arising from the parenchymal tissue of the (minor) salivary glands (see also Chap. 2).

Etiology

There are no known etiologic factors.

Epidemiology

The estimated incidence is approximately 3 per 100,000 population per year for all benign and malignant salivary gland tumors together, including those of the major salivary glands.

Clinical Aspects

Clinically, salivary gland tumors of the intraoral salivary glands present as a slowly growing, non-ulcerative swelling of the mucosa, being asymptomatic otherwise. The palate is the site of preference for tumors of the minor salivary glands, particularly at the junction of the hard and soft palate (Figs. 6.12 and 6.13). In general, CT scanning is advised to look for possible destruction of the palatal bone. Occasionally, a palatal swelling is just representing the tip of an iceberg from a large lesion in the maxillary sinus.

Long duration of the swelling and absence of pain are no proof of a benign histologic type of a salivary gland tumor. Approximately 50 % of the palatal salivary gland tumors are malignant. In small lesions, an excisional biopsy is justified. In case of a malignancy, particularly in adenoid cystic carcinoma, additional surgery will be required. In larger tumors, an incisional biopsy should be taken, preferably in the center of the swelling and deep enough to obtain representative tumor tissue.

Histopathology
Palatal salivary gland tumors may be benign or malignant. It is sometimes difficult for the pathologist to provide a firm diagnosis based on an incisional biopsy.

Treatment
Surgical removal is the treatment of choice; postoperative radiotherapy may be indicated in case of a malignant salivary gland tumor.

6.9 Stomatitis Nicotina

Definition
Benign lesion of the palatal mucosa caused by smoking ("smoker's palate"), particularly pipe smoking.

Clinical Aspects
Whitish aspect of the palatal mucosa, particularly of the hard palate, with presence of tiny red dots, apparently representing the orifices of the minor salivary gland ducts (Fig. 6.14).

Histopathology
Mild hyperkeratosis without signs of epithelial dysplasia and focal presence of inflamed excretory ducts of the minor salivary glands (Fig. 6.15).

Treatment
After cessation of the smoking habits, the mucosal changes will regress within several months.

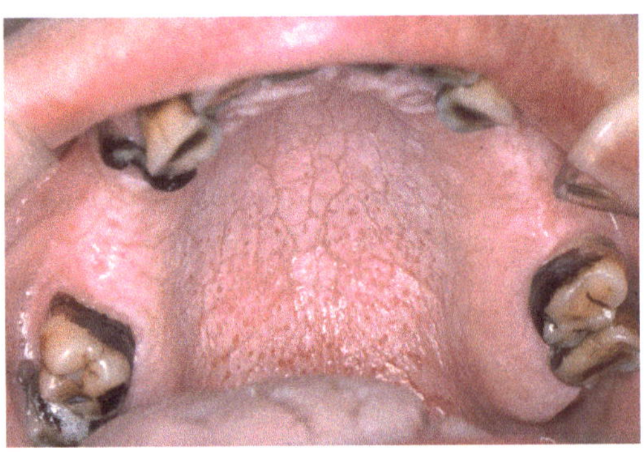

Fig. 6.14 Stomatitis nicotina

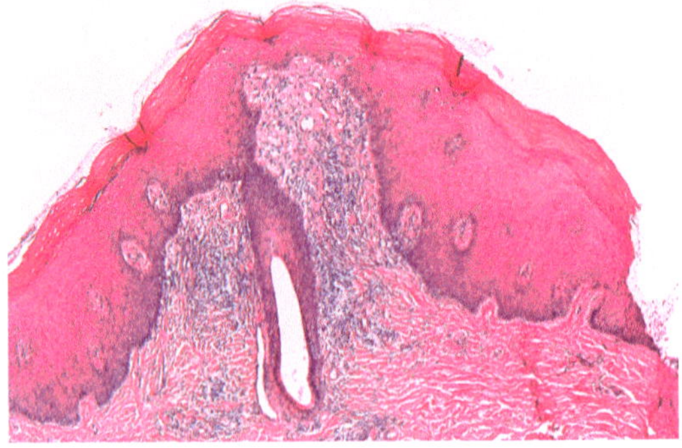

Fig. 6.15 Low-power view of stomatitis nicotina. Notice the excretory salivary duct surrounded by inflammatory cells

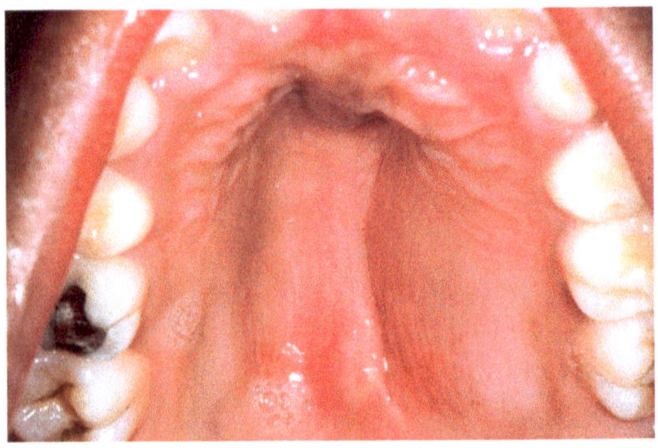

Fig. 6.16 Palatal swelling, painful, of some weeks duration. The biopsy showed the presence of subacute necrotizing sialoadenitis

6.10 Subacute Necrotizing Sialoadenitis (SANS)

Definition
Subacute inflammation of the intraoral salivary glands.

Etiology
The etiology is unknown.

Epidemiology
Occurs mainly in children and adolescents.

Clinical Aspects
SANS is more or less limited to the hard palate (Fig. 6.16). Presents as a unilateral, painful swelling, often rather rapidly arising in a matter of a week.

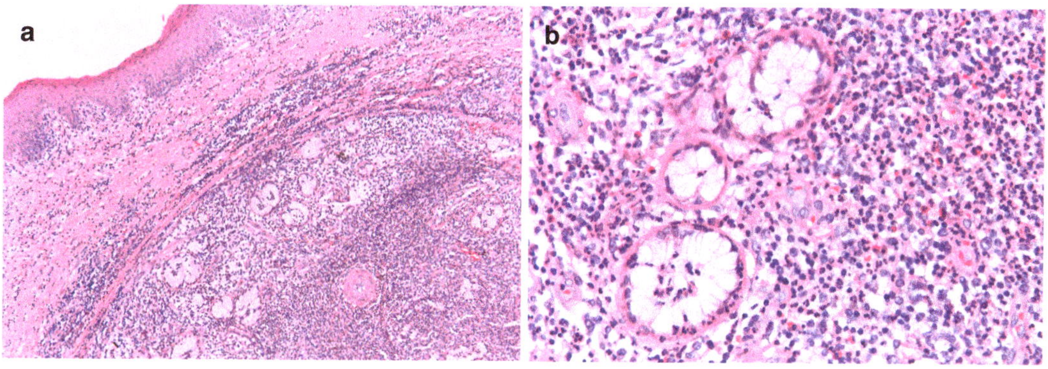

Fig. 6.17 (**a**) Low-power view of subacute necrotizing sialoadenitis. (**b**) Remnants of salivary glands surrounded by inflammatory cells in subacute necrotizing sialoadenitis

Histopathology
Subacute inflammatory changes in the minor salivary glands (Figs. 6.17a, b). Necrosis may be observed. There is no squamous ductal metaplasia as is observed in necrotizing sialometaplasia.

Treatment
Not required; regression of the swelling takes plays in 2–4 weeks.

6.11 Torus Palatinus

Definition
Exostosis in the midline of the hard palate (see also Chap. 7).

Epidemiology
Mainly seen in middle-aged persons.

Clinical Aspects
Bony hard, otherwise asymptomatic swelling in the midline of the hard palate; may be lobulated (Fig. 6.18).

Treatment
Surgical correction is only indicated in case of interference with the wearing of an upper denture. In case of intended removal, a preoperative CT scan may be helpful for assessment of the thickness of the torus in order to prevent a nasal perforation during surgery.

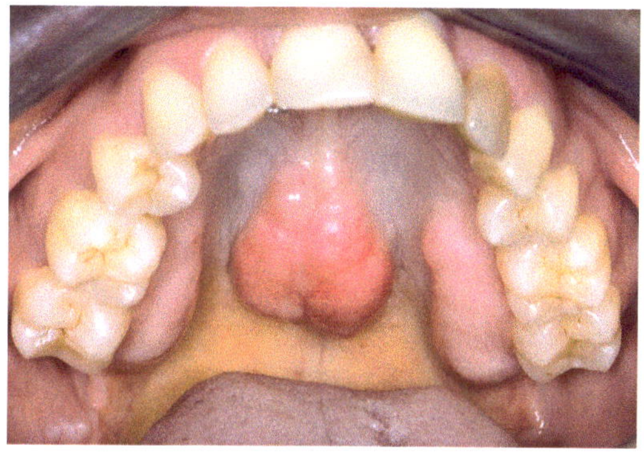

Fig. 6.18 Torus palatinus, bony hard, asymptomatic otherwise

6.12 Some Other Lesions of the Palate

6.12.1 Candidiasis

Some Characteristics
Candidiasis may involve the palate, both in the pseudomembranous form and in the erythematous form (Fig. 6.19) (see also Chaps. 2 and 4). May be associated with candidal infection of the dorsal surface of the tongue ("kissing lesion"). Palatal candidiasis often causes a burning sensation.

Local causes may include smoking, ill-fitting dentures ("stomatitis prothetica"), and steroid-containing inhalers. Possible systemic causes include an underlying HIV infection.

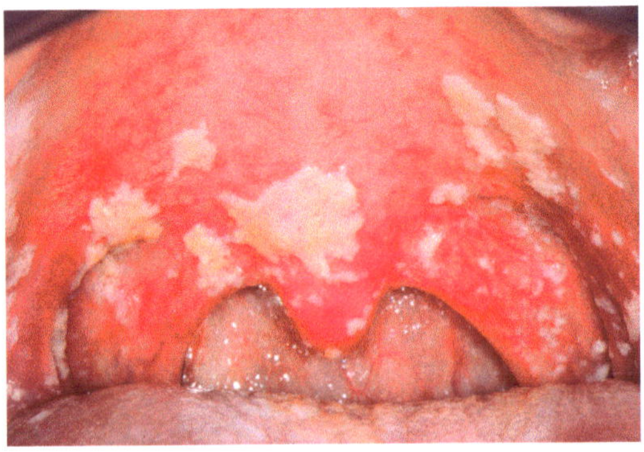

Fig. 6.19 Pseudomembranous candidiasis

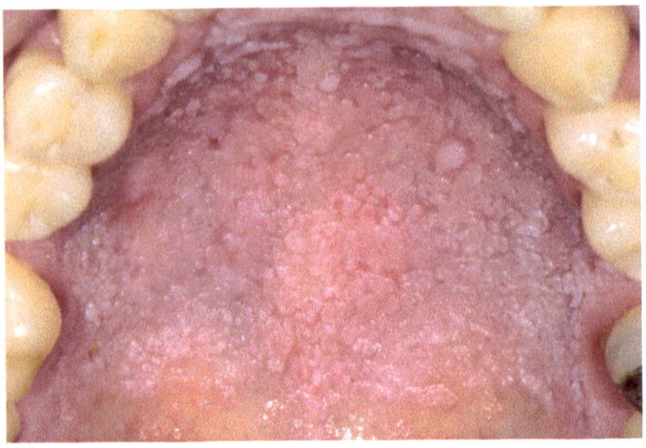

Fig. 6.20 Palatal aspect in patient suffering from Darier-White disease

6.12.2 Darier-White Disease

Some Characteristics

Hereditary benign mucocutaneous diseases characterized by mucocutaneous papules and nail disturbances. The oral mucosa lesions may have a leukoplakialike appearance (Fig. 6.20). Treatment of the oral lesions is not required.

6.12.3 Fellatio

Some Characteristics

In orogenital sex, solitary and sometimes multiple, red and somewhat painful erosions may occur on the hard palate (Fig. 6.21). Healing will usually take place in a matter of a week.

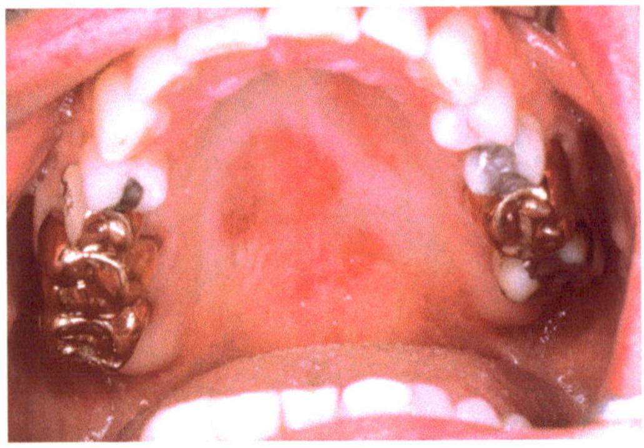

Fig. 6.21 Erythematous lesion due to fellatio

6.12.4 Langerhans Cell Histiocytosis

Some Characteristics

Langerhans cell histiocytosis has been discussed in Chap. 7. In case of oral involvement, mainly the mandibular bone is affected and the patients are usually children or young adults. Occurrence at an older age and involvement of the palatal mucosa is extremely rare (Fig. 6.22a, b).

6.12.5 Leukoplakia and Erythroplakia

Some Characteristics

Leukoplakia rarely involves the hard palate in contrast to involvement of the soft palate.

Palatal involvement occurs almost exclusively in smokers (Fig. 6.23a–d (see also Chap. 2).

Erythroplakia rarely involves the hard palate and is more common on the soft palate (see also Chap. 2) (Fig. 6.24). Bilateral, symmetrical red changes of the palatal mucosa are most likely the result of erythematous candidiasis. Redness in the midline of the hard palate may be the result of fellatio.

6.12.6 Lichen Planus

Some Characteristics

Lichen planus involvement of the palate is relatively rare (Fig. 6.25); see also Chap. 2. In this event, there are always lichenoid lesions present elsewhere in the oral cavity.

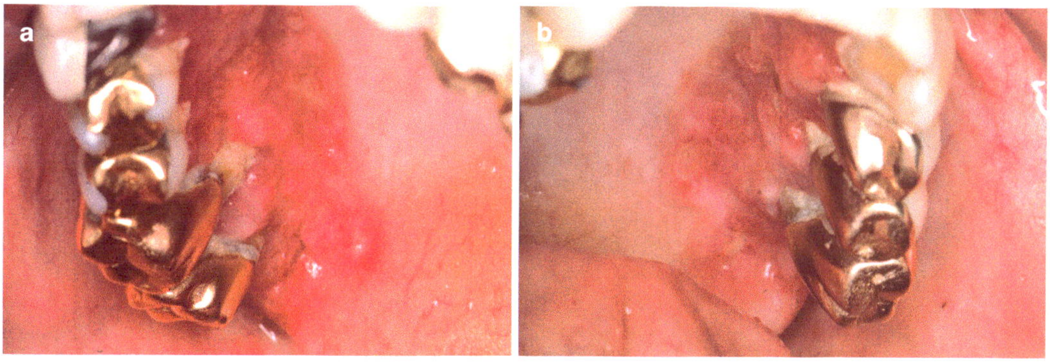

Fig. 6.22 (**a**) Langerhans cell histiocytosis of the palatal mucosa in an elderly patient. (**b**) Bilateral involvement; unusual presentation

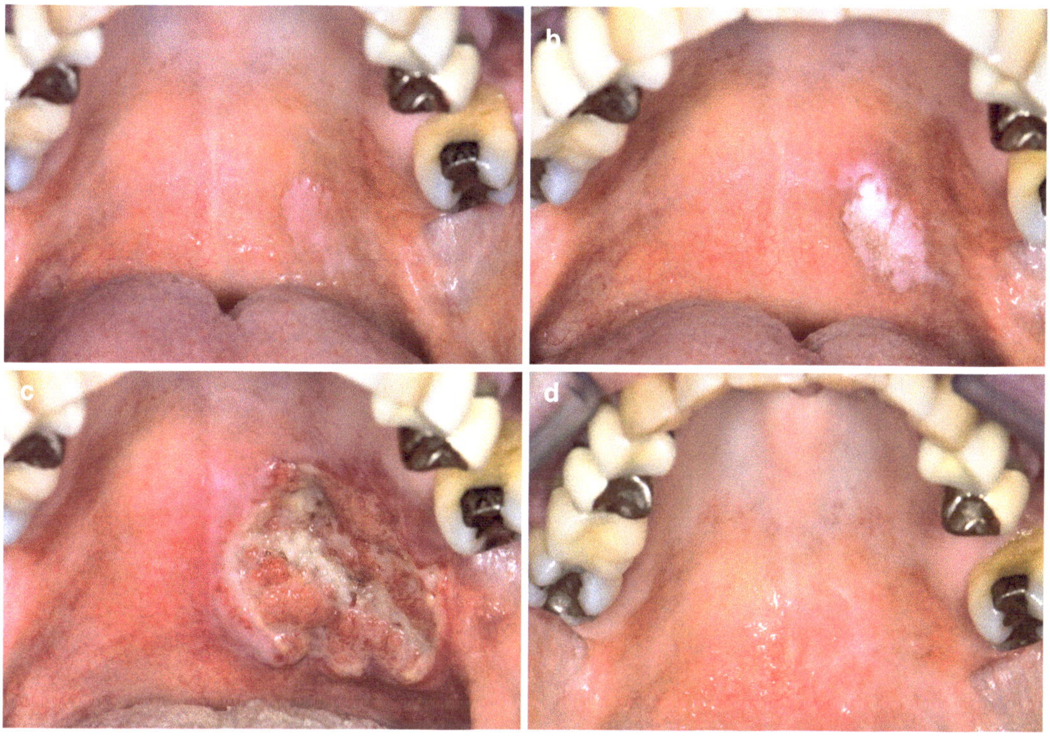

Fig. 6.23 (**a**) Leukoplakia at the junction of the hard and soft palate. (**b**) Six months later; the leukoplakia has changed somewhat in size and texture. (**c**) Clinical aspect 1 week after surgical excision. (**d**) Clinical aspect 1 year after removal; no signs of local recurrence

6.12.7 Metastases

Some Characteristics

Metastases of tumors located elsewhere in the body may occur in the palatal mucosa (Fig. 6.26). In most instances, the primary is known already.

6.12.8 Multiple Myelomas (Kahler's Disease)

Some Characteristics

Multiple myelomas, as being mentioned in Chap. 2, mainly involve the mandibular bone. Occurrence in the oral soft tissues, such as on the palate, is rare (Fig. 6.27).

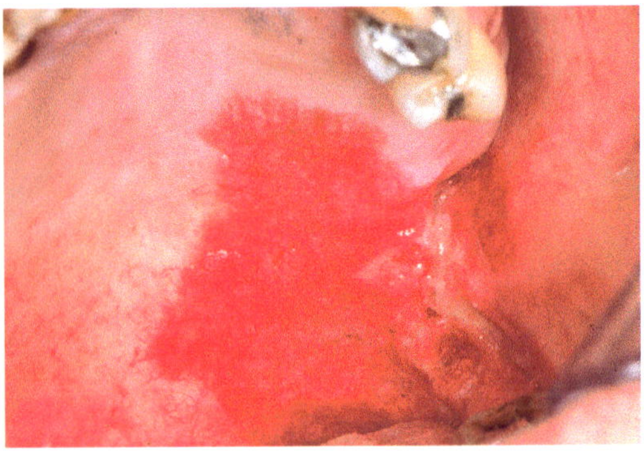

Fig. 6.24 Erythroplakia of the palate

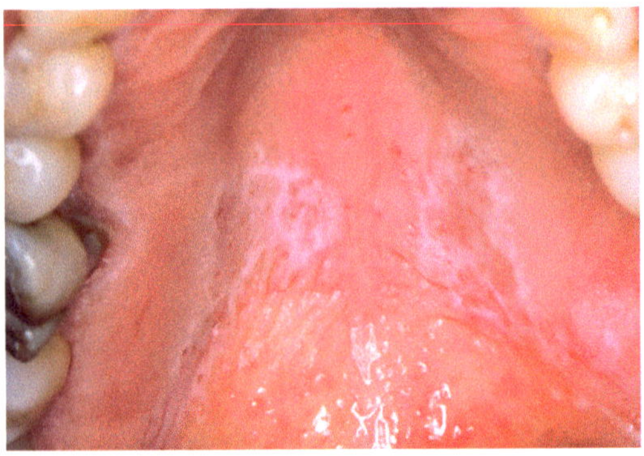

Fig. 6.25 Reticular lichen planus of the palate; rare site

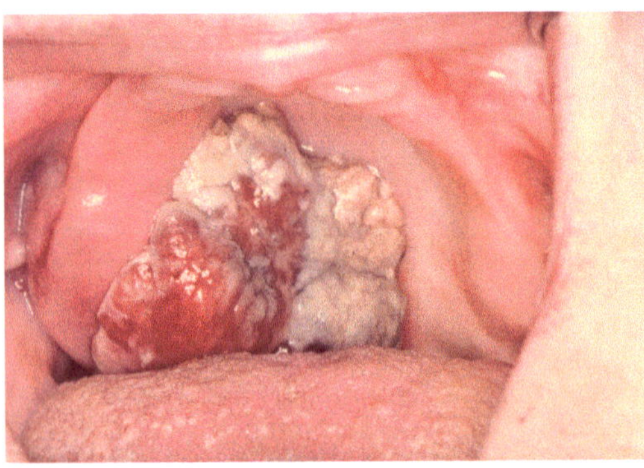

Fig. 6.26 Metastasis from a renal cell carcinoma

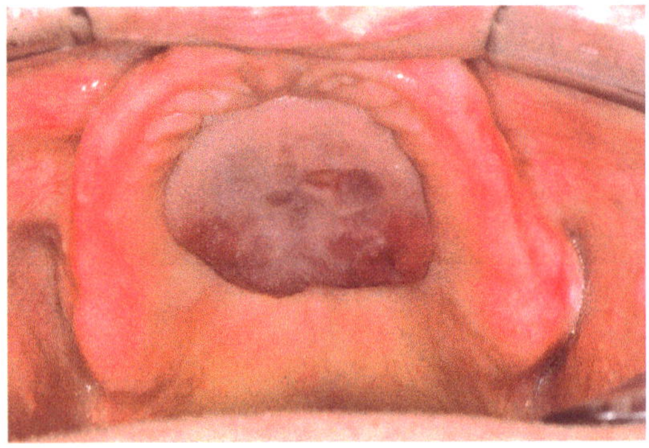

Fig. 6.27 Unusual swelling of the palate based on multiple myeloma

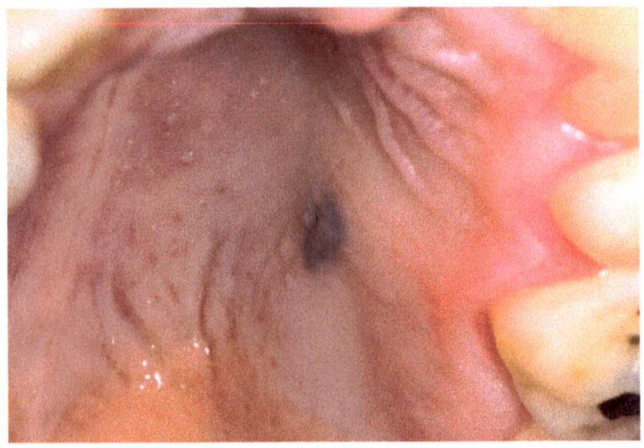

Fig. 6.28 Pigmented lesion, asymptomatic. The excisional biopsy showed the presence of a "blue nevus"

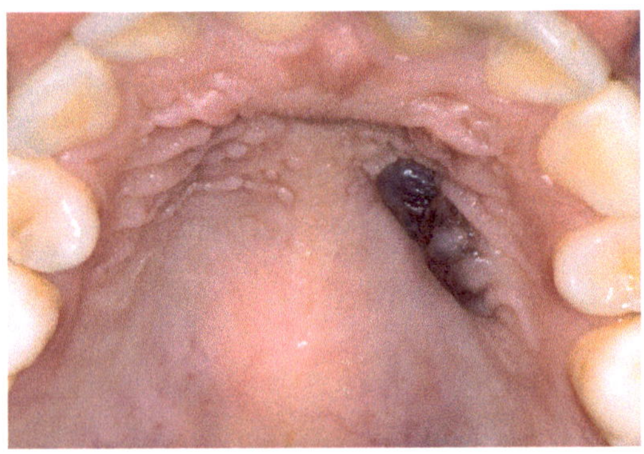

Fig. 6.29 Bluish lesion on the palate mimicking melanoma. The biopsy showed the presence of an intramucosal nevus

6.12.9 Nevus Pigmented

Some Characteristics

Benign neoplasm of melanin-producing nevus cells (see also Chap. 2). The hard palate is the site of preference (Figs. 6.28 and 6.29). A nevus is asymptomatic otherwise and may mimic early melanoma. A final diagnosis of pigmented nevus can only be made by histopathologic examination. In the past, a nevus was regarded to be

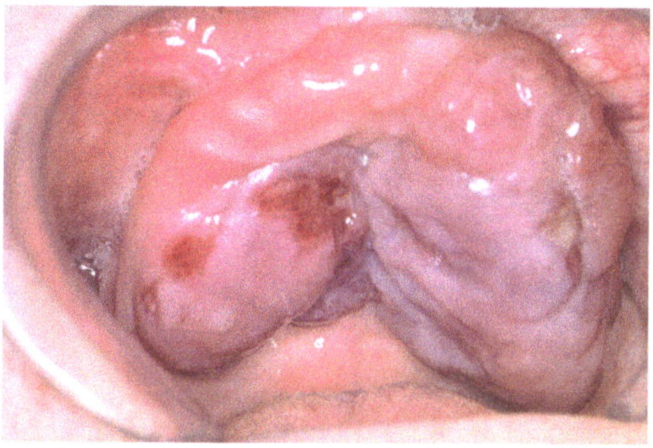

Fig. 6.30 Bilateral swelling of the palatal mucosa caused by a non-Hodgkin lymphoma. The tumor has probably been present for some years

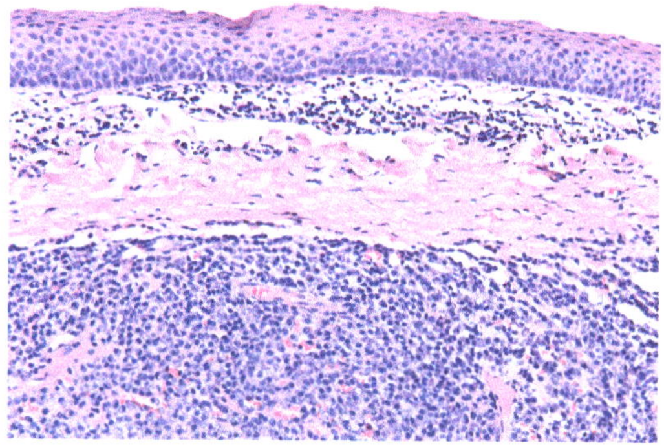

Fig. 6.32 Low-power view of non-Hodgkin lymphoma

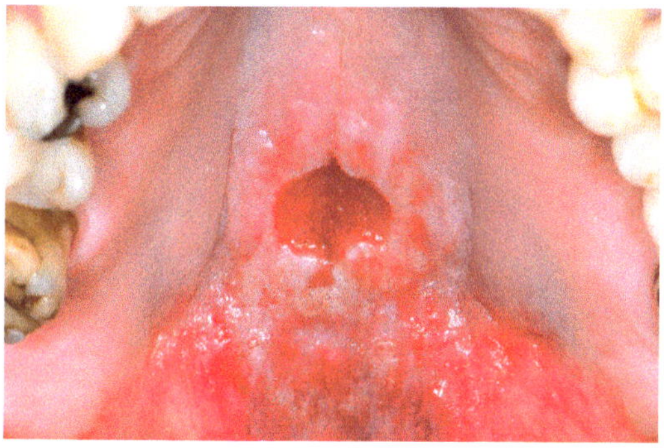

Fig. 6.31 Ulcerative manifestation of palatal non-Hodgkin lymphoma

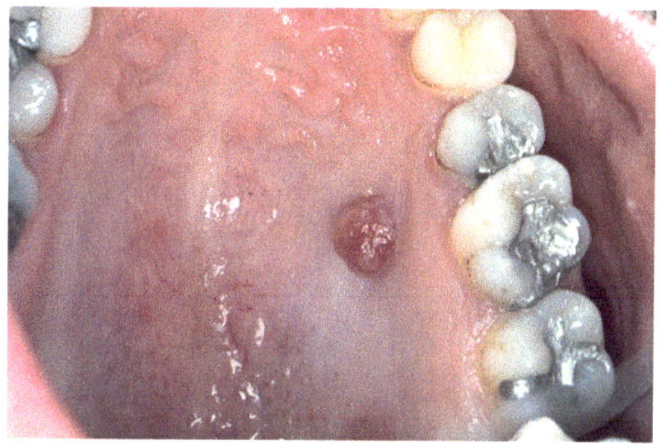

Fig. 6.33 Odontogenic fistula; may mimic a salivary gland tumor

potentially malignant, but this has never been proven.

6.12.10 Non-Hodgkin Lymphoma (Incl. Lymphoid Hyperplasia)

Some Characteristics

A non-Hodgkin lymphoma can be the first and only manifestation of the disease (see also Chap. 7). The palate is the site of preference for oral non-Hodgkin lymphomas of the soft tissues. May present as a slowly growing non-ulcerative and otherwise asymptomatic swelling but may also present as a fast-growing and painful ulcerative lesion (Figs. 6.30, 6.31 and 6.32).

Occasionally, one is dealing with a pseudolymphoma ("lymphoid hyperplasia of the palate").

6.12.11 Odontogenic Fistula

Some Characteristics

Periapical inflammation around the palatal apices of the upper bicuspids and molars may give rise to a palatal fistula (Fig. 6.33). Such fistula may mimic a salivary neoplasm or a squamous cell carcinoma.

6.12.12 Palatal Perforation Due to Cocaine Abuse

Some Characteristics

The use of cocaine may result in atrophy of the mucosal lining of the nasal cavity, which in a late stage may result in necrosis of the palatal bone (Fig. 6.34).

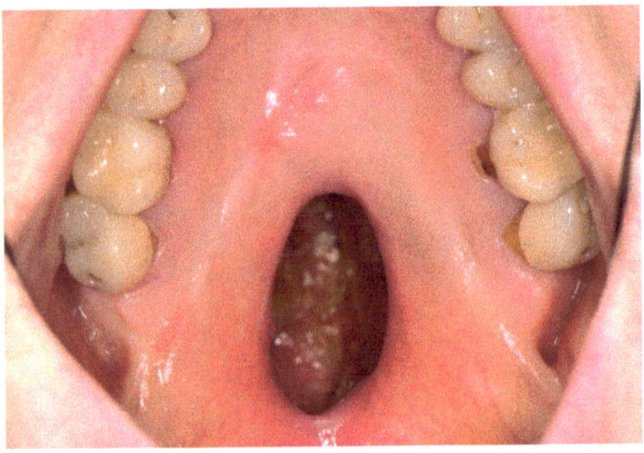

Fig. 6.34 Palatal defect due to the use of cocaine

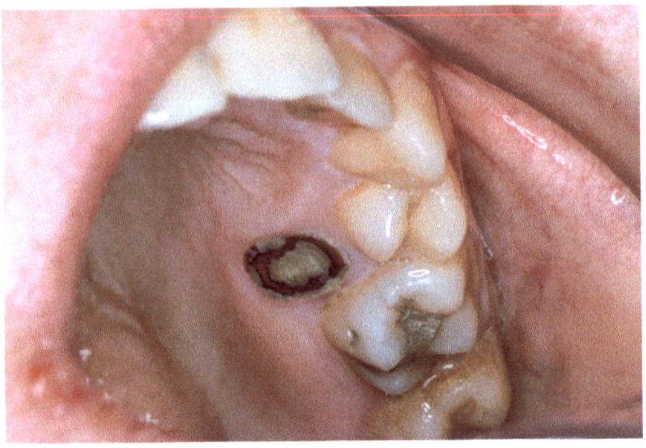

Fig. 6.35 Palatal "lesion" based on eruption of a deeply decayed bicuspid (25)

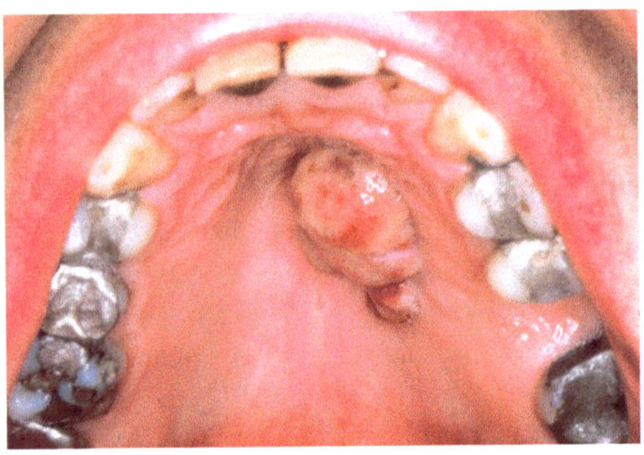

Fig. 6.36 Pyogenic granuloma of the palate

6.12.13 Palatal Tooth Eruption

Some Characteristics

Particularly upper canines and occasionally also second bicuspids may erupt on the palatal side of the maxilla (Fig. 6.35).

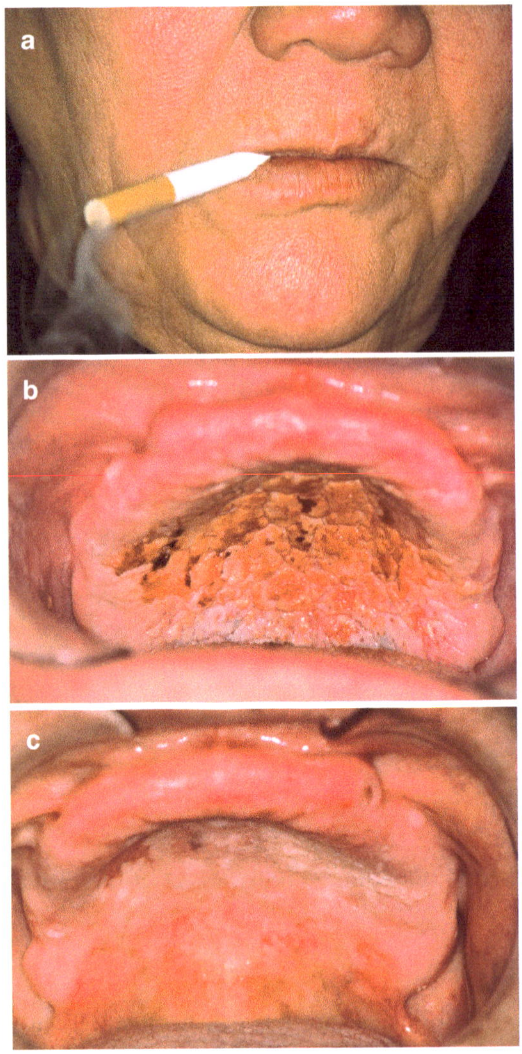

Fig. 6.37 (**a**) "Reverse smoking". (**b**) The clinical aspect somewhat resembles stomatitis nicotina. (**c**) Clinical aspect six months after cessation of the reverse smoking habit

6.12.14 Pyogenic Granuloma

Some Characteristics

Occurs relatively seldom on the palate (Fig. 6.36) (see also Chap. 2).

6.12.15 Reverse Smoking

Some Characteristics

In "reverse smoking," the glowing end of a cigarette is kept inside the mouth (Fig. 6.37a–c);

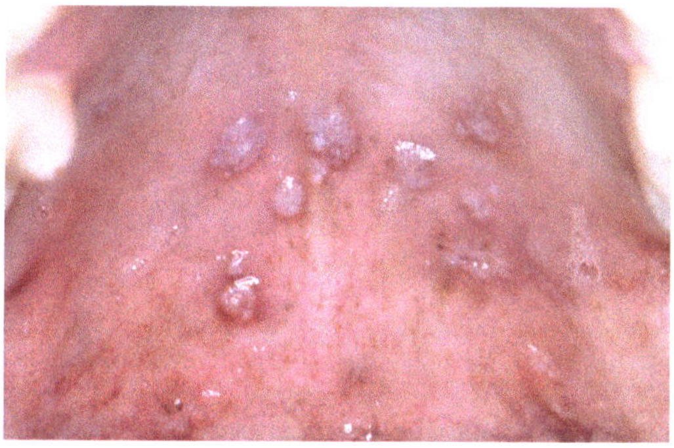

Fig. 6.38 Multiple nodules on the palate caused by sarcoidosis

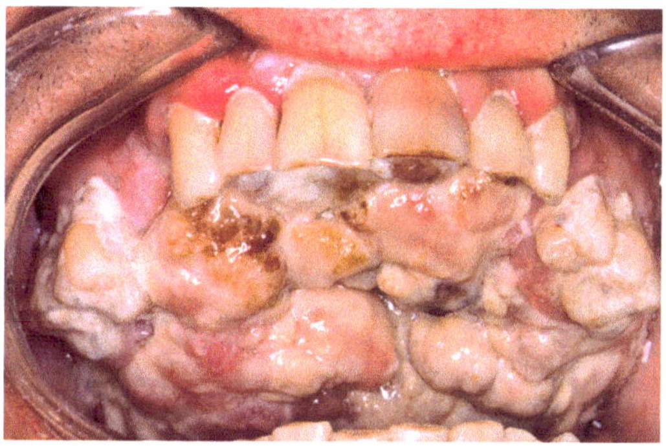

Fig. 6.39 Neglected squamous cell carcinoma

this habit is found in some parts of India and also in some parts of South America. The resulting palatal lesions may mimic leukoplakia or erythroplakia; occasionally, a nicotinic stomatitislike aspect can be observed. After cessation of the habit, regression will take place in a matter of a few months. In case of persisting habits, a squamous cell carcinoma may develop.

6.12.16 Sarcoidosis

Some Characteristics

Sarcoidosis may cause solitary or multiple nodules in any part of the oral mucosa, including the palate (Fig. 6.38) (see also Chap. 2).

6.12.17 Squamous Cell Carcinoma

Some Characteristics

Oral squamous cell carcinoma rarely involves the hard palate (Fig. 6.39); involvement of the soft palate is more common (see also Chap. 2).

7 Diseases of the Jaw Bones

7.1 Introduction

In this chapter lesions and disorders are dealt with that may occur in the jaw bones. A distinction can be made between osseous lesions and lesions that are of odontogenic origin, such as odontogenic infections, cysts, and tumors. Furthermore, the jaw bones may be involved in a number of systemic diseases and syndromes.

7.2 Cysts of the Jaw Bones

The nasopalatine duct cyst has been dealt with in the chapter of diseases of the palate (Chap. 6), since the clinical presentation, if applicable, is almost invariably a swelling of the palate. Because of its extremely rare occurrence, the intraosseous dermoid cyst is not discussed here.

7.2.1 Aneurysmal Bone Cyst

Definition
Entity of which occurrence in the jaw bones is somewhat disputed. An aneurysmal bone cyst of the jaw bones may actually represent cyst formation in a preexistent osseous lesion such as a central giant cell lesion.

Etiology
The etiology is unknown.

Clinical Aspects
Usually located in the lower jaw; presents itself as a swelling.

Radiographic Aspects
Uni- or multilobular well-defined radiolucent lesion (Fig. 7.1).

Histopathology
The histopathology shows connective tissue with lacunae and clefts filled with blood. Occasional multinucleated giant cells and osteoid formation are observed (Fig. 7.2).

Treatment
Enucleation. Because of the scarcity of reported cases, no information is available about possible recurrences.

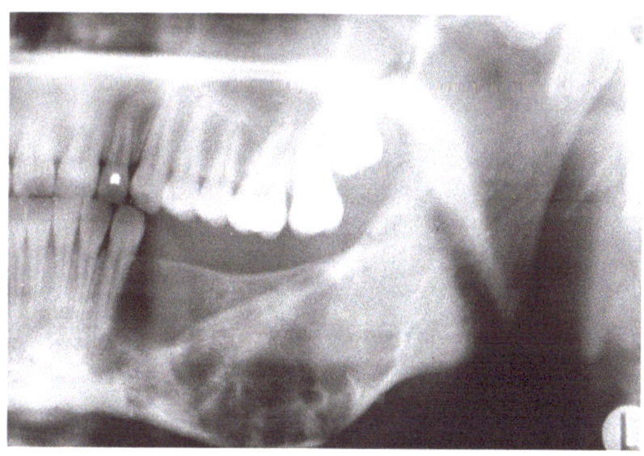

Fig. 7.1 Radiographic aspect of a possible aneurysmal bone cyst of the mandible

I. van der Waal, *Atlas of Oral Diseases: A Guide for Daily Practice*,
DOI 10.1007/978-3-662-48122-6_7

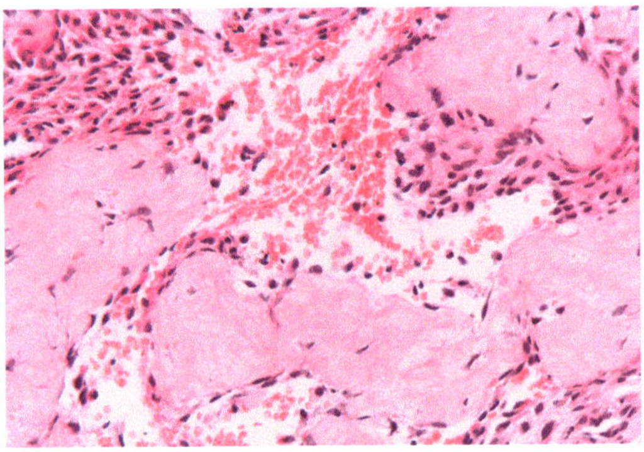

Fig. 7.2 Histopathologic aspect compatible with a diagnosis of aneurysmal bone cyst

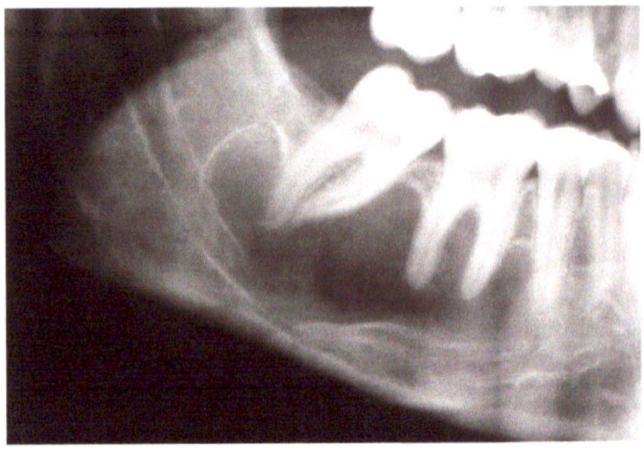

Fig. 7.3 Radiographic aspect compatible with, but not diagnostic of a simple bone cyst

7.2.2 Simple Bone Cyst

Definition

Intraosseous cavitation of unknown origin. May also occur elsewhere in the skeleton.

Synonyms are hemorrhagic bone cyst, traumatic bone cyst, and solitary bone cyst.

Due to the absence of cyst epithelium, it is in fact incorrect to use the term "cyst."

Epidemiology

Only occurs in young people.

Clinical Aspects

When occurring in the jaw only, the mandible is affected. Usually an incidental finding on a radiograph without any symptoms. There is no swelling. The teeth in the affected area of the jaw remain vital.

Radiographic Aspects

Well-defined ("corticated"), often lobulated radiolucency around and between the roots of the teeth (Fig. 7.3). The nondistinctive radiographic aspect gives room for an extensive differential diagnosis such as keratocystic odontogenic tumor, ameloblastoma, and giant cell lesion.

Diagnosis

The diagnosis "simple bone cyst" is based on the finding of an empty cavity on exploration, occasionally being filled with some fluid and being lined by delicate fibrous tissue without epithelial lining (Fig. 7.4).

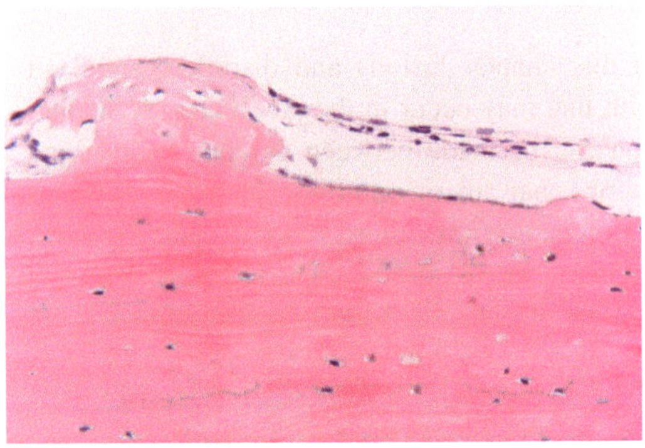

Fig. 7.4 Delicate fibrous lining of a simple bone cyst; no epithelial lining

Treatment

The surgical exploration that is required to obtain a diagnosis at the same time represents the treatment. There is no need to insert any type of implant material in the empty cavity. Recurrence (persistence) is rare. In such event one may choose just to follow the patient instead of repeating an exploration.

7.2.3 Latent Bone Cyst (Stafne's Bone Cyst)

Definition

The latent bone cyst is actually based on an impression of the lingual cortex of the mandible, usually in the region of the angle (Fig. 7.5). In fact the term "cyst" is incorrect as there is no cavity lined with epithelium. Some prefer the term "lingual cortical mandibular defect."

Epidemiology
The estimated prevalence is less than 0.1 %. The defect rarely becomes visible under the age of 40 years and is more common in men than in women. Bilateral occurrence is extremely rare.

Radiographic Aspects
Well-circumscribed round or oval radiolucency near the angle of the mandible, below the level of the mandibular canal (Fig. 7.6). The absence of symptoms, the localization, and the radiographic image usually allow to make a final diagnosis. In case of doubt, a CT scan can be performed in order to demonstrate the mandibular lingual defect.

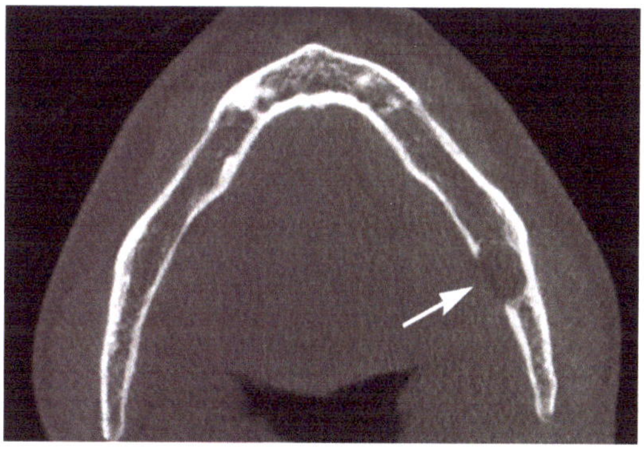

Fig. 7.5 CT scan shows the lingual depression in the mandible; not a true cyst

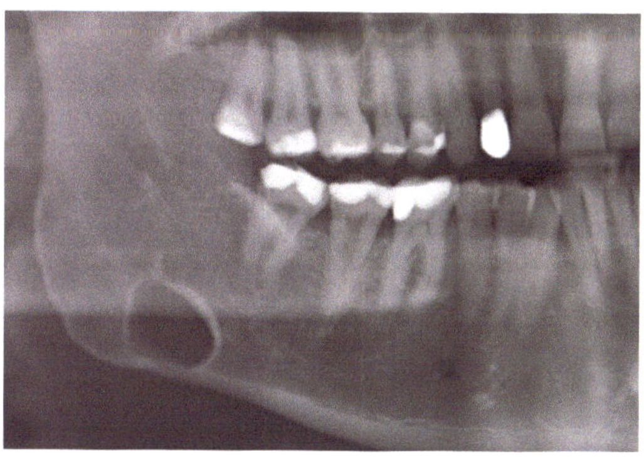

Fig. 7.6 Latent bone cyst below the mandibular canal; incidental finding

Treatment
Exploration is only indicated in case of doubt. It is interesting to mention that after having made a window in the intact buccal cortical bone, one, sometimes somewhat confusing, immediately enters the floor of the mouth and not an intraosseous cavity.

7.3 Cysts and Tumors of Odontogenic Origin

General Aspects
Cysts lined by odontogenic epithelium. Some cysts are caused by an inflammatory stimulus (inflammatory cysts), while for other cysts such a stimulus is unknown, being referred to as developmental cysts (Table 7.1). Odontogenic cysts may become symptomatic but may also be detected as an incidental finding on a radiograph. Malignant changes in the epithelium of odontogenic cysts are exceedingly rare. Odontogenic cysts are treated by enucleation or, occasionally, by marsupialization (see for explanation Chap. 2).

Table 7.1 Classification of odontogenic cysts

1 Developmental cysts
1.1 Dental lamina cyst (gingival cyst) in the newborn
1.2 Gingival cyst in the adult
1.3 Primordial cyst
1.4 Eruption cyst
1.5 Follicular (dentigerous) cyst
1.6 Lateral periodontal cyst
1.7 Keratinizing odontogenic cyst
1.8 Sialo-odontogenic cyst ("glandular odontogenic cyst")
2 Inflammatory cysts
2.1 Radicular cyst
2.2 Residual (radicular) cyst
2.3 Paradental cyst (including the mandibular buccal infected cyst)

The lesion previously known as odontogenic keratocyst is currently designated "keratocystic odontogenic tumor," being classified as an odontogenic tumor

7.3.1 Odontogenic Cysts

7.3.1.1 Developmental Odontogenic Cysts

The dental lamina cyst of the newborn, the gingival cyst in adults, and the eruption cyst are located in the soft tissues and are discussed in Chap. 5.

Primordial Cyst

Definition

Cystic change in a developing tooth germ before formation of dentin or enamel matrix. Can, theoretically, also arise in a supernumerary tooth germ. It is a somewhat debatable entity, by many considered to always be based histopathologically on a keratocystic odontogenic tumor.

Epidemiology

Extremely rare odontogenic cyst.

Clinical Aspects

Incidental finding on a radiograph. Rarely, if ever, causes symptoms.

Radiographic Aspects

Well-defined radiolucency in an area of a missing tooth (and a negative history of a previous tooth extraction) (Fig. 7.7).

Histopathology

Often, according to some authors, always lined by epithelium that shows the characteristic features of a keratocystic odontogenic tumor.

Treatment

Enucleation.

Follicular (Dentigerous) Cyst

Definition

Cyst development in a follicle of an unerupted tooth.

Epidemiology

Quite common odontogenic cyst that almost exclusively occurs in the permanent dentition.

Clinical Aspects

Incidental finding on a radiograph, mainly related to mandibular and maxillary wisdom teeth and upper canines.

Radiographic Aspects

Well-defined radiolucency around the crown of an impacted tooth (Fig. 7.8). The differential diagnosis includes, among others, a keratocystic odontogenic tumor and an ameloblastoma. When the radiolucency surrounding the crown measures more than 2–3 mm, somewhat arbitrarily chosen, the term follicular cyst is used instead of "enlarged" tooth follicle.

Histopathology

The lining of a follicular cyst consists of two or more layers of squamous epithelium without characteristic features (Fig. 7.9). Occasional "goblet cells" may be observed (Fig. 7.10).

Histopathologically, no distinction can be made between the lining of a follicular cyst and the

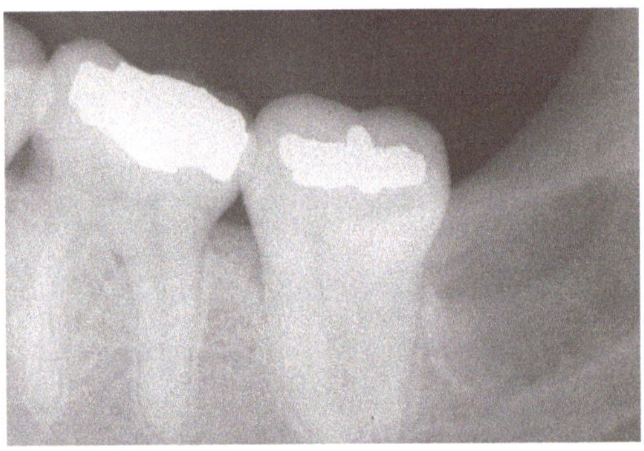

Fig. 7.7 Radiographic aspect distally of 37 compatible with a primordial cyst; no history of removal of 38

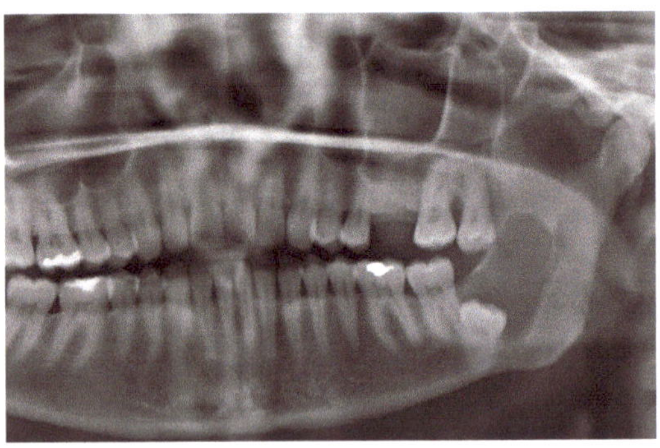

Fig. 7.8 Radiographic aspect compatible with the diagnosis of follicular cyst of 38

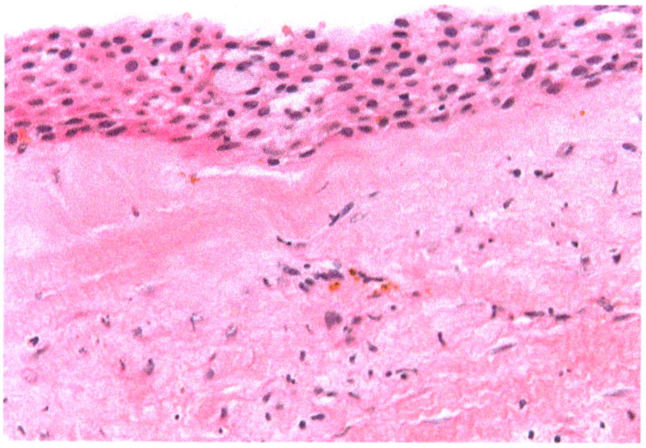

Fig. 7.9 Histopathologic aspect compatible with but not diagnostic of a follicular cyst

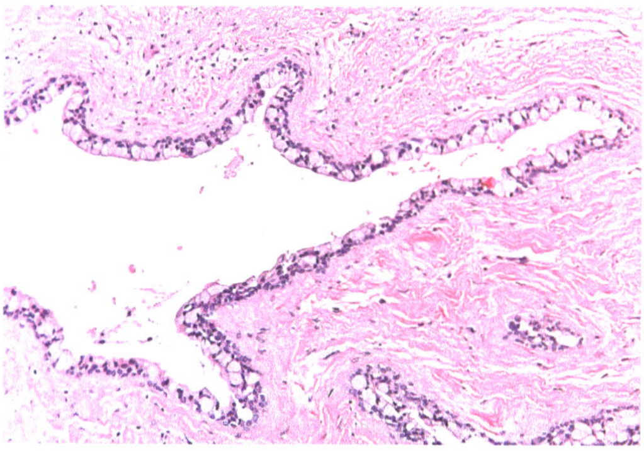

Fig. 7.10 Goblet cells in the lining of a follicular cyst

lining of an (enlarged) tooth follicle. In tooth follicles embryonal rests of odontogenic epithelium may be encountered, sometimes mimicking ameloblastomatous cells. Furthermore, myxoid changes in the stroma can be observed, mimicking to some extent the features of an odontogenic myxoma.

Treatment

Enucleation and removal of the associated tooth. Recurrences are extremely rare.

Lateral Periodontal Cyst (Incl. Botryoid Odontogenic Cyst)

Definition

In the past, a lateral periodontal cyst has been defined clinicoradiographically as a cyst located between the roots of two vital teeth. At present, the definition has been extended by certain histopathological characteristics. A botryoid odontogenic cyst shows the same histopathological characteristics as a lateral periodontal cyst but extends over an area of several teeth.

Clinical Aspects

The lateral periodontal cyst is almost exclusively found in the premolar area of the mandible, usually being an accidental finding on a radiograph.

Radiographic Aspects

Well-defined radiolucency between the roots of two vital teeth (Fig. 7.11a). In case of a lobular radiolucency, extending over an area of several teeth, the term "botryoid odontogenic cyst" is applied. The differential diagnosis includes, among others:

- Ameloblastoma
- Keratocystic odontogenic tumor
- Central giant cell lesion
- Ossifying fibroma
- Langerhans cell histiocytosis
- Simple bone cyst

Histopathology

The histopathology shows an epithelial lining of just a few cell layers thick with characteristic epithelial plaques (Fig. 7.11b). In fact, a more or less similar lining is seen in the gingival cyst of the

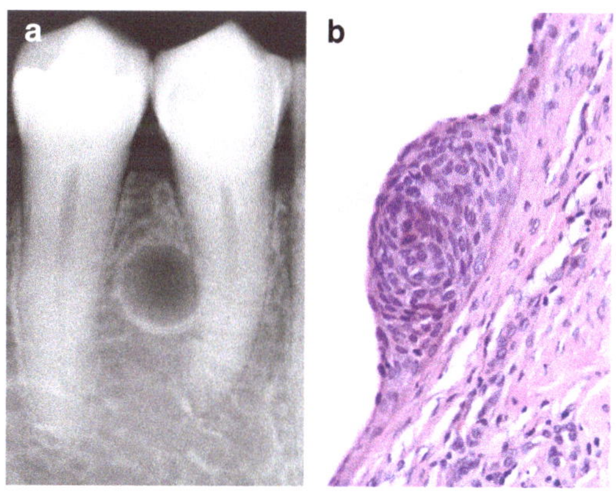

Fig. 7.11 (**a**) The radiographic aspect is compatible with a diagnosis of a lateral periodontal cyst. (**b**) Epithelial "plaque", more or less diagnostic of the diagnosis lateral periodontal cyst

adult. The latter cyst is by many authors regarded as the extraosseous counterpart of the intraosseous lateral periodontal cyst.

Treatment
Enucleation; especially the botryoid odontogenic cyst has a tendency to recur.

Keratinizing Odontogenic Cyst

Definition
The keratinizing odontogenic cyst (KOC) is a developmental odontogenic cyst, presenting clinicoradiographically as a follicular cyst (Fig. 7.12). The diagnosis is based on histopathologic features only. These features consist of an epithelial cyst lining showing hyperkeratosis without the characteristic epithelial architecture of a keratocystic odontogenic tumor (KCOT) (Fig. 7.13). In the past this cyst was for many years regarded as the orthokeratotic variant of a KCOT, that, in contrast to the parakeratotic variant of a KCOT, rarely recurred after removal.

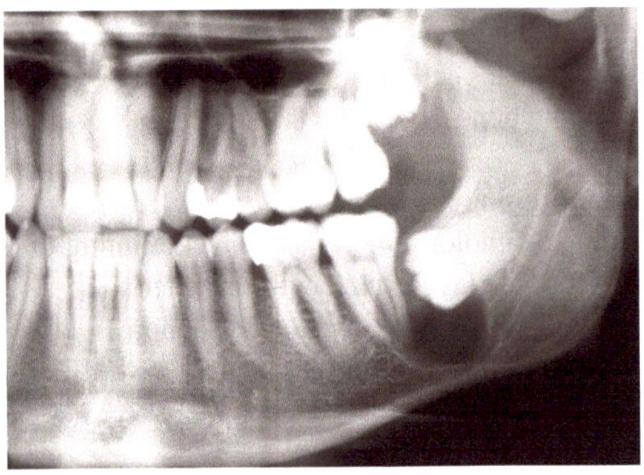

Fig. 7.12 Non-characteristic radiograph of a keratinizing odontogenic cyst

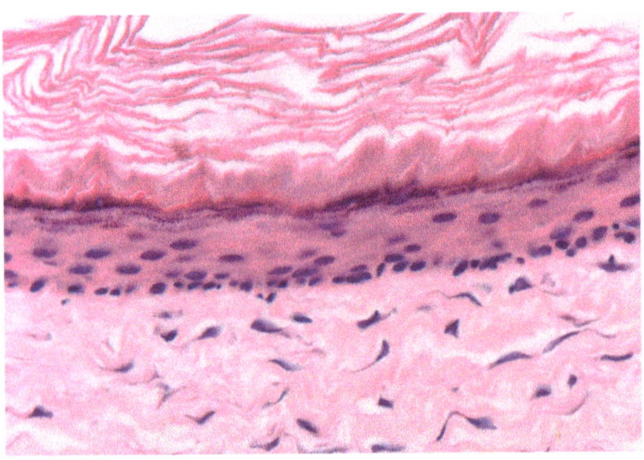

Fig. 7.13 Keratinizing odontogenic cyst somewhat mimicking a keratocystic odontogenic tumor

Radiographic Aspects
There are no specific radiographic features.

Treatment
The diagnosis KOC is always a postsurgical, histopathologic diagnosis. There is no tendency for recurrences and follow-up is not indicated.

Sialo-odontogenic Cyst

Definition
Rare developmental cyst with tubular-like structures in the epithelial lining which resemble salivary gland tissue.

Epidemiology
Usually in middle-aged persons.

Clinical Aspects
Usually located in the anterior part of the lower jaw.

Radiographic Aspects
Unilobular or multilobular radiolucency, indistinguishable from a keratocystic odontogenic tumor or ameloblastoma (Fig. 7.14).

Histopathology
Apart from squamous epithelium also tubular structures and mucous producing cells are encountered (Fig. 7.15); can somewhat resemble mucoepidermoid carcinoma.

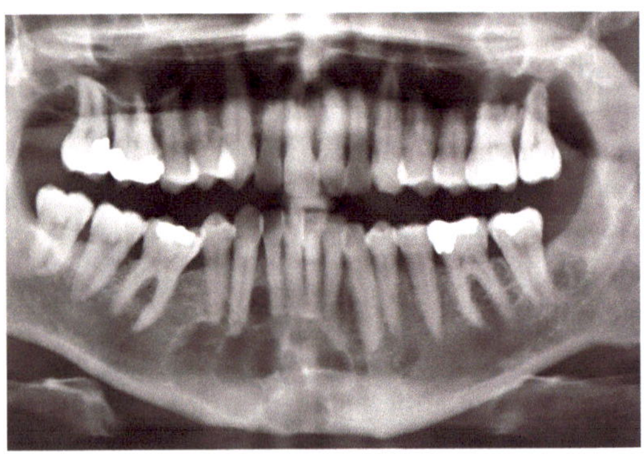

Fig. 7.14 Non-characteristic radiograph of a sialo-odontogenic cyst in the 43–44 region

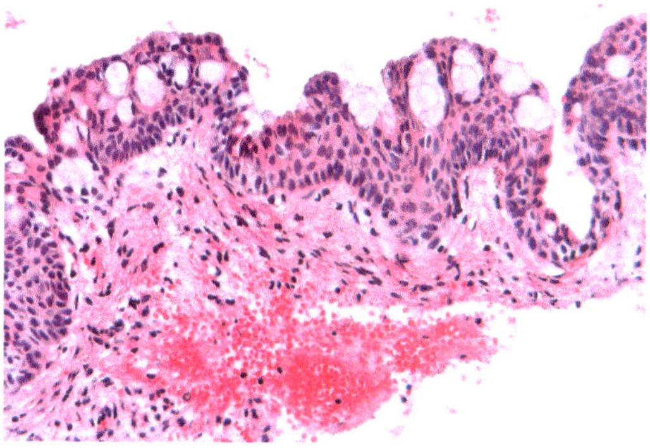

Fig. 7.15 Low-power view of the epithelial lining of the wall of a sialo-odontogenic cyst

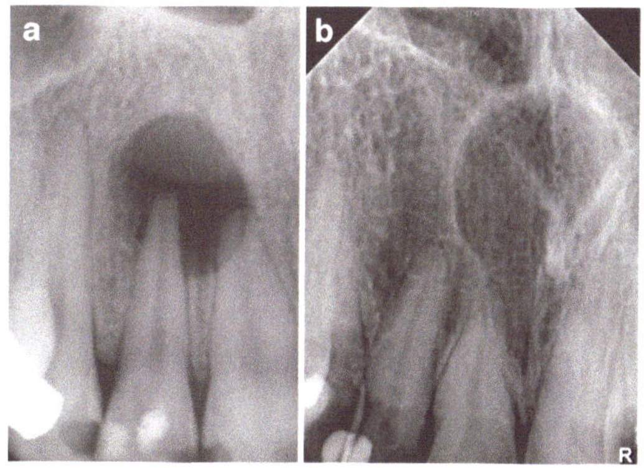

Fig. 7.16 (**a**) Radiolucency at the apex of the non-vital 12. (**b**) A nasopalatine duct cyst may somewhat resemble a radicular cyst of an upper central incisor

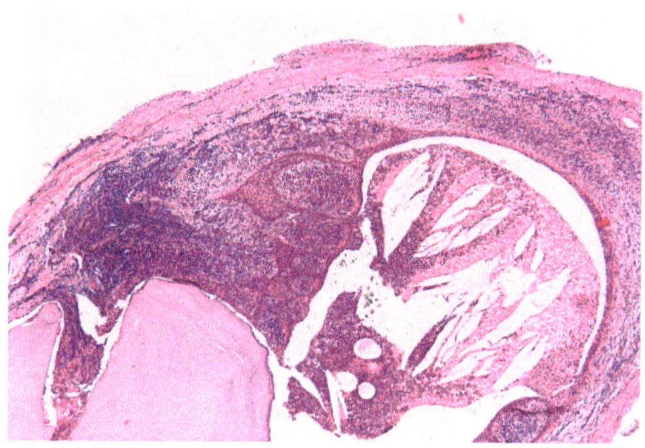

Fig. 7.17 Radicular cyst at the apex of a non-vital tooth

Treatment
Enucleation; recurrences have been reported.

7.3.1.2 Inflammatory Odontogenic Cysts

Radicular Cyst

Definition
Cyst around the apex of a root of a non-vital tooth.

Clinical Aspects
Rarely occurs in the temporary dentition. Occasionally causes a swelling or an abscess.

Radiographic Aspects
Well-defined radiolucency around the apex of a root (Fig. 7.16a). Occasionally root resorption may be observed. Cannot be distinguished radiologically from a periapical granuloma, although the presence of a surrounding cortical line and large size are indicative of a radicular cyst. The radiographic aspect of a nasopalatine duct cyst may somewhat mimic a radicular cyst (Fig. 7.16b). However, in a nasopalatine duct cyst, the vitality of the teeth remains intact.

Histopathology
Non-characteristic lining with stratified squamous epithelium (Fig. 7.17).

Treatment
Endodontic treatment, sometimes in combination with apicoectomy. If necessary extraction of the tooth and enucleation of the cyst may be considered.

Residual (Radicular) Cyst

Definition
(Radicular) cyst left behind after a tooth extraction.

Clinical Aspects
A residual may give rise to a swelling of the bone.

Radiographic Aspects
Well-defined radiolucent lesion in an edentulous part of lower or upper jaw (Fig. 7.18a, b). The differential diagnosis includes, a.o., ameloblastoma, keratocystic odontogenic tumor, and other non-odontogenic tumors. In an edentulous part of the dorsal part of the maxilla, it might be difficult to distinguish a residual cyst from an extension of the maxillary sinus (Fig. 7.19).

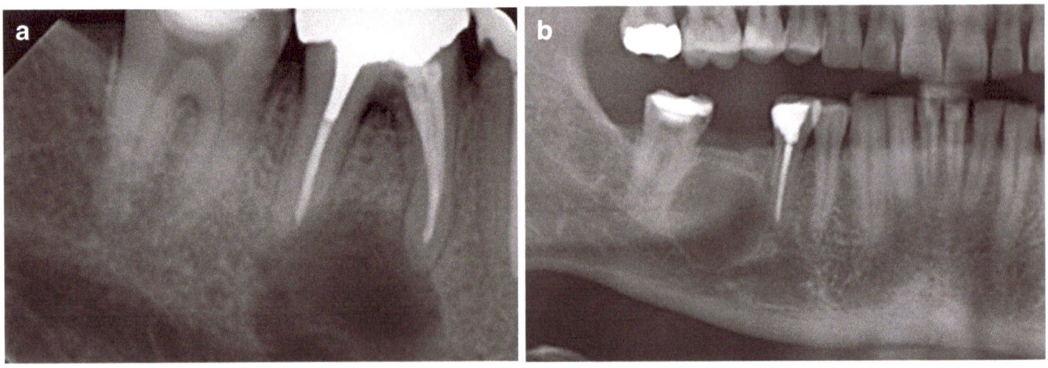

Fig. 7.18 (**a**) The radiographic aspect is suggestive of a radicular cyst. (**b**) After extraction of 46 two years ago, the cyst has apparently persisted (residual cyst)

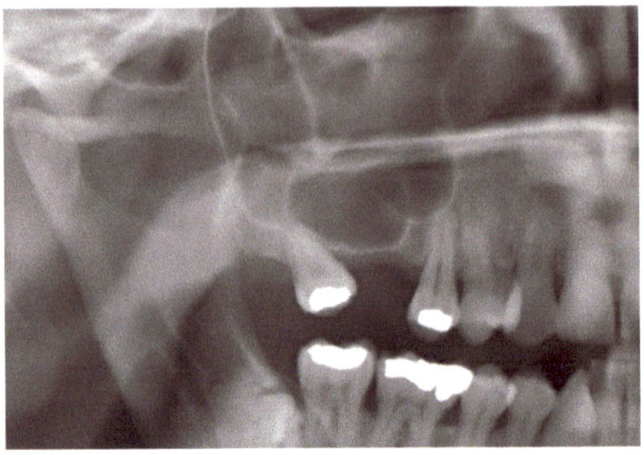

Fig. 7.19 Expansion of the maxillary sinus may mimic a residual cyst

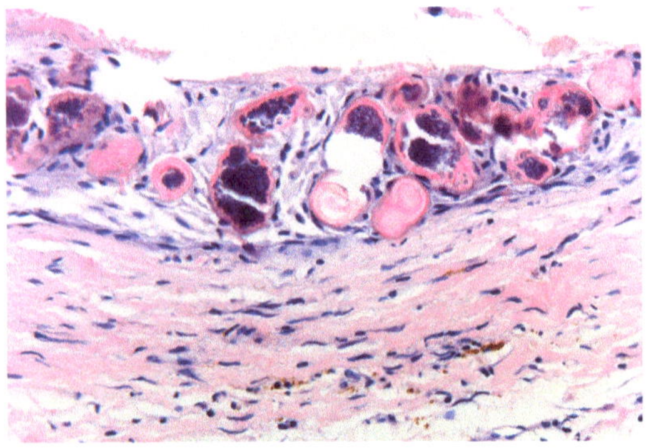

Fig. 7.21 Rushton bodies in the lining of a residual cyst

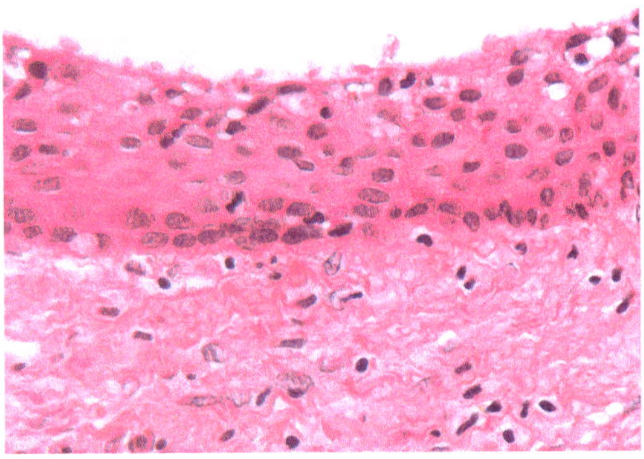

Fig. 7.20 Non-characteristic squamous epithelium lining of a residual cyst

Histopathology
Non-characteristic lining with squamous epithelium (Fig. 7.20). Occasional presence of calcifications in the lining epithelial cells, called "Rushton bodies" (Fig. 7.21). Rushton bodies may be misinterpreted as part of a cystic calcifying odontogenic tumor, a rare odontogenic tumor that will not be discussed here any further.

Treatment
Enucleation or, if indicated, marsupialization (Fig. 7.22a–d).

Paradental Cyst (Incl. Mandibular Buccal Infected Cyst)

Definition
Cyst formation in a persisting follicle of an erupted tooth; the mandibular buccal infected cyst is a rare subtype.

Clinical Aspects
Usually incidental finding on a radiograph. Occasionally pocket formation and mild symptoms of gingival discharge of fluid.

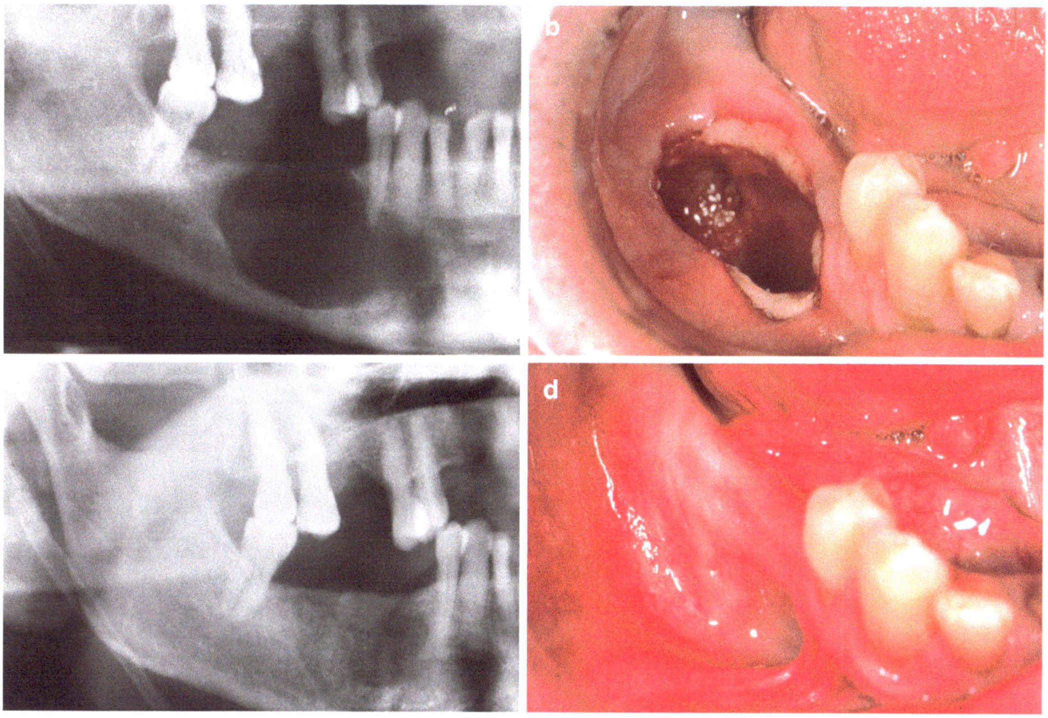

Fig. 7.22 (**a**) Radiographic aspect compatible with a diagnosis of a residual cyst. (**b**) Clinical aspect immediately after marsupialization. (**c**) Radiographic aspect one year postoperatively. (**d**) Clinical aspect one year postoperatively

Radiographic Aspects

The paradental cyst presents as a circumscribed radiolucency, distally of an erupted tooth, often a lower wisdom tooth. The mandibular buccal infected cyst may be accompanied by a periapical radiolucency around a vital tooth (Fig. 7.23).

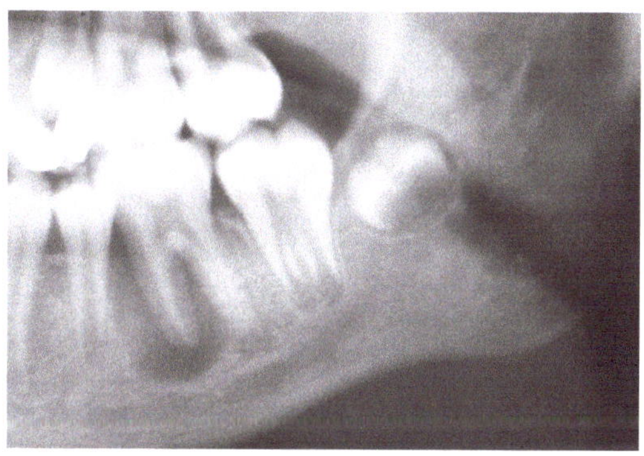

Fig. 7.23 Paradental cyst ("mandibular buccal infected cyst") of a vital 36 in a young patient

Histopathology

Non-characteristic epithelial lining of the cyst wall.

Treatment

Enucleation (Fig. 7.24a–d). In some cases the tooth is lost due to periodontal problems.

7.3.2 Odontogenic Tumors

Introduction

Odontogenic tumors are made up of one or more dental tissues, such as enamel, dentin, and cementum. Some of these tumors are to be regarded as developmental disorders; others do have neoplastic properties. The 2005 classification by the World Health Organization distinguishes benign and some extremely rare malignant tumors. Here we will limit our discussion to the most common benign odontogenic tumors, being:

- Ameloblastoma and ameloblastoma-like tumors
- Cementoblastoma
- Keratocystic odontogenic tumor

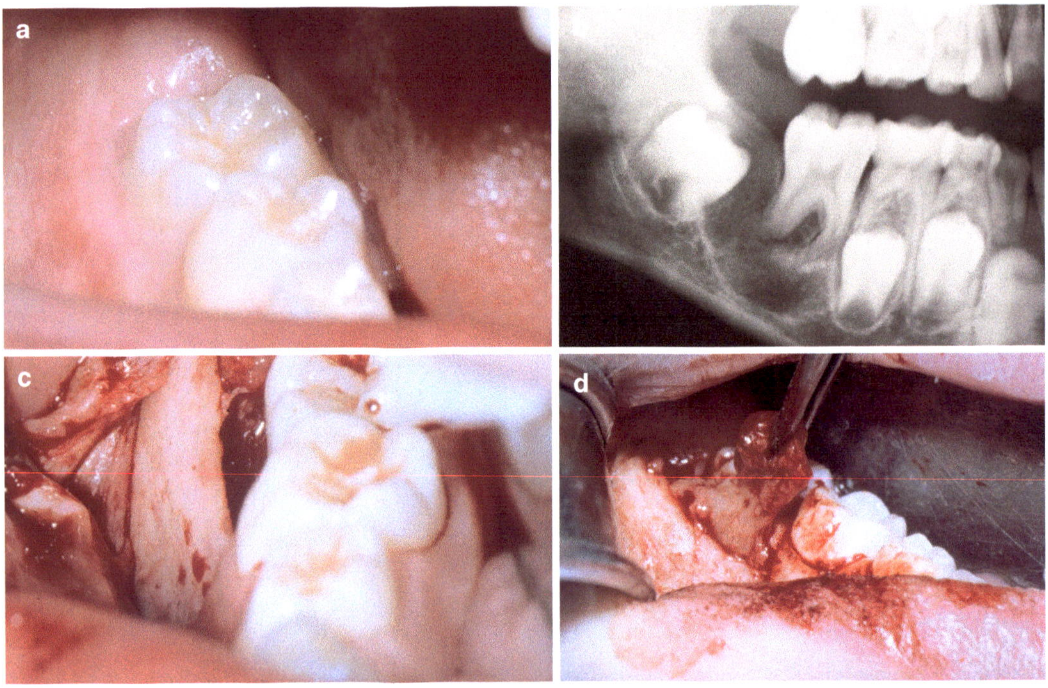

Fig. 7.24 (**a**) Mild periodontal complaints of vital 46; buccal pocket at probing. (**b**) Radiolucency around 46, compatible with a diagnosis of mandibular buccal infected cyst. (**c**) After reflecting a mucoperiosteal flap, a gap is observed between the alveolar bone and 46. (**d**) Removal of the cyst at the buccal aspect of 46

- Myxoma
- Odontoma

7.3.2.1 Ameloblastoma

Definition

Nearly always histologically benign tumor consisting of ameloblast-like epithelial cells.

Is characterized by a high rate of recurrence. An ameloblastoma with histopathological malignant characteristics such as cellular or nuclear polymorphism, mitotic activity, and invasive growth is extremely rare. A histologically benign ameloblastoma may in rare instances metastasize to the cervical lymph nodes or to sites elsewhere in the body, being referred to as metastasizing ameloblastoma.

Etiology

There are no known etiologic factors.

Epidemiology

The estimated incidence is one per million population per year. Sometimes diagnosed at a young age. The average age at the time of diagnosis is around 30 years.

Clinical Aspects

The tumor nearly always develops in the jaw bone (intraosseous ameloblastoma), probably from residual epithelium of the dental lamina. Occasionally the tumor arises from odontogenic epithelium of the alveolar mucosa (peripheral ameloblastoma).

An ameloblastoma is often diagnosed after histopathological evaluation of a lesion that clinicoradiographically looked like a cyst. Sometimes an ameloblastoma presents as an intraoral or extraoral swelling (Fig. 7.25a, b). Occasionally causes disturbed tooth eruption.

Radiographic Aspects

Unilobular or multilobular radiolucency, sometimes surrounded by a cortical line. May cause resorption of teeth (Fig. 7.26). Often expansion of the jaw bone. May mimic, a.o., a residual cyst, a follicular cyst, or a keratocystic odontogenic

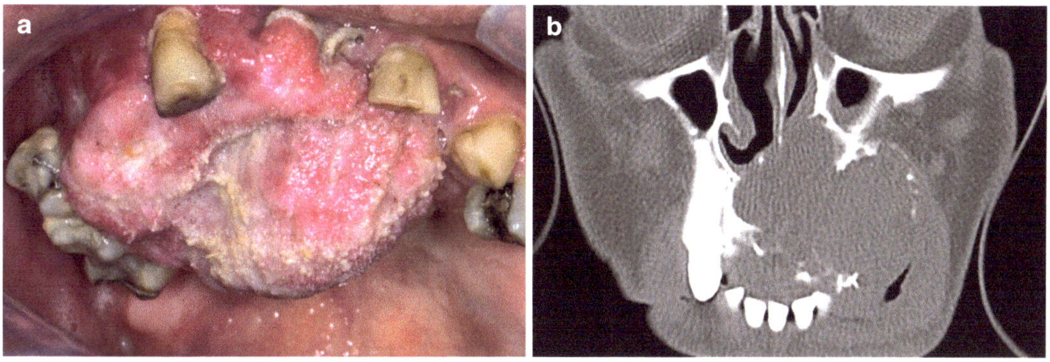

Fig. 7.25 (a) Example of a neglected ameloblastoma in the anterior part of the mandible. (b) A CT scan shows the extent of the tumor

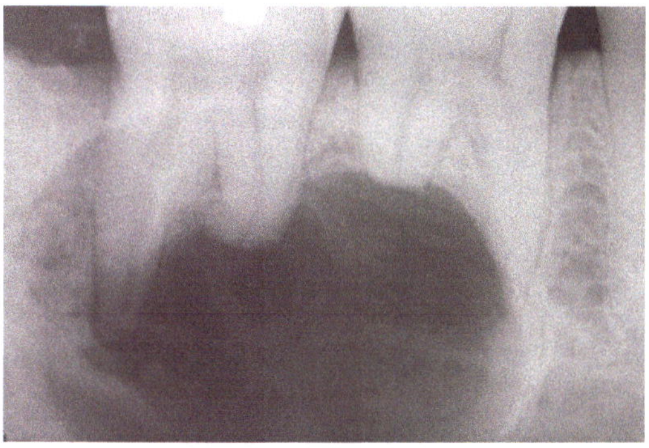

Fig. 7.26 Resorption of the roots of 46 and 47 caused by an ameloblastoma

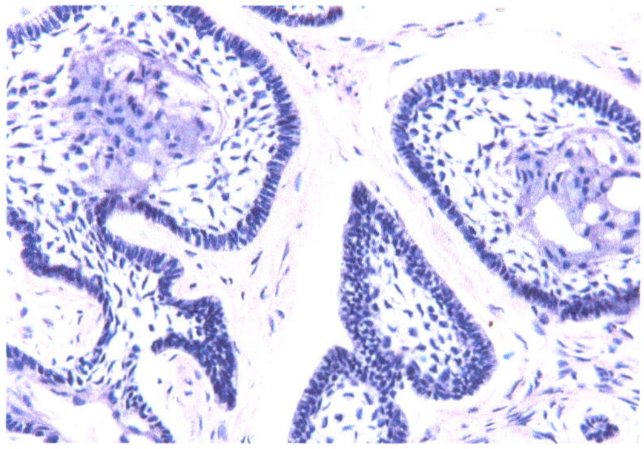

Fig. 7.28 Histopathologic aspect of ameloblastoma, follicular type

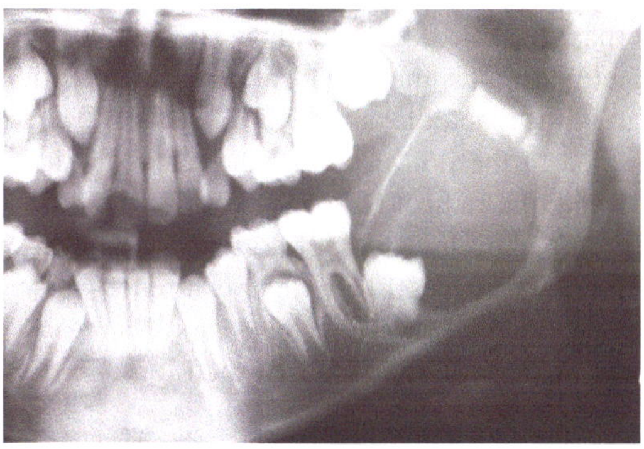

Fig. 7.27 Non-diagnostic radiograph of a radiolucency caused by an ameloblastoma

tumor (Fig. 7.27). Particularly in the upper jaw but also in the mandible, additional CT scans are required in order to get better information about the extent of the lesion and the integrity of the cortical plates of the jaw bones.

Histopathology

Almost all ameloblastomas are histopathologically benign. The diagnosis "malignant" ameloblastoma is justified only in case of cellular and nuclear polymorphism and/or mitotic activity. Most ameloblastomas are histopathologically easy to diagnose, especially in case of the common follicular type (Fig. 7.28). However, some histopathologic subtypes, such as the plexiform type and the granular cell type, may be difficult to recognize as such (Fig. 7.29). Furthermore, it may be difficult to distinguish an acanthomatous ameloblastoma from a squamous odontogenic tumor, another extremely rare but less aggressive odontogenic tumor.

The unicystic ameloblastoma is a rare variant, being characterized macroscopically as a cystic lesion and microscopically by a lining with ameloblastomatous epithelial cells (Fig. 7.30). The

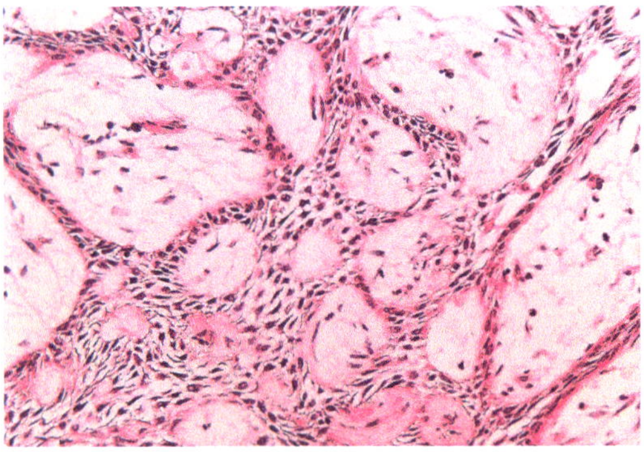

Fig. 7.29 Ameloblastoma, plexiform type. This subtype can be misinterpreted as epithelial proliferation

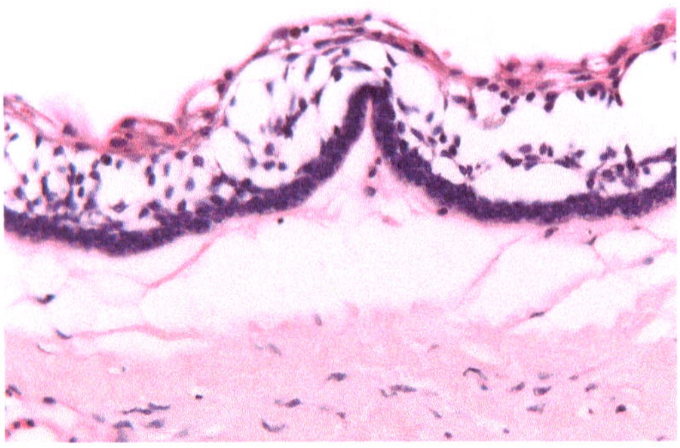

Fig. 7.30 Low-power view of an ameloblastomatous lining in a unicystic ameloblastoma

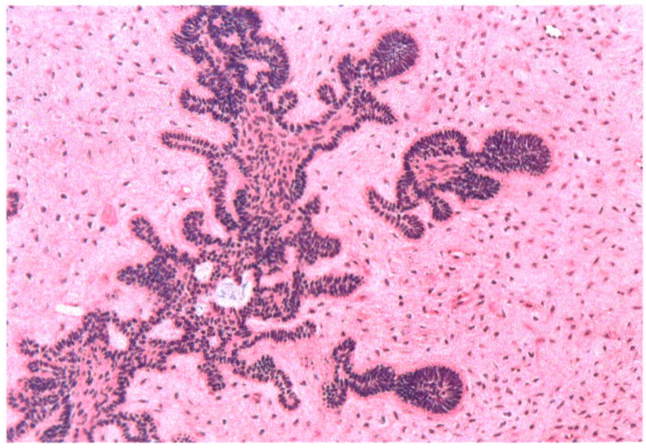

Fig. 7.31 Ameloblastic fibroma; the stroma resembles pulpal tissue

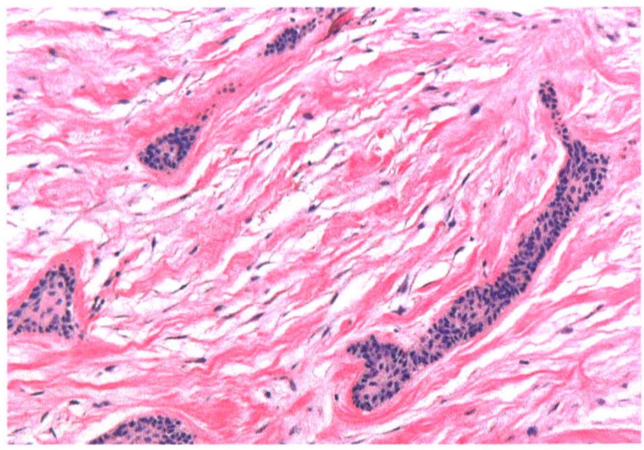

Fig. 7.32 Epithelial nests in a tooth follicle resembling ameloblastomatous proliferations

diagnosis "unicystic ameloblastoma" cannot be made on the basis of radiographic aspects.

The histopathological differential diagnosis of an ameloblastoma may include a number of other odontogenic, somewhat ameloblastoma-like tumors, such as the already mentioned squamous odontogenic tumor, the ameloblastic fibroma (Fig. 7.31), the ameloblastic fibrodentinoma, and the ameloblastic fibro-odontoma, having generally a less aggressive behavior than an ameloblastoma.

Note: in follicular tissue of impacted teeth, epithelial proliferations may occur that might be misdiagnosed histopathologically as part of an ameloblastoma (Fig. 7.32).

Treatment

Preferably wide surgical excision with a margin of surrounding clinically normal bone, if necessary sacrificing the continuity of the mandible. In children a more conservative approach is perhaps justified; this possibly also applies to ameloblastomas that are located in the anterior part of the mandible or maxilla. Especially when located in the dorsal part of the mandible and the maxilla, radical removal has to be pursued, since a recurrence in that location will be difficult to treat successfully. Most recurrences after enucleation do so within a few years. Therefore, strict annual follow-up is indicated for, e.g., 10 years.

7.3.2.2 Cementoblastoma

Definition

A benign tumor consisting of cementum.

Epidemiology

Rare tumor; the estimated incidence is less than one per million population per year. Is usually diagnosed before the age of 25 years.

Clinical Aspects

Usually relates to the mandibular molars. Fast-growing swelling, painful.

Radiographic Aspects

Well-circumscribed opacity attached to the root of a tooth (Fig. 7.33).

Histopathology

Cementum and cementum-like tissue attached to the root of a tooth (Fig. 7.34a, b).

Treatment

Extraction or surgical removal of the tooth together with the attached cementoblastoma. Recurrences are not uncommon.

7.3.2.3 Keratocystic Odontogenic Tumor ("Keratocyst")

Definition

The diagnosis keratocystic odontogenic tumor (KCOT) is based exclusively on histopathologic criteria. In the past, the lesion was classified as an odontogenic cyst. Worldwide there is a debate among (oral) pathologists about the correctness of "upgrading" the odontogenic keratocyst to a keratocystic odontogenic tumor.

Clinical Aspects

Intraoral or extraoral swelling; sometimes an incidental finding on a radiograph.

Radiographic Aspects

Unilobular or multilobular well-defined radiolucency (Fig. 7.35); sometimes expansion of the bone (Fig. 7.36). A KCOT rarely causes tooth resorption. The radiographic aspect is not pathognomonic and may resemble, a.o., a residual cyst, an ameloblastoma, a central giant cell lesion, and other odontogenic and non-odontogenic lesions.

Multiple KCOTs, not necessarily present simultaneously, are indicative of the hereditary basal cell nevus syndrome (Gorlin syndrome); the other aspects of this syndrome are, a.o., the

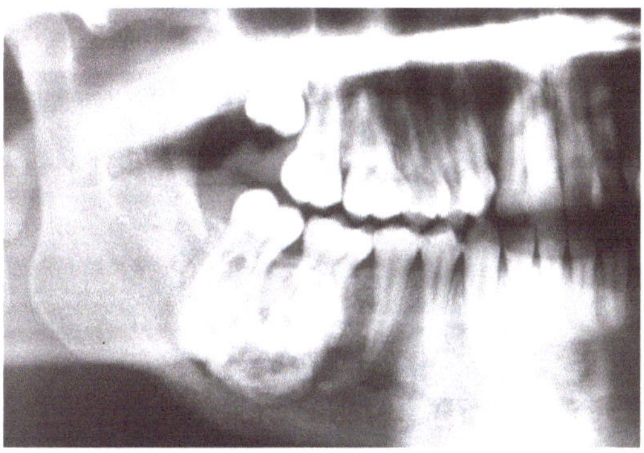

Fig. 7.33 Radiographic aspect of cementoblastoma of 46 in a 22-year-old man

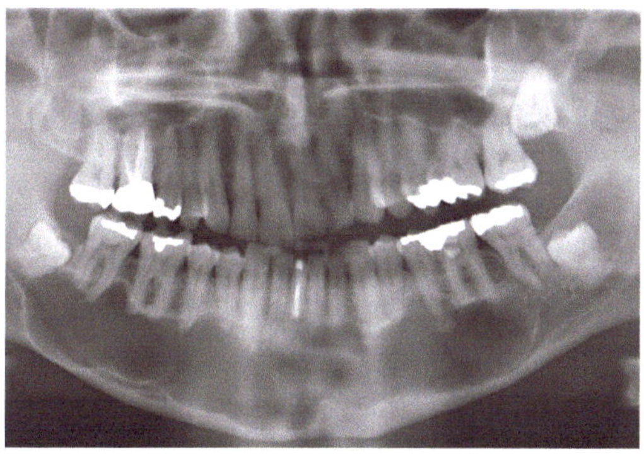

Fig. 7.35 Multilobular radiolucency extending bilaterally in the mandible; keratocystic odontogenic tumor

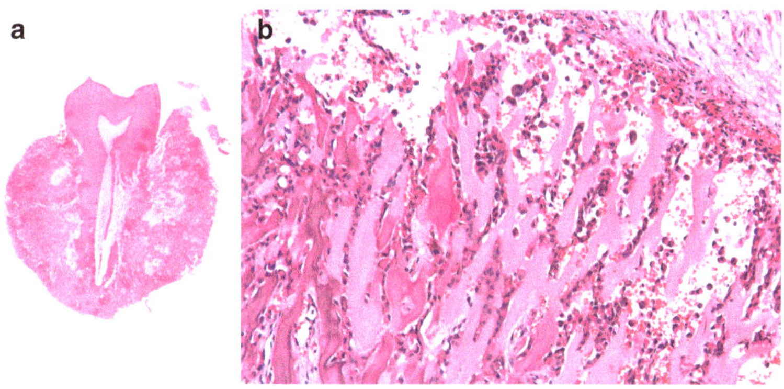

Fig. 7.34 (**a**) Gross specimen of a cementoblastoma attached to the roots. (**b**) Histopathologic aspect of cementoblastoma; viewed "in isolation" the differential diagnosis includes an osteosarcoma

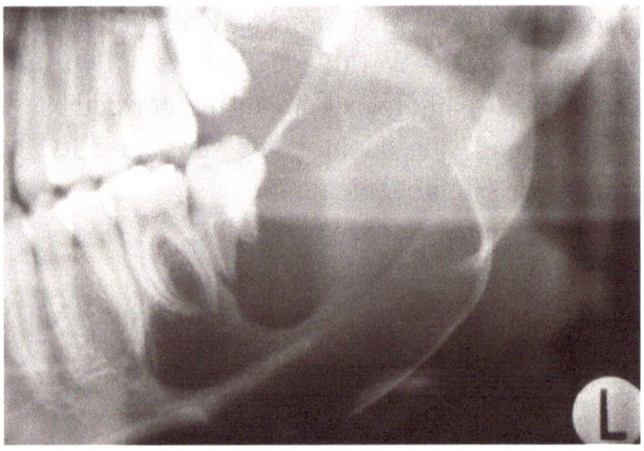

Fig. 7.36 Multilobular radiolucency; keratocystic odontogenic tumor

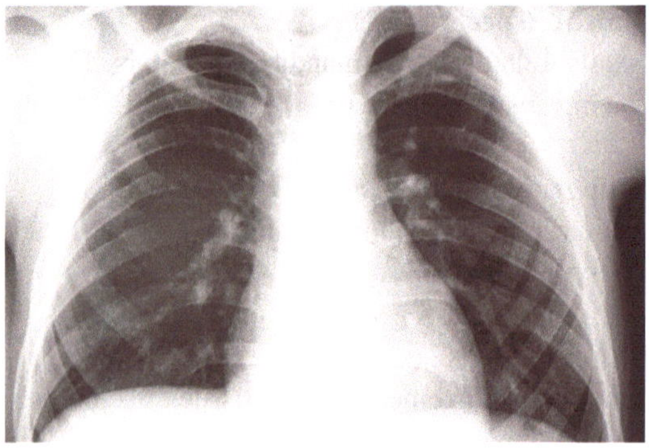

Fig. 7.38 The chest X-ray shows two bifid ribs on the left side

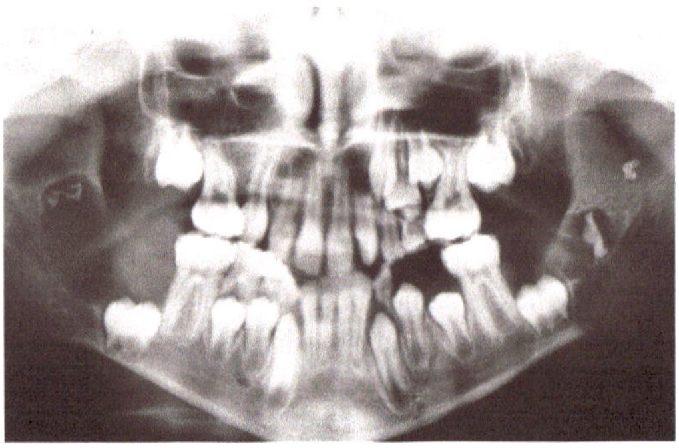

Fig. 7.37 Keratocystic odontogenic tumor bilateral in the mandible in a patient suffering from the basal cell nevus syndrome

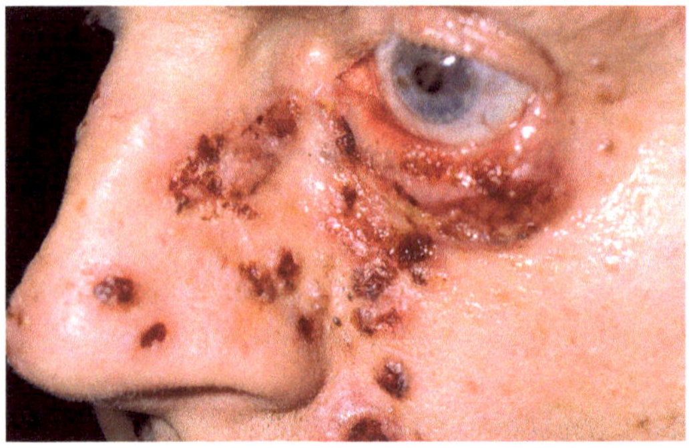

Fig. 7.39 Multiple basal cell carcinomas immediately after treatment in a patient with basal cell nevus syndrome

presence of one or more bifid ribs, pits in the skin of the hand palms, calcifications of the falx cerebri, and, most important, multiple basal cell carcinomas of the skin, often located in the head and neck area and occurring already at an early age (Figs. 7.37, 7.38, and 7.39).

Histopathology

KCOT has characteristic histopathologic aspects consisting among others of an epithelial lining of 6–8 cell layers thick, palisade arrangement of the basal cells, corrugated surface of the epithelium, and a parakeratotic, often corrugated surface (Fig. 7.40a, b). The characteristic features may partly disappear when the cyst becomes secondary inflamed. In case of distinct hyperkeratosis, one is most likely dealing with a keratinizing odontogenic cyst (see before).

Treatment

Enucleation and, if possible, removal of the overlying mucosa. In some cases marsupialization or decompression is to be preferred, usually requiring enucleation at a later stage. Some clinicians use the "fixation before and/or after enucleation technique," applying Carnoy's fixative solution before and/or after enucleation.

The recurrence rate of KCOTs depends on the extent of the surgical removal and may be up to 25 % or more during a follow-up period of five years after just enucleation. Because of the risk of recurrence, annual follow-up is advised for at least five years. Although the recurrence rate after enucleation is lower than in ameloblastomas, one may consider to perform radical surgery for KCOTs located in the posterior part of the jaws, particularly when located in the ascending ramus of the mandible since recurrences at that side may be difficult to treat successfully.

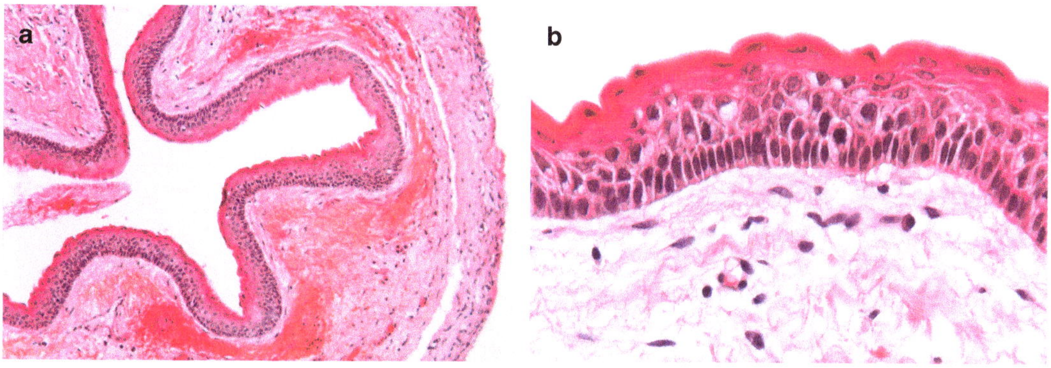

Fig. 7.40 (**a**) Rather typical folding of the wall of a keratocystic odontogenic tumor (KCOT). (**b**) Characteristic epithelial lining of a KCOT; notice the palisade arrangement of the basal cell layer

In case of suspicion of the basal cell nevus syndrome, referral to a department of clinical genetics is indicated.

7.3.2.4 Odontogenic Myxoma

Definition

Odontogenic tumor of mesenchymal tissue of the tooth bud.

Epidemiology

The estimated incidence is less than one per million population per year. The tumor is usually diagnosed at the age of 20–30 years.

Clinical Aspects

The odontogenic myxoma almost exclusively occurs within the bone of the upper or the lower jaw. Sometimes, the tumor gives rise to an intraoral or extraoral swelling, usually being asymptomatic otherwise.

Radiographic Aspects

Unilobular or multilobular radiolucency with sometimes a "honeycomb" aspect (Fig. 7.41); sometimes associated with an impacted tooth. The radiographic differential diagnosis includes, among others, ameloblastoma, keratocystic odontogenic tumor, central giant cell lesion, and a central arteriovenous malformation.

Histopathology

Circumscribed loose, fibromyxoid tissue containing stellate or sometimes rounded cells (Fig. 7.42). Cellular and nuclear polymorphism or mitotic activity is rarely observed. Sometimes the presence of nests of odontogenic epithelium, but this is not a requirement for the diagnosis of odontogenic myxoma.

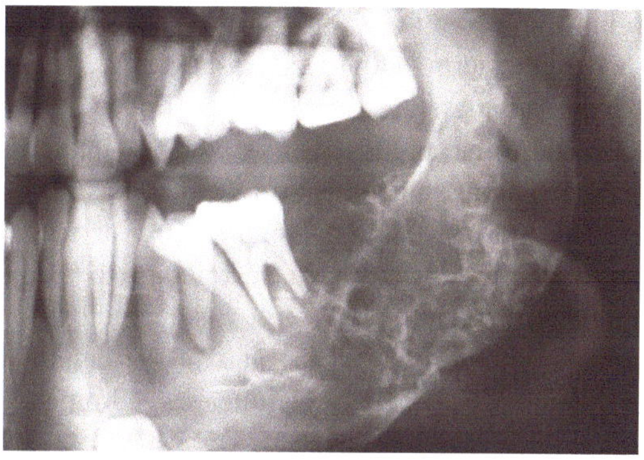

Fig. 7.41 Honeycomb radiolucency compatible with a diagnosis of odontogenic myxoma

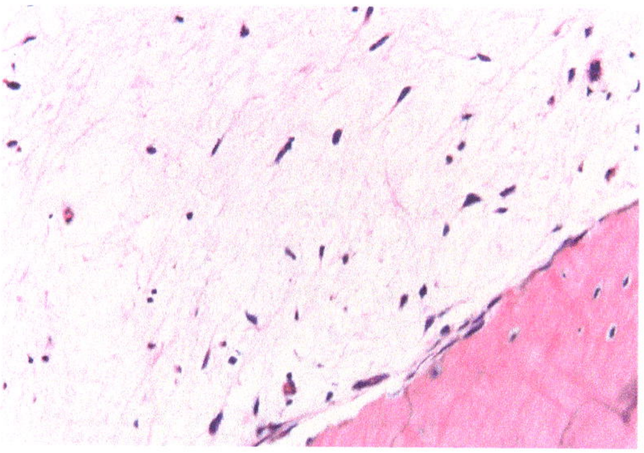

Fig. 7.42 Histopathologic aspect of odontogenic myxoma within the jaw bone

Myxoid changes in a tooth follicle may be misinterpreted as an odontogenic myxoma. Dental pulp tissue dropped off from a surgically removed not yet fully developed tooth (e.g., a mandibular wisdom tooth) can be misinterpreted as an odontogenic myxoma.

Treatment
Radical surgical excision, comparable with the recommendations for the treatment of an ameloblastoma. Long-term follow-up up to 10 years is recommended.

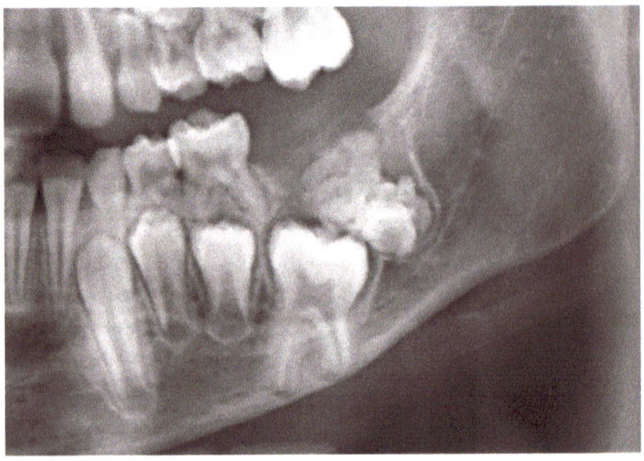

Fig. 7.43 Odontoma preventing the eruption of 36

7.3.2.5 Odontoma

Definition
Though the term odontoma is suggestive of a (benign) neoplasm, an odontoma can be regarded as a hamartoma composed of varying amounts of enamel, dentin, and cementum. Odontomas may resemble normal (supernumerary) teeth or malformed teeth and may also be referred to as a compound odontoma (see histopathology). Multiple odontomas may be part of the hereditary familial polyposis ("Gardner's syndrome") (see elsewhere in this chapter).

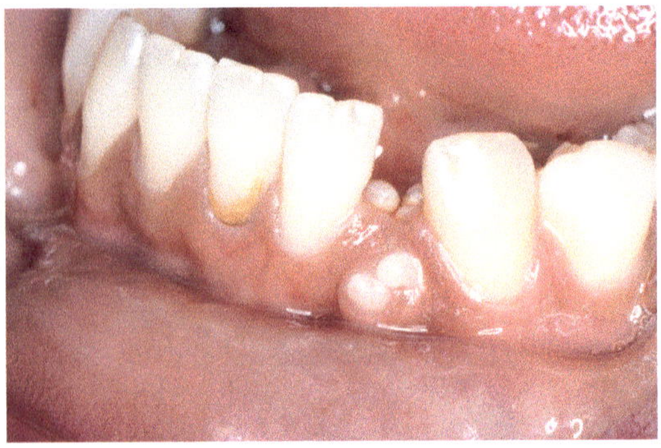

Fig. 7.44 Erupting odontoma consisting of multiple toothlike structures

Etiology
Unknown; possibly caused by trauma, particularly when located in the upper or lower front region.

Clinical Aspects
In most cases an intraosseous odontoma is an incidental finding on a radiograph. In some cases an odontoma is diagnosed because of disturbed eruption of a tooth (Fig. 7.43). On rare occasions, parts of an odontoma erupt into the mouth (Fig. 7.44).

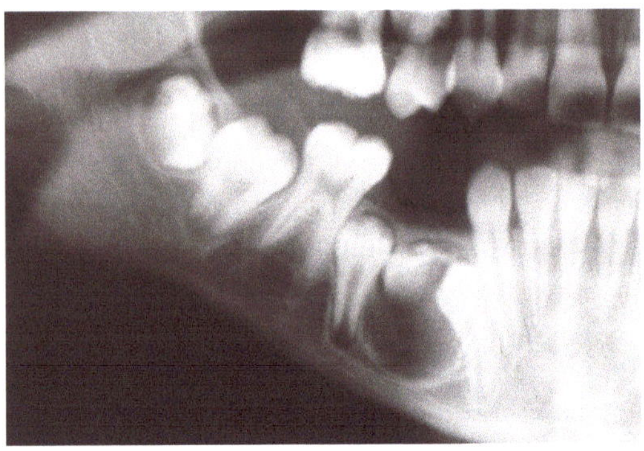

Fig. 7.45 Early stage of odontoma around 44

Radiographic Aspects
At the initial stage the radiographic aspect consists of a non-characteristic well-circumscribed radiolucency (Fig. 7.45). At a later stage there is an opaque structure, usually surrounded by a radiolucent zone. Sometimes one or more tooth structures are recognizable (Fig. 7.46).

Histopathology
Enamel, dentin, and cementum are found in varying amounts (Fig. 7.47). When there are toothlike structures, the term "compound" odontoma is used, while in the presence of an irregular, haphazard architecture, the term "complex" odontoma is applied. This distinction does not have any clinical relevance. In exceptionally rare circumstances, an associated ameloblastoma may be observed, being referred to as odontoameloblastoma

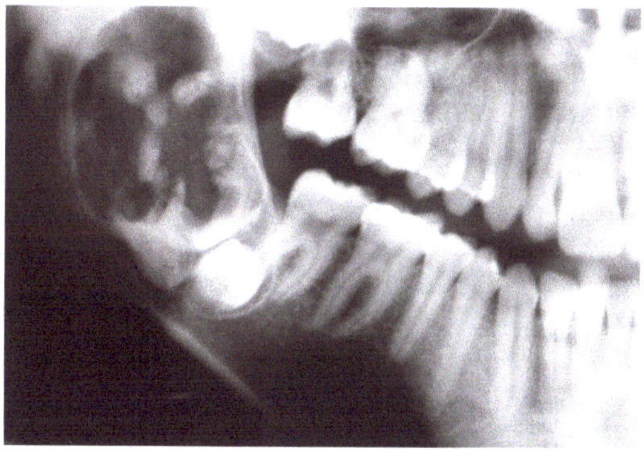

Fig. 7.46 Early stage of odontoma in the mandibular ramus; incidental finding

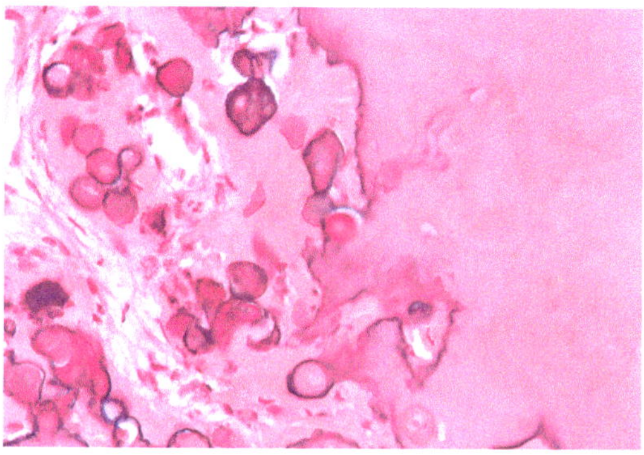

Fig. 7.47 Histopathology of complex odontoma

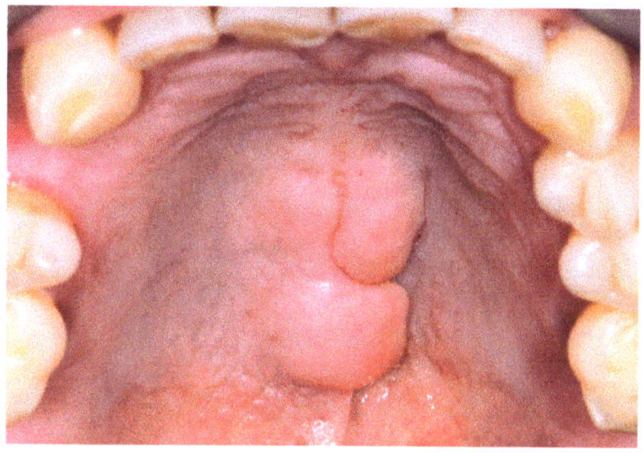

Fig. 7.48 Torus palatinus

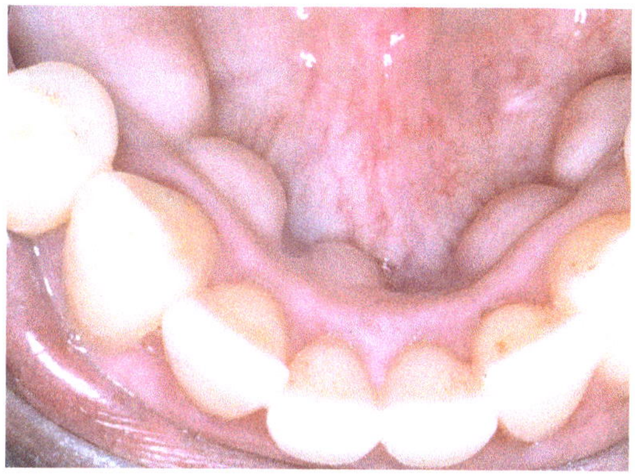

Fig. 7.49 Bilateral tori mandibulares at the lingual aspect of the mandible; no symptoms

and requiring treatment according to the previously mentioned guidelines for ameloblastoma.

Treatment

When the eruption of a tooth is prevented by an odontoma, removal is indicated, leaving the associated tooth in situ when appropriate. When there is no eruption disturbance, treatment is not truly indicated unless the correctness of the diagnosis is questioned.

7.4 Exostoses

Definition

Benign local excrescences of bone. Three groups of exostoses are recognized, being:

- Torus palatinus (see also Chap. 6)
- Torus mandibularis
- Multiple (buccal) exostoses (see also Chap. 5)

Etiology

Developmental phenomenon, although multiple buccal exostoses may perhaps be caused by chronic periodontal irritation.

Epidemiology

Rather common phenomenon. The various types of exostoses usually appear at adulthood.

Clinical Aspects

Usually lobulated, bony hard swelling, being asymptomatic otherwise. A torus palatinus is located in the midline of the hard palate (Fig. 7.48, see also Chap. 6). A torus mandibularis has almost always a bilateral distribution, being located on the lingual aspect in the bicuspid region (Figs. 7.49 and 7.50). Multiple buccal exostoses may occur both in the maxilla and the mandible.

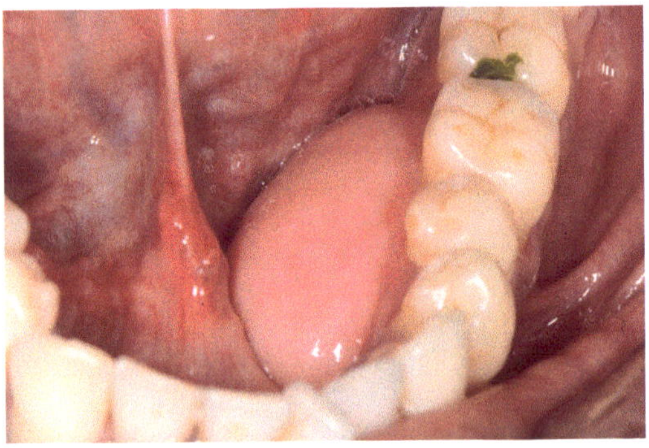

Fig. 7.50 Unusual unilateral presentation of torus mandibularis; no symptoms

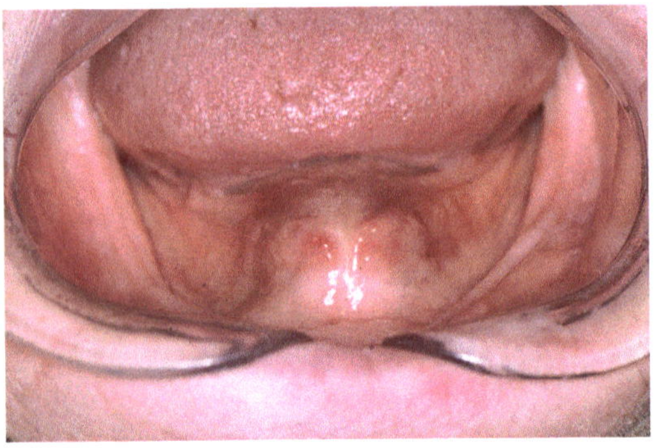

Fig. 7.51 Prominent spina mentalis, bony hard, after resorption of the alveolar ridge. No symptoms

Differential Diagnosis
In case of a palatal swelling, the possibility of a salivary gland tumor has to be taken into account, as well a disease that extends from the nasal or maxillary sinus into the mouth. In case of a mandibular torus, the possibility of a supernumerary impacted bicuspid should be considered. A bony hard swelling in an edentulous mandible on the lingual aspect of the midline usually represents the spina mentalis (Fig. 7.51).

Radiographic Aspects
Only mandibular tori may be visible on routine radiographs. Additional imaging such as (cone beam) CT imaging is only indicated in case of surgical correction of a palatine torus.

Histopathology
On histopathologic examination, normal vital bone tissue is encountered.

Treatment
Treatment is only indicated when the exostosis interferes with the wearing of a full or partial denture.

7.5 Fibro-osseous Diseases

7.5.1 Fibrous Dysplasia

Definition and Terminology
Fibrous dysplasia is a benign condition, presumably developmental in nature, characterized by the presence of fibrous connective tissue with a characteristic whorled pattern and containing trabeculae of immature non-lamellar bone. The term "dysplasia" has, indeed, a different (benign) meaning in relation to bone disorders than in epithelial mucosal lesions, where it indicates an increased risk of malignant transformation.

Fibrous dysplasia may be monostotic or polyostotic. The prefix "monostotic" is also used in case of involvement of multiple craniofacial bones, i.e., maxillary and frontal bone, and also in case of simultaneous occurrence in the mandible and maxilla in the absence of lesions elsewhere in the skeleton, being referred to as craniofacial fibrous dysplasia.

The polyostotic type can be subdivided into (1) Jaffe's type, with skin pigmentations (café au lait spots), and (2) Albright or McCune-Albright syndrome, a more severe type, in which skin pigmentations are accompanied by endocrine disturbances of the pituitary gland, the thyroid gland, the parathyroid glands, and the ovaries. Because of its rare occurrence, the polyostotic type will not be further discussed here.

Etiology
A postzygotic mutation in the guanine nucleotide-binding protein, alpha-stimulating activity polypeptide 1 plays an important role in the histogenesis of fibrous dysplasia.

Epidemiology
The monostotic type of fibrous dysplasia is relatively rare but is much more common than the polyostotic type. The estimated incidence of

monostotic fibrous dysplasia of the jaws is one per million population per year. Monostotic fibrous dysplasia shows no preference for males or females and occurs particularly in children and young adults.

Clinical Aspects

The first sign of fibrous dysplasia is a non-tender slow-growing swelling of the bone, unilateral and not crossing the midline, either in the mandible or the maxilla (Fig. 7.52a, b). The consistency of the swelling may vary from firm elastic to bony hard. There is usually no displacement of teeth, and the dental occlusion remains undisturbed. Although the history, the clinical findings, and the radiographic aspects are more or less diagnostic, it is safe practice to confirm the diagnosis by a biopsy.

Laboratory Findings

Serum values of calcium, phosphate, and alkaline phosphatase remain unchanged.

Radiographic Aspects

In the immature stage, monostotic fibrous dysplasia may be a multilobular radiolucent lesion with ill-defined borders. In the mature stage, a more or less distinct trabecular pattern may be recognized. The lesion may also be opaque with or without a ground-glass appearance. Resorption of teeth is rare. The cortical bone may become extremely thin due to the expansive nature of the lesion. However, true perforation of the cortical bone seldom occurs. There is usually no distinct periosteal reaction. Particularly in case of maxillary involvement, the extent of the disease should be made visible by CT scans (Fig. 7.53a–d).

Scintigraphic Aspects

Scintigraphy usually shows an increased accumulation which is by some interpreted as "activity" of the disease process. A more likely explanation is that the increased accumulation is the result of the increased thickness of the involved bone. Such accumulation remains unchanged at an older age.

Histopathology

The histopathologic features may vary widely. Classically, a cellular fibrous connective tissue is seen, sometimes showing a whorled pattern (Fig. 7.54a, b). There may be an abundance of connective tissue with little formation of bone, while in other cases the formation of bone is more prominent, with little stroma present. The bony trabeculae have an irregular outline and are often referred to as "Chinese characters." The bony trabeculae mainly consist of plexiform (woven) bone but may occasionally show a lamellar architecture, sometimes being arranged in a parallel fashion. In contrast to fibrous dysplasia elsewhere in the skeleton, osteoblastic rimming of the trabeculae is generally accepted as part of the histopathologic spectrum of fibrous dysplasia of the jaws. In addition to signs of bone formation, there are also signs of resorption with

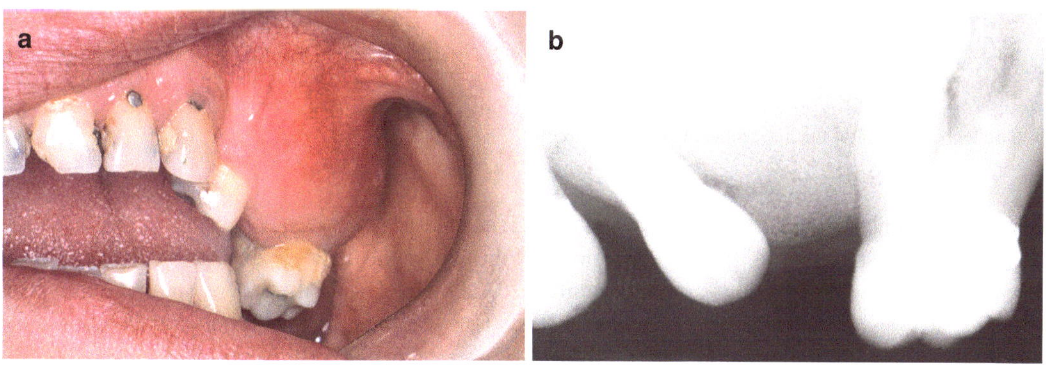

Fig. 7.52 (**a**) Bony hard swelling of the maxilla present since childhood; asymptomatic otherwise. (**b**) The radiograph shows a ground-glass appearance suggestive of fibrous dysplasia

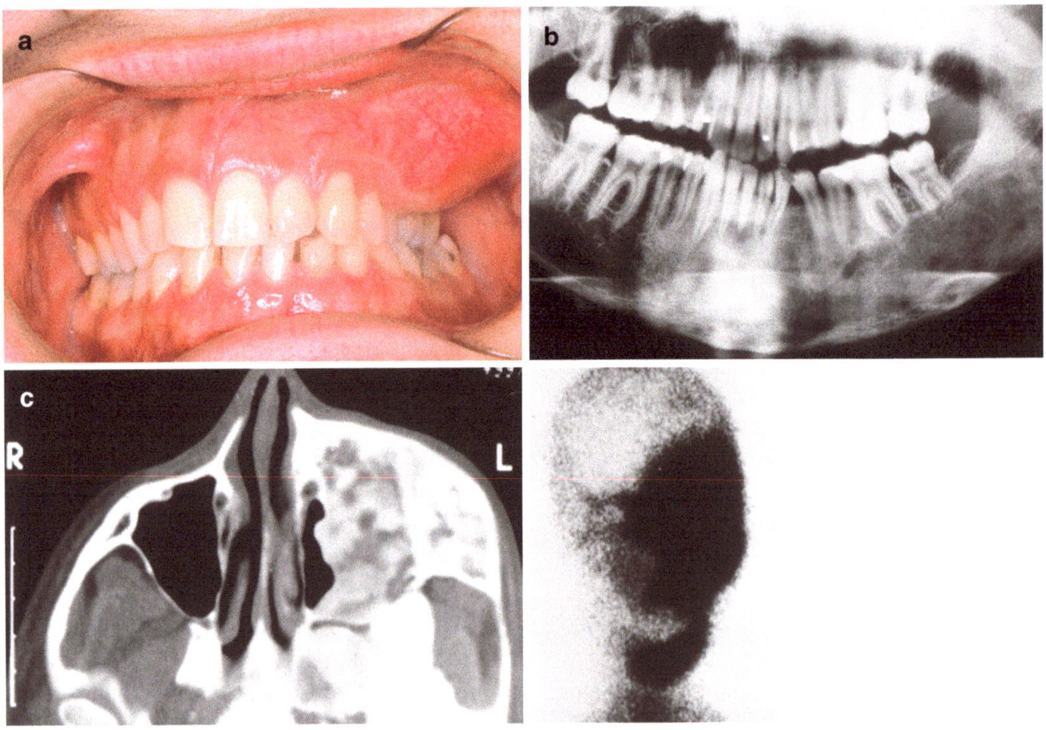

Fig. 7.53 (**a**) Bony hard swelling of the left maxilla in an adolescent caused by fibrous dysplasia. (**b**) On the panoramic view, the maxillary lesion is hardly visible; also involvement of the mandible. (**c**) The CT scan and the bone scan show the extent of the disorder, even extending into the base of the skull

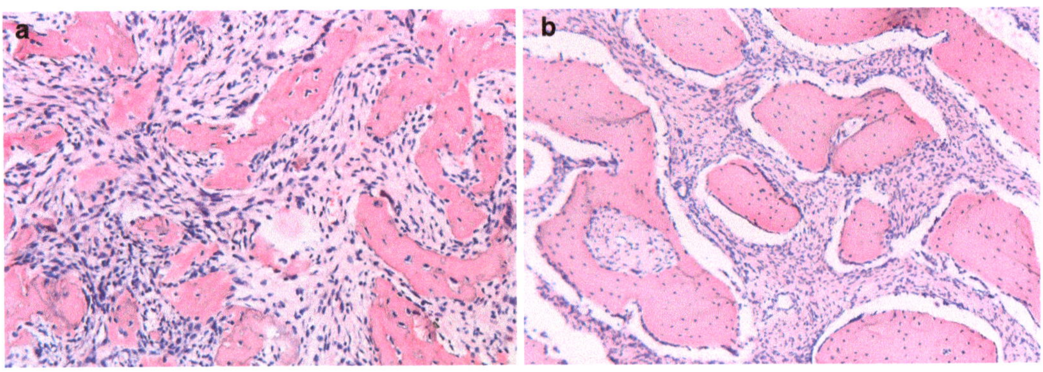

Fig. 7.54 (**a**) "Chinese characters" in fibrous dysplasia; is compatible with ossifying fibroma and osseous dysplasia. (**b**) Parallel orientation of the trabeculae in an other patient

sometimes distinct osteoclasts present, even to the extent of resembling a giant cell lesion. Occasionally, cementum-like structures are observed. "Cyst" formation in fibrous dysplasia is rare. The histopathologic features are more or less indistinguishable from those of ossifying fibroma and osseous dysplasia.

Treatment

Fibrous dysplasia usually becomes inactive at age 20–25 years. Due to its tendency to blend into the adjacent normal bone, fibrous dysplasia of the jaws can actually never be removed in toto. When a surgical, modeling correction is performed during childhood, recurrence is to be expected within a short period of time, sometimes even in a matter of months. In asymptomatic patients in whom the lesions are slow-growing or have stopped growing, a wait-and-see policy is advised. In case of orbital involvement, there are opposing views with regard to the usefulness of decompression of the optical canal in order to prevent blindness.

Occasionally, the successful use of calcitonin or bisphosphonates has been reported in the treatment of fibrous dysplasia. Irradiation is contraindicated because of the potential risk of inducing malignant changes at a later age.

Malignant transformation into an osteosarcoma has been reported but is extremely rare in the monostotic type. In such instances, the correctness of the original diagnosis of fibrous dysplasia should be questioned.

7.5.2 Osseous Dysplasia (Incl. Periapical Osseous Dysplasia)

Introduction

The present view is that cementum and bone are indistinguishable from each other from a histological point of view. Therefore, it is recommended to apply the term cementum only for tissue that is attached to the dentin of a root of a tooth. As a result, the previous terminology of cemento-osseous lesions has been adjusted, deleting the "cementum" part.

Definition and Terminology

Osseous dysplasia (OD) is a nonneoplastic lesion that often, but not exclusively, affects the periapical region of one or more teeth. The histopathologic features are similar to those of fibrous dysplasia and ossifying fibroma. For osseous dysplastic lesions present in multiple quadrants of the mandible and maxilla, either in a periapical or a non-periapical position, the term florid osseous dysplasia (FOD) may be used, while others remain using, somewhat inconsistently, the traditional term "gigantiform cementoma."

Epidemiology

In general, osseous dysplastic lesions have a preference for middle-aged women and occur especially in the dark-skinned population.

Etiology

The etiology of osseous dysplasia is unknown.

Clinical Aspects

Clinically, there are rarely any signs or symptoms. The disorder does not cause any symptoms and is usually diagnosed as an incidental on a radiograph. The vitality of the teeth remains intact.

Radiographic Aspects

Osseous dysplasia is often located at the apices of one or more lower incisors (Fig. 7.55), but the mandibular premolar-molar regions may be involved as well. Usually, there is a symmetrical mandibular distribution. Maxillary lesions can easily be overlooked since the regular radiographs are not very suitable for the identification of a jaw lesion in the maxilla.

Osseous dysplastic lesions do not cause resorption of apices. In the initial stage, there is a rather ill-defined radiolucent area; at this stage a solitary lesion cannot clearly be distinguished from a periapical granuloma or a simple bone cavity. With time, central calcification takes place, resulting in a dense opaque lesion with often a radiolucent peripheral rim, which is of help in differentiating the lesion from a dense bone island. Occasionally, osseous dysplastic lesions are mistaken for root remnants (Fig. 7.56).

In florid osseous dysplasia ("gigantiform cementoma"), there may be a swelling of the affected area of the jaws (Fig. 7.57a–c).

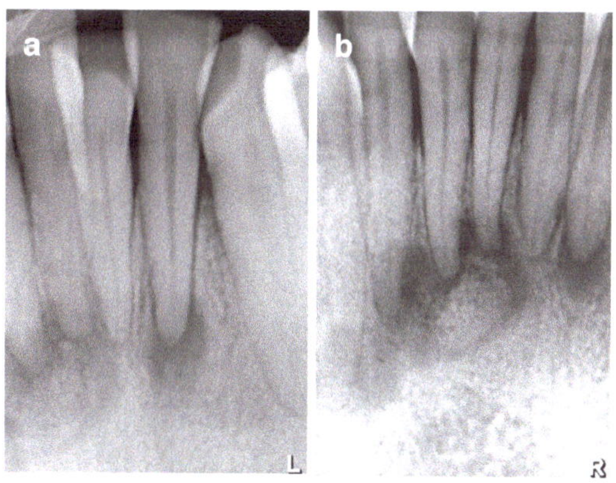

Fig. 7.55 (**a**) Incidental finding of periapical osseous dysplasia; all teeth are vital. (**b**) Same patient as shown in (a)

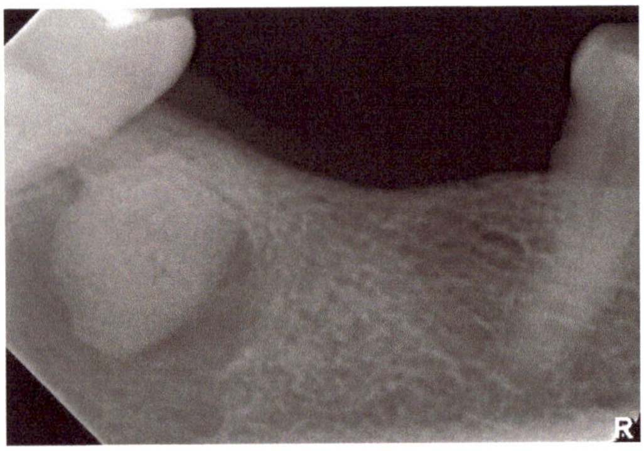

Fig. 7.56 Late stage of osseous dysplasia; no symptoms. Not to be mistaken for a root remnant

Histopathology

The histopathologic features are indistinguishable from fibrous dysplasia and ossifying fibroma. In case of an oral communication, varying amounts of inflammatory cells may be present (Fig. 7.58).

Treatment

Treatment is not required unless there is doubt about the diagnosis. Radiographic follow-up every five years may be considered for reassurance of the patient.

7.5.3 Ossifying Fibroma

Definition

An ossifying fibroma (OF) is a benign, intraosseous, well-demarcated osteogenic neoplasma consisting of fibrous tissue containing varying amounts of bone. There is also the peripheral ossifying fibroma that occurs as a localized swelling ("epulis") of the gingiva (see Chap. 5). This entity should not be regarded as the extraosseous counterpart of intraosseous OF.

Etiology

Unknown; ossifying fibroma lacks the genetic alterations observed in fibrous dysplasia.

Epidemiology

The estimated incidence is less than one per million population per year. Most lesions are encountered in patients above 40 years of age.

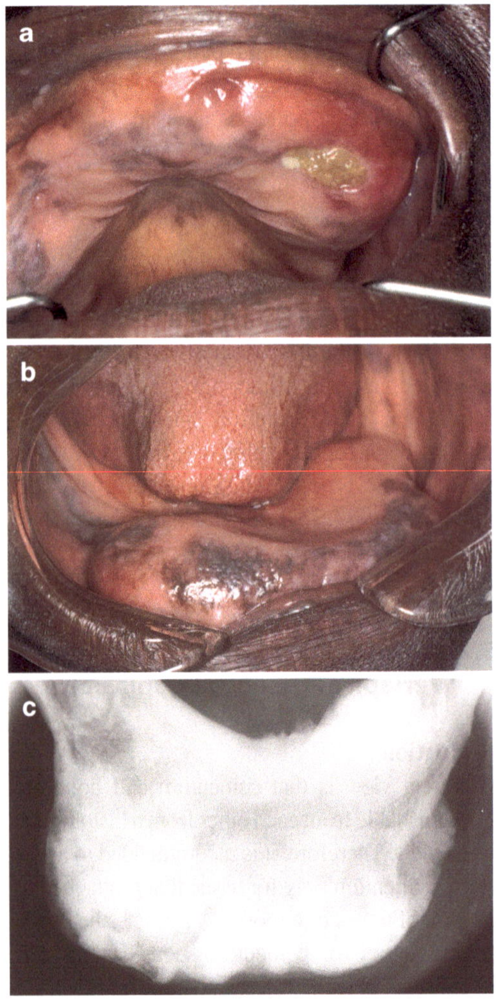

Fig. 7.57 (**a**) Expansion of the maxilla in florid osseous dysplasia; notice the secondary ulceration of the alveolar mucosa. (**b**) Also the alveolar ridge in the mandible has expanded. (**c**) Occlusal view of the anterior part of the mandible showing the extent of the lesion

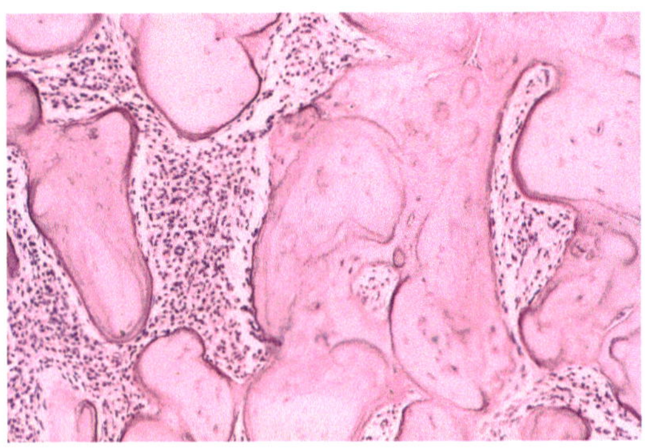

Fig. 7.58 Histopathologic aspect of florid osseous dysplasia ("gigantiform cementoma") with signs of secondary inflammation

Clinical Aspects

The most common clinical presentation of OF is a painless, slowly increasing swelling of the jaw (Fig. 7.59a). Occasionally, OF causes paresthesia or hyperesthesia. In some cases, particularly in children, an aggressive behavior may be observed ("juvenile aggressive ossifying fibroma"). The size of an OF may vary from one to several centimeters. In the maxilla, the antrum may become involved. The relative ease with which an OF will shell out from its bony bed is the most important factor in differentiating this lesion from fibrous dysplasia.

Radiographic Aspects

Radiographically, OF is, by definition, well circumscribed and is located in the tooth-bearing

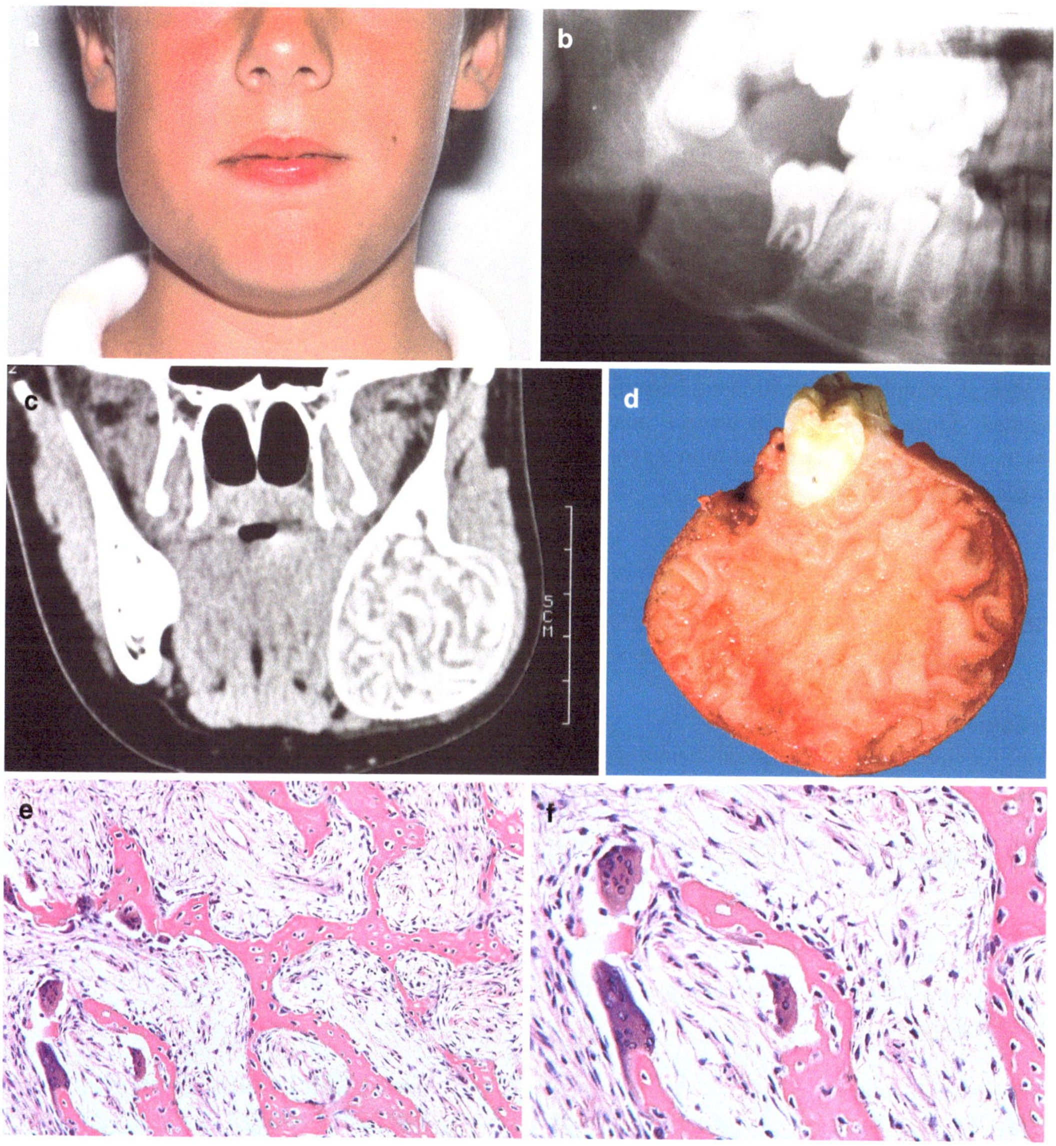

Fig. 7.59 (**a**) Swelling of the right cheek caused by an ossifying fibroma. No intraoral abnormalities. (**b**) Noncharacteristic aspect of ossifying fibroma. Notice displacement of 48. (**c**) The CT scan shows expansion of the mandible; notice the trabecular pattern. (**d**) Gross specimen of (trabecular) ossifying fibroma. (**e**) Histopathology of (trabecular) ossifying fibroma. (**f**) Notice the presence of some osteoclasts

regions of the jaws. The lesion may be radiolucent with or without central opacities (Fig. 7.59b, c). The pattern may be either unilobular or multilobular. Teeth adjacent to or involved in the lesion may be displaced. In a few percent of cases, root resorption does occur. The radiographic differential diagnosis includes some other bone diseases and a number of odontogenic cysts and tumors.

Histopathology

The histopathologic features of OF very much resemble those of fibrous dysplasia and osseous dysplasia (Fig. 7.59d–f). There may be a trabecular type ("trabecular" type) or a so-called psammomatoid type. It is somewhat questionable whether the histopathologic pattern of OF allows for prognostication. Some authors identify a separate, more aggressive (juvenile) variant based on histopathologic criteria. Malignant transformation rarely, if ever, occurs.

Treatment

In general, complete enucleation has been recommended. Occasionally, a recurrence may be observed, even to the extent that more aggressive surgery is required.

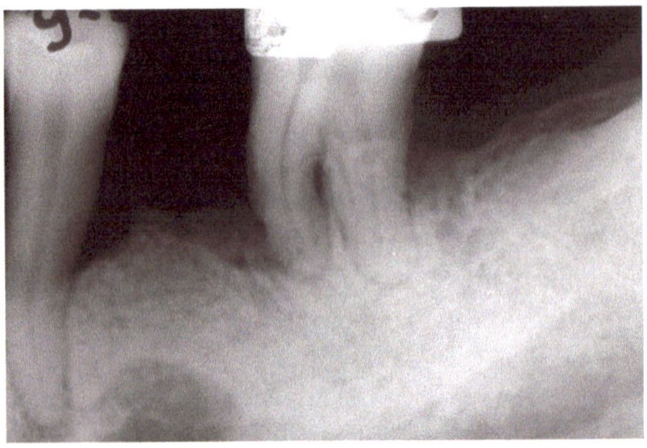

Fig. 7.60 Somewhat circumscribed radiolucency based on a focal osteoporotic bone marrow defect

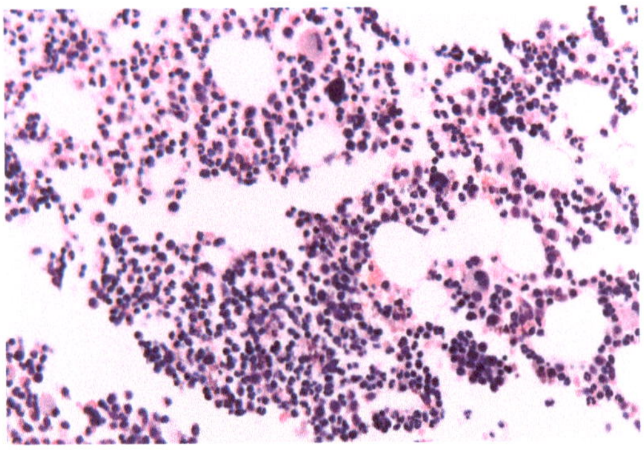

Fig. 7.61 Normal hematopoietic bone marrow consistent with the diagnosis of focal osteoporotic bone marrow defect

7.6 Focal Osteoporotic Bone Marrow Defect

Definition

Bone cavity containing normal hematopoietic marrow mimicking an intraosseous lesion.

Epidemiology

Rare phenomenon.

Clinical Aspects

There are no abnormal clinical findings nor any symptoms.

Radiographic Aspects

Often circumscribed, but sometimes ill-defined radiolucency occurring in the mandible, usually in an area of a missing tooth (Fig. 7.60). The size may vary from a few millimeters up to a few centimeters. Because of the non-characteristic radiographic features, the differential diagnosis consists of a number of odontogenic and non-odontogenic lesions.

Histopathology

Normal hematopoietic marrow (Fig. 7.61).

Treatment

The diagnosis is always a retrospective one, established after removal and histopathologic examination of the intraosseous tissue. Follow-up is not indicated.

7.7 Giant Cell Lesion, Central (Intraosseous)

Definition

A central giant cell lesion is a benign lesion that is more or less limited to the jaws, usually intraosseous, being characterized by the presence of multinucleated giant cells. The multinucleated giant cells probably are derived from endothelial cells. When occurring outside the bone, presenting as an epulis-like lesion of the gingiva or as a swelling of the alveolar mucosa in an edentulous part of the jaws, the term peripheral giant cell lesion is applied (see Chap. 5).

The previously used term "granuloma" has been deleted since there is no formation of true granulomas. Also the previously used adjective "reparative" (granuloma) has been deleted since the lesion is actually a destructive lesion rather than a reparative one.

Epidemiology
The estimated incidence is one per million population per year. Occurs mainly in children and young adults.

Clinical Aspects
Occurs only in the tooth-bearing part of the mandible or maxilla. The clinical presentation is a slowly enlarging swelling, sometimes accompanied by increased mobility of teeth (Figs. 7.62 and 7.63), usually being asymptomatic otherwise.

Radiographic Aspects
Well-circumscribed unilobular or multilobular radiolucency. Occasionally displacement of adjacent teeth and root resorption. The radiographic differential diagnosis includes, a.o., keratocystic odontogenic tumor, ameloblastoma, and fibro-osseous lesions.

Histopathology
The presence of variable multinucleated giant cells in a fibrous and often well-vascularized fibrous stroma (Fig. 7.64). The histopathologic

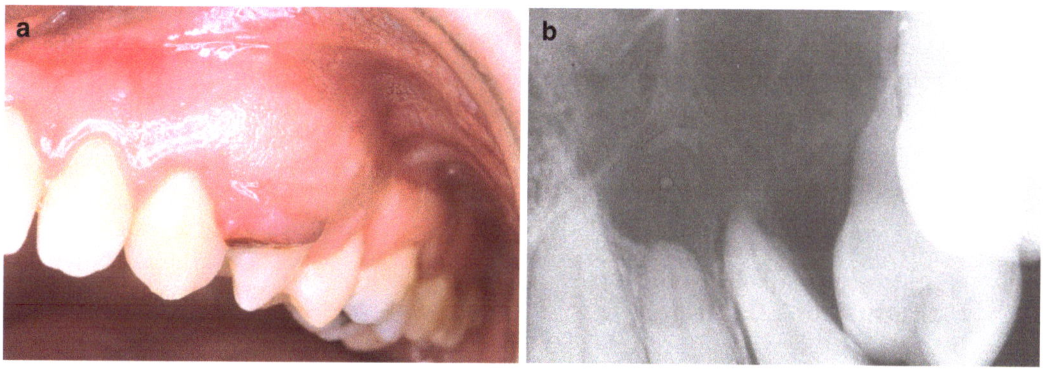

Fig. 7.62 (**a**) Bony hard swelling of the maxilla. (**b**) The radiolucency is based on a giant cell lesion

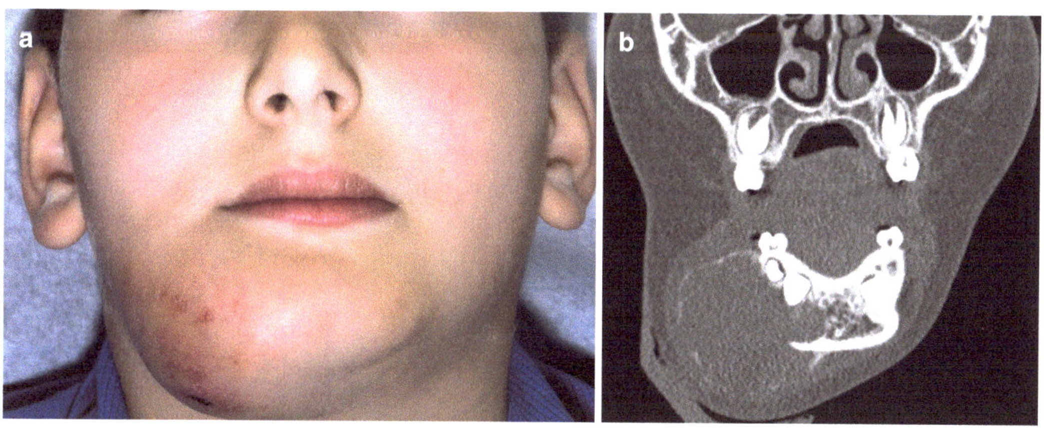

Fig. 7.63 (**a**) Swelling of the mandible caused by a central giant cell lesion. (**b**) The CT scan shows the extent of the lesion

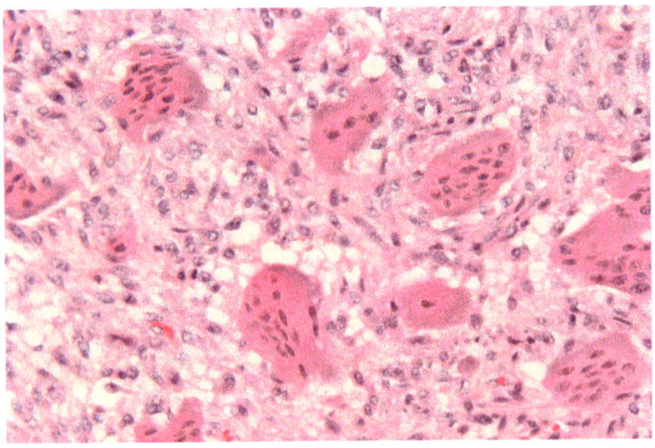

Fig. 7.64 Low-power view of (central) giant lesion

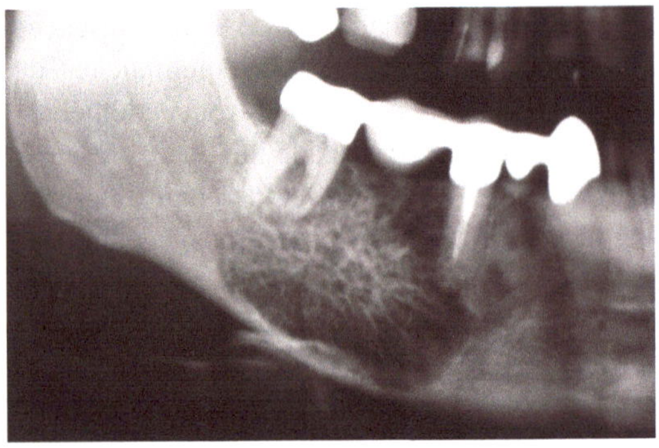

Fig. 7.65 Feathery pattern suggestive of a venous malformation of the mandible

differential diagnosis includes, a.o., other giant cell containing osseous lesions such as cherubism, fibro-osseous lesions, and osteosarcoma. In rare instances, a central giant cell lesion is caused by hyperparathyroidism.

Treatment
Thorough enucleation and curettage are usually sufficient. Occasionally, the lesion recurs and may behave in a more aggressive way; in such instances, other treatment modalities, such as the daily use of calcitonin, should be considered.

7.8 Hemangioma (Arteriovenous Malformation), Central/Intraosseous

Definition
Intraosseous presence of a hemangioma, usually in the form of an arteriovenous malformation (see also Chap. 2).

Etiology
Unknown.

Clinical Aspects
May occur everywhere in the skeleton; rarely occurs in the jaw bones. May present as a slow-growing, otherwise asymptomatic swelling. May be an incidental finding on the radiograph. May cause persistent gingival bleeding, either spontaneously or after a tooth extraction.

Radiographic Aspects
Well-demarcated radiolucency, occasionally showing a feathered radiopaque pattern (Fig. 7.65). The differential diagnosis includes, a.o., ameloblastoma, keratocystic odontogenic tumor, odontogenic myxoma, and central giant cell lesion.

Treatment
In the presence of a pulsatile lesion, MRI imaging and arteriography are indicated (Fig. 7.66a–c). In the absence of pulsations, a biopsy may be required to confirm the diagnosis. Depending on the result of the imaging procedures, one may decide whether or not to treat. Treatment may vary from intralesional injection with a sclerosing agent or enucleation in case of a venous malformation to artificial embolization followed by surgery in case of an arterial malformation.

7.9 Langerhans Cell Histiocytosis (LCH)

Definition
Nonneoplastic proliferation of Langerhans cells originating from the bone marrow, possibly as a result of a deficiency of T-suppressor cells. May occur everywhere in the skeleton either in a single bone (monostotic) or in multiple bones (polyostotic). May also occur in the soft tissues or in parenchymal organs, such as the lungs.

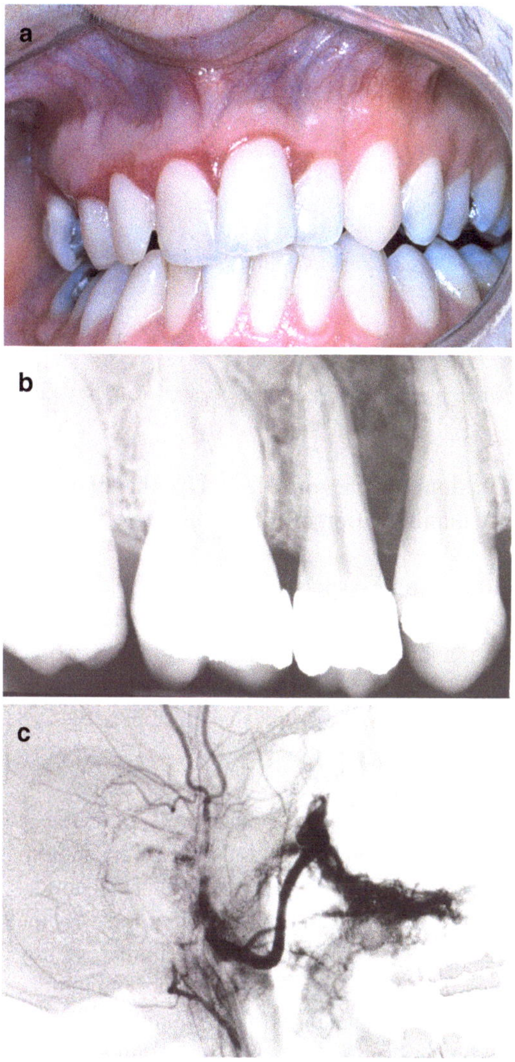

Fig. 7.66 (a) Gingivitis-like aspect caused by an underlying arterial malformation. (b) Radiolucency between 14 and 15 caused by an arterial malformation. (c) Arteriography confirms the presence of an arterial malformation

Epidemiology
Rare disease; usually becomes manifest already during early childhood.

Etiology
Unknown.

Clinical Aspects
May occur in the mandible or maxilla (Fig. 7.67a, b). First manifestation may be ulceration or retraction of the gingiva (see Chap. 5).

Radiographic Aspects
Solitary or multiple, somewhat circumscribed radiolucency. May mimic inflammatory periodontal bone loss.

Histopathology
Proliferation of histiocytic cells and often the presence of numerous eosinophilic granulocytes. The presence of Langerhans cells can be demonstrated by the use of the immunohistochemical marker CD1A (Fig. 7.68) or electron microscopy demonstrating Birbeck granules.

Treatment
A solitary intraosseous lesion can be treated by thorough excochleation. Multiple lesions may be successfully treated by intralesional injections of corticosteroids but often require systemic corticosteroid treatment. On the other hand, spontaneous remission may occur (Fig. 7.69a, b).

7.10 Lymphoreticular Diseases

7.10.1 Hodgkin and Non-Hodgkin Lymphoma

Definition
Lymphomas consist of neoplastic proliferations of the lymphopoietic part of the reticuloendothelial system (see also Chap. 2). Lymphomas and leukemias of the lymphocytic or histiocytic type are essentially the same type of disease; abnormalities in the peripheral blood cells, as is the case in leukemia, are the result of involvement of the bone marrow. Based on histopathologic features, lymphomas are subdivided in Hodgkin lymphomas and non-Hodgkin lymphomas. Since Hodgkin lymphoma rarely involves the oral cavity or the jaws, this subtype will not be discussed here any further.

Non-Hodgkin lymphomas may arise in lymph nodes (nodular type) or outside of the lymph nodes (extranodal type). Non-Hodgkin lymphomas of the oral mucosa and the jaw bones are examples of the extranodal type.

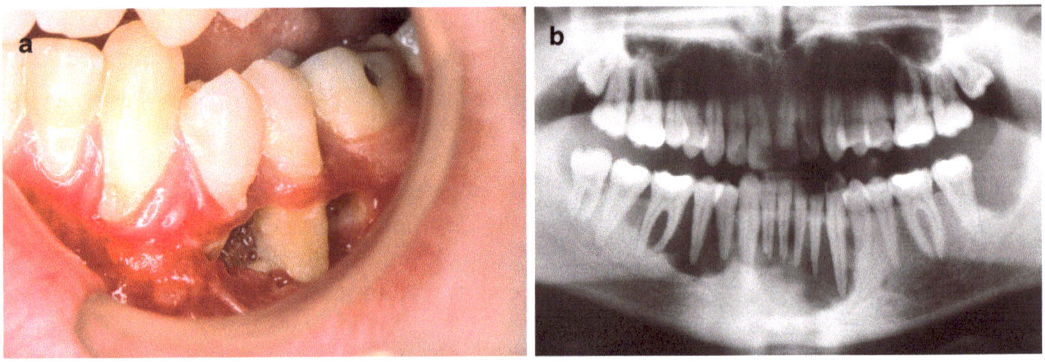

Fig. 7.67 (**a**) Defect of the mandible in an 18-year-old boy caused by Langerhans cell histiocytosis. (**b**) The defect reaches from 33 to 46; notice also a lesion in the region of 38

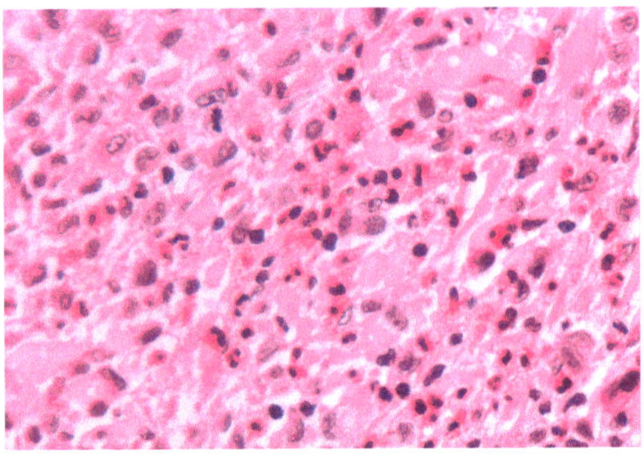

Fig. 7.68 Low-power view of Langerhans cell histiocytosis, being positive for CD1A

Epidemiology

The incidence of all types of lymphomas that may occur in the body amounts approximately 15 new patients per 100,000 population per year. With regard to oral manifestations as being the first sign of the disease, the estimated incidence is approximately one per million population per year.

Clinical Aspects

The palate is the site of preference in case of soft tissue involvement by a non-Hodgkin lymphoma (see Chap. 6). In case of jaw bone involvement, it mainly concerns the mandible. Unilateral paresthesia or anesthesia, sometimes running a recurrent course, of the mental nerve may be the first symptom of the disease. There may be an associated swelling of the affected bone (Figs. 7.70a, b and 7.71a, b). Occasionally, the oral lesion is the first and only manifestation of the disease.

Radiographic Aspects

Often ill-defined radiolucency. In dentate parts of the mandible, the lamina dura may become blurred (Fig. 7.72). In unerupted teeth the cortication of the apical crypts may disappear.

Histopathology

The non-Hodgkin lymphomas are subdivided in a B-cell type and a T-cell type, as can be demonstrated by the use of immunohistochemical stains. Intraoral lymphomas often are of the B-cell type (Fig. 7.73). There are numerous histologic subtypes of non-Hodgkin lymphomas, e.g., diffuse large B-cell type, mantle cell lymphoma, and follicular lymphoma. With regard to their biological behavior, non-Hodgkin lymphomas are grouped into an indolent type, an aggressive type, and a highly aggressive type.

Staging

Staging of the disease will be performed according to the Ann Arbor staging system, in which a distinction is made in the number of involved sites and the localization of the lesion on either side or at both sides of the diaphragm.

Treatment

Treatment depends on the histologic subtype and the stage of the disease and may consist of

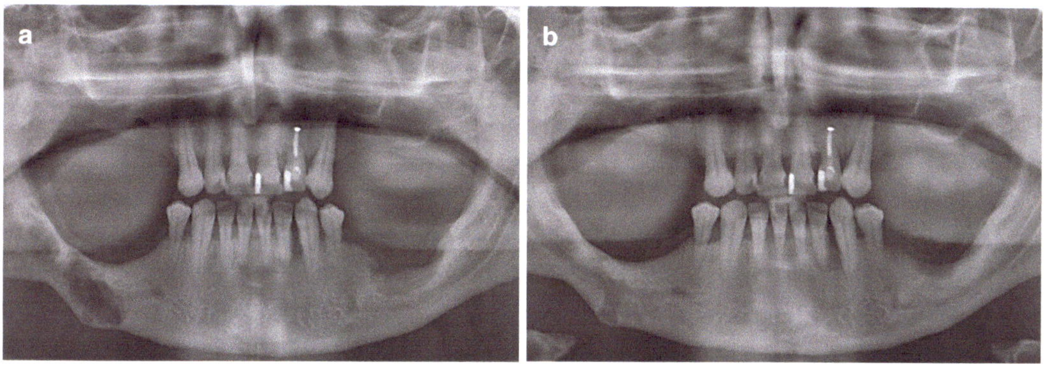

Fig. 7.69 (**a**) Bilateral mandibular defects caused by LCH; no symptoms. No treatment instituted. (**b**) Radiograph taken 6 months later shows spontaneous regression of the lesions

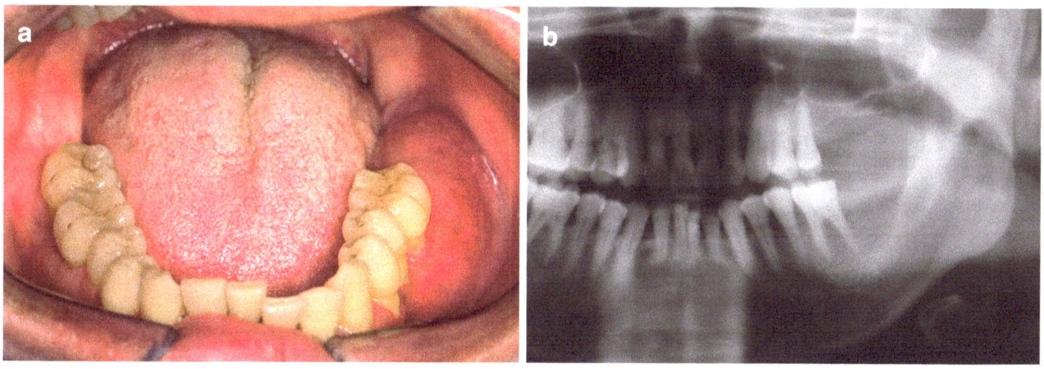

Fig. 7.70 (**a**) Swelling of the mandibular bone at the left side due to an underlying non-Hodgkin lymphoma. (**b**) On the panoramic view, only subtle changes of the mandibular bone can be observed

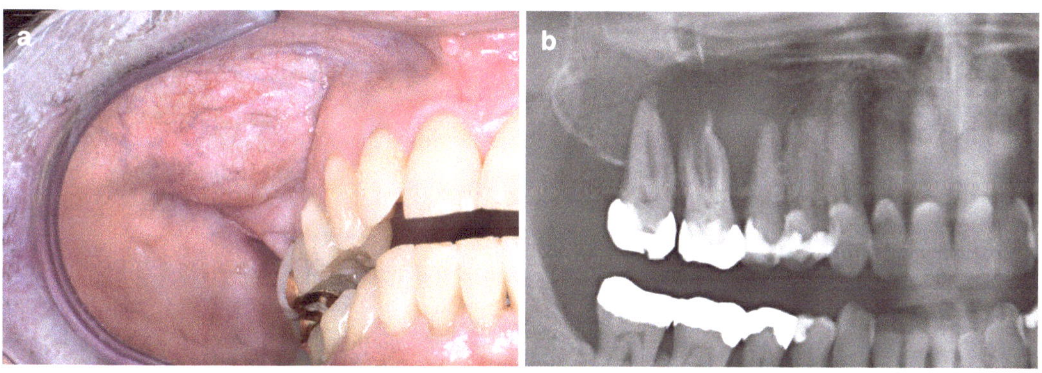

Fig. 7.71 (**a**) Non-Hodgkin lymphoma of the maxillary bone or extending from the maxillary sinus. (**b**) Radiolucency based on non-Hodgkin lymphoma extending from 14 to 17

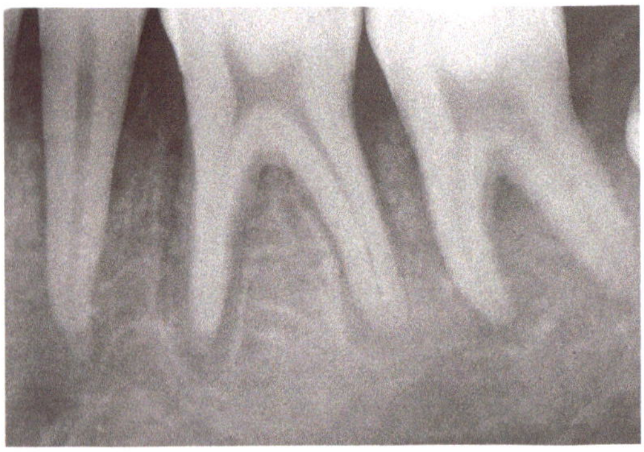

Fig. 7.72 Loss of the lamina dura in a patient suffering from leukemia

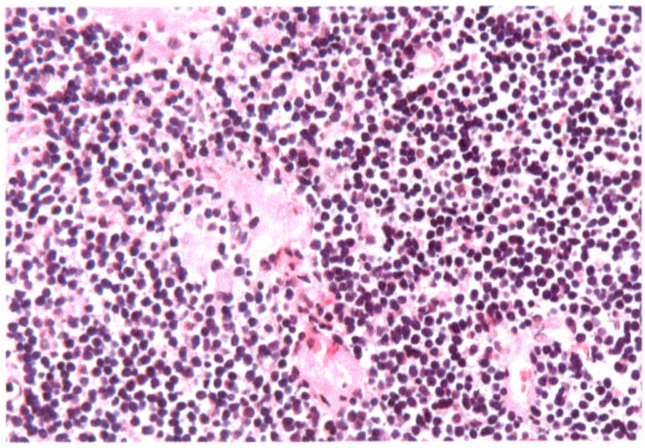

Fig. 7.73 Low-power view of B-cell non-Hodgkin lymphoma of the mandible

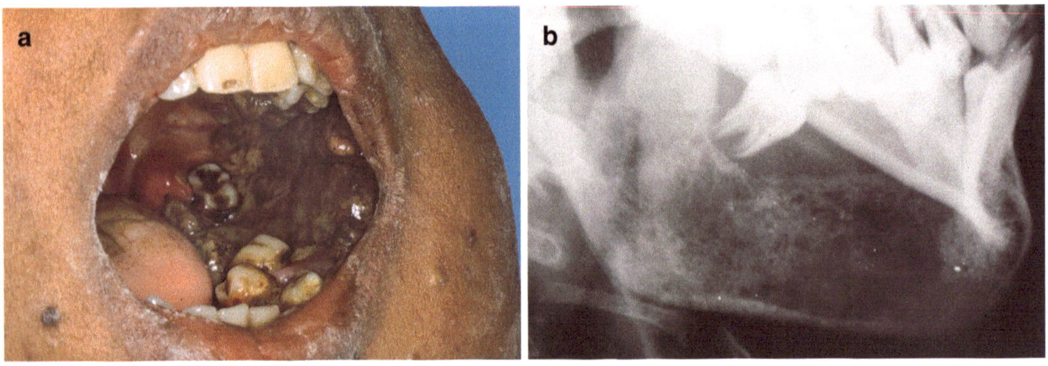

Fig. 7.74 (**a**) Burkitt's lymphoma of the mandible in an 18-year-old boy. (**b**) Destructive radiolucency of the mandibular bone

radiotherapy, chemo-immunotherapy, and stem cell transplantation.

Prognosis

While today the prognosis of Hodgkin lymphoma is rather favorable, the prognosis of non-Hodgkin lymphomas has not much improved over the years and depends largely on the histopathologic subtype and the stage of the disease.

7.10.2 Burkitt's Lymphoma

Definition

Special subtype of B-cell lymphoma that mainly occurs in certain parts of Africa.

Etiology

Apparently, the Epstein-Barr virus plays an important role in the etiology.

Epidemiology

Mainly in children, particularly in young boys.

Clinical Aspects

Is usually located in the abdomen. Is relatively common in the jaws. Signs and symptoms consist of swelling, pain, and increased mobility of teeth (Fig. 7.74a).

Radiographic Aspects

Poorly delineated radiolucency; not characteristic (Fig. 7.74b).

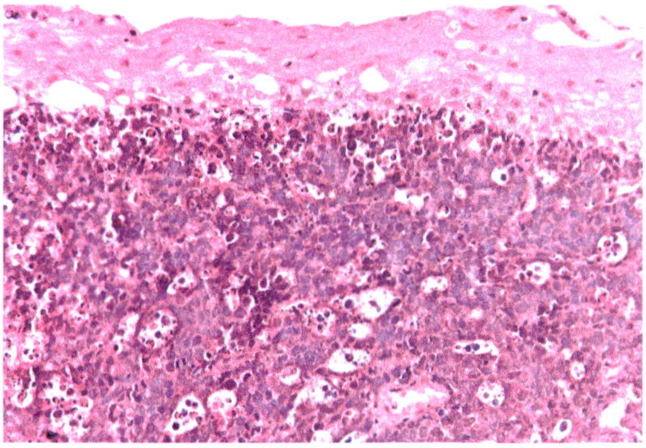

Fig. 7.75 "Starry sky" pattern almost diagnostic of Burkitt's lymphoma

Histopathology

Proliferation of B-cells, showing numerous macrophages that result in a rather typical "starry sky" pattern (Fig. 7.75).

Treatment

Treatment consists of systemic chemotherapy; the prognosis depends on the stage of the disease.

7.10.3 Multiple Myeloma (Kahler's Disease)

Definition

Intraosseous malignant proliferation of plasma cells, often multicentric, formerly referred to as Kahler's disease.

Epidemiology

Of all cancers that may arise in the body, some 1 % consists of multiple myelomas. Occurs almost exclusively in the adult population.

Clinical Aspects

Often occurs in the spine, being painful and sometimes causing pathologic fractures. May also affect the jaws, particularly the mandible, thereby causing anesthesia of the inferior alveolar nerve. Occasionally presentation in the oral soft tissues. May cause amyloid depositions in the tongue.

Radiographic Aspects

Multiple, ill-defined radiolucencies in the mandible (Fig. 7.76).

Laboratory Findings

In the urine special proteins, the "Bence Jones" proteins are present. Serum protein and urine protein immunoelectrophoresis will show the presence of myeloma protein (M-component).

Histopathology

Monoclonal proliferation of plasma cells (Fig. 7.77).

Treatment

Treatment consists of chemotherapy; if indicated, stem cell transplantation. Systemic

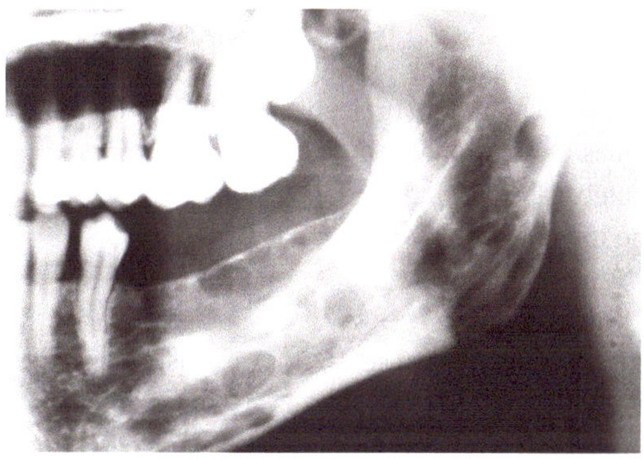

Fig. 7.76 Multiple radiolucencies caused by multiple myelomas

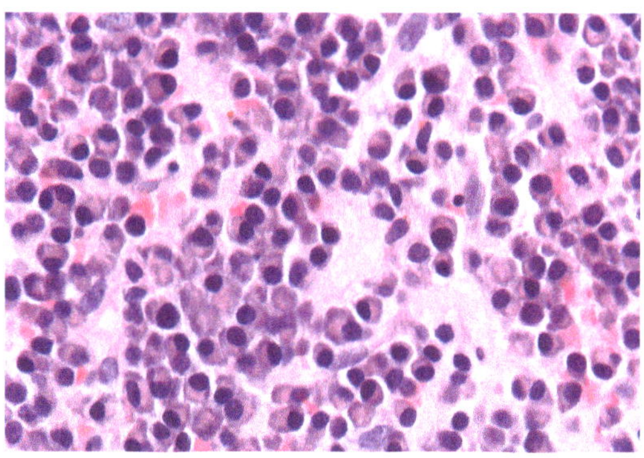

Fig. 7.77 Low-power view of multiple myelomas; notice the numerous plasma cells

bisphosphonates are rather effective in delaying the disease process and may prevent pathologic fractures. As has been discussed elsewhere in this chapter, the use of bisphosphonates carries the risk of inducing osteonecrosis of the jaws.

Radiotherapy is applied in cases of severe pain. The prognosis largely depends on the stage of the disease at the time of diagnosis.

7.11 Metastases

Definition

Malignant neoplasm derived from a primary tumor located elsewhere in the body. Metastases occurring in the oral soft tissues are dealt with in Chap. 2.

Epidemiology

Metastases in the oral soft tissues or the jaw bones are extremely rare and constitute approximately 1 % of all malignancies that may occur in the mouth.

Clinical Aspects

Intraosseous metastases almost exclusively occur in the mandible. In most cases the primary is known already. The primaries are located in the most common cancer sites, such as the breast, prostate, lungs, and kidney. The first symptom may be one-sided anesthesia of the lower lip. May also be detected in case of disturbed healing after tooth extraction.

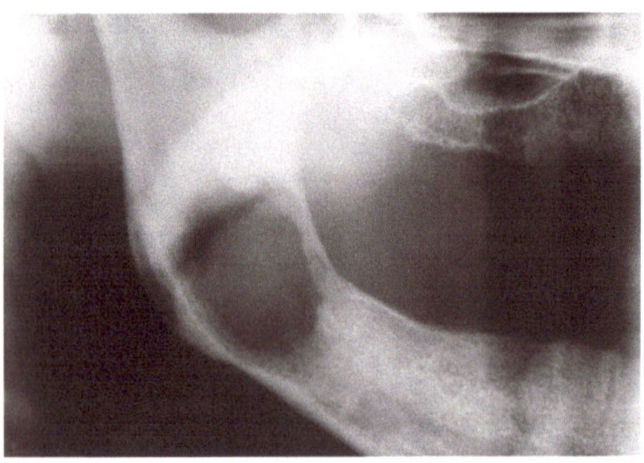

Fig. 7.78 Radiolucent defect in the angle of the mandible caused by a lung metastasis

Radiographic Aspects

Usually ill-defined radiolucency; occasionally an opacity (Figs. 7.78 and 7.79a, b).

Histopathology

Obviously, the histopathologic aspects depend on the histopathology of the primary, if identified already (Fig. 7.79c). Immunohistochemical markers, e.g., prostate-specific antigen, may be of help in identifying the primary, if not known already.

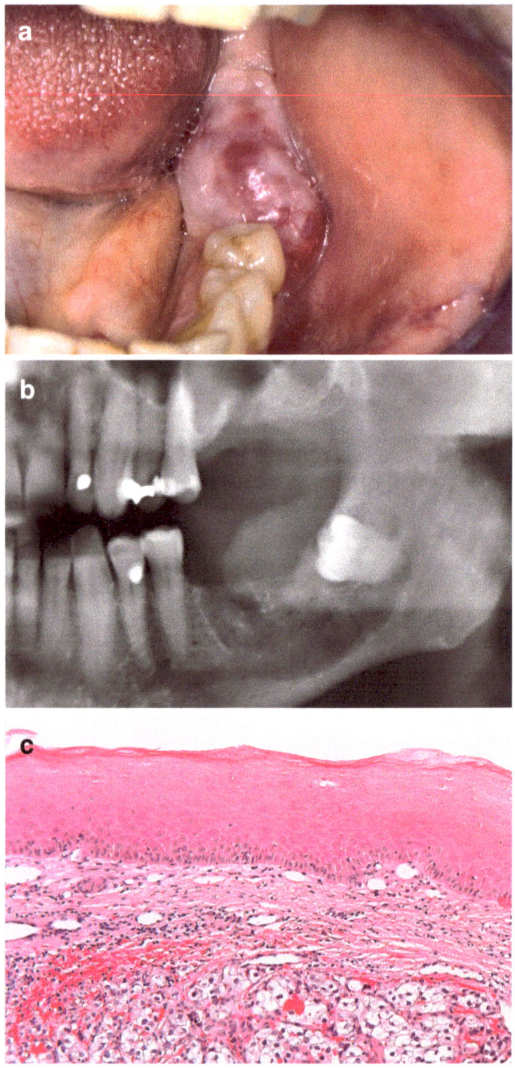

Fig. 7.79 (**a**) Disturbed wound healing after extraction of 36 and 37. The medical history was negative. (**b**) Diffuse lucent changes in the region of 36–37. The biopsy showed a metastasis of a renal carcinoma. (**c**) Low-power view of renal carcinoma. Notice the intact overlying oral mucosa

Treatment

Only in the absence of other metastases, treatment with a curative intent may be considered.

7.12 Osteoma

Definition

Benign neoplasm of bone. Multiple osteomas of the jaws are indicative of the hereditary Gardner's syndrome (familial polyposis) being discussed elsewhere in this chapter.

Epidemiology

Osteomas rarely occur in the jaws, the estimated incidence being less than one per million population per year.

Clinical Aspects

Slowly enlarging, bony hard swelling, being asymptomatic otherwise (Fig. 7.80a, b). Although the history and the clinicoradiographic features are rather diagnostic, it is safe practice to have the diagnosis confirmed by a biopsy.

Radiographic Aspects

Well-circumscribed opaque pattern, not diagnostic. The differential diagnosis may include complex odontoma, fibrous dysplasia, and osteosarcoma.

Histopathology

Histopathologically, vital compact osseous tissue is observed (Fig. 7.81). There may be a fluent transition between the aspects of an osteoma and a low-grade osteosarcoma.

Treatment

Surgical removal, if feasible.

7.13 Osteomyelitis and Allied Inflammatory Lesions and Disorders

7.13.1 Alveolitis

Definition

Local inflammation of the alveolar bone after a tooth extraction; can be regarded a localized form of osteomyelitis.

Etiology

Probably the result of precocious disintegration of the blood clot. Smoking may be a predisposing factor.

Clinical Aspects

Alveolitis typically causes severe pain that starts a few days after the tooth extraction. Occurs almost exclusively in the mandibular bicuspid and molar region (Fig. 7.82a, b). The clinical presentation is an empty alveolus ("dry socket"). In case of doubt about the completeness of the tooth extraction, the taking of a radiograph may be considered. Occasionally, there may be a need for histopathologic verification to exclude any other disease.

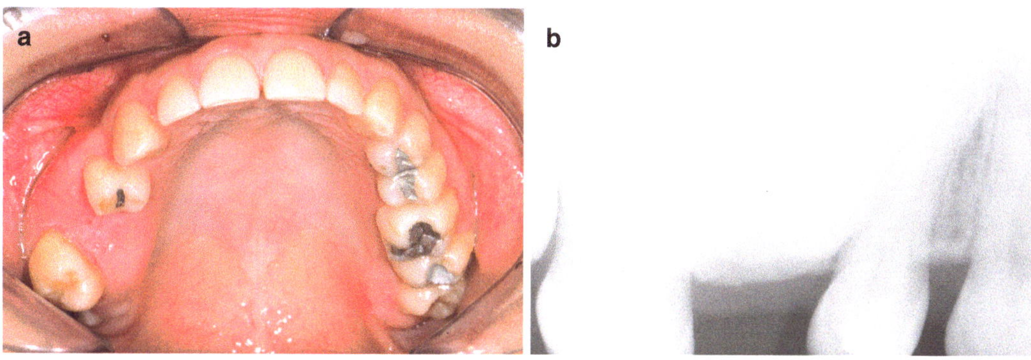

Fig. 7.80 (a) Bony hard swelling in the 15–17 region, asymptomatic otherwise, caused by an osteoma. (b) Well-circumscribed opacity compatible with but not diagnostic of osteoma

Treatment

Wound rinsing with saline after meals may speed up healing. Wound dressings are usually not very effective in reducing the pain. Prescription of analgesics for at least a week or often even for a longer period of time is indicated. Reassurance of the patient is an important part of the management in case of alveolitis.

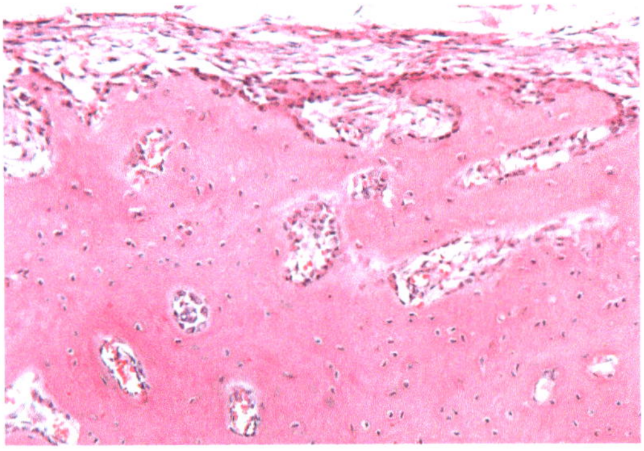

Fig. 7.81 Low-power view of an osteoma

7.13.2 Lingual Sequestrum

A lingual sequestrum is a rather rare, idiopathic (perhaps of traumatic origin), painful exposure of the lingual aspect of the posterior mandible. Healing usually takes place within a few weeks (Fig. 7.83a, b). Removal of the sequestrum may speed up healing, but is not really necessary.

7.13.3 Osteomyelitis (Incl. Periostitis, Osteoradionecrosis, and Medication-Related Osteonecrosis)

Definition

Inflammation of the bone and/or periosteum (periostitis).

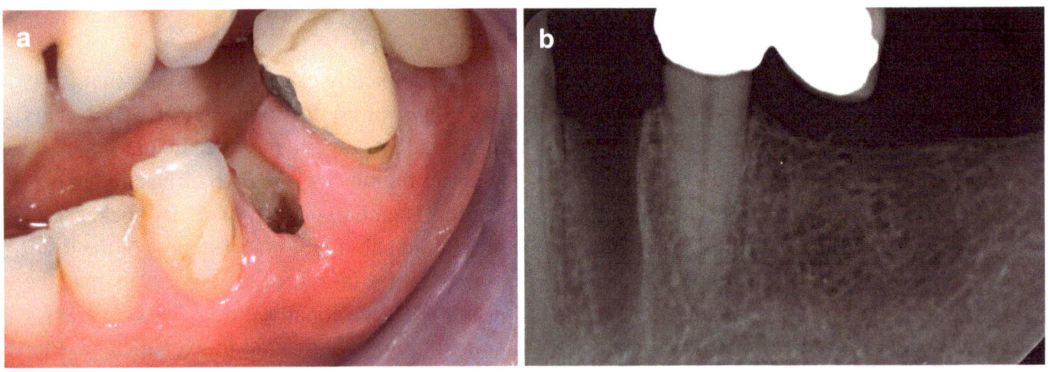

Fig. 7.82 (a) Clinical aspect of alveolitis ("dry socket"). (b) The periapical film does not show anything abnormal

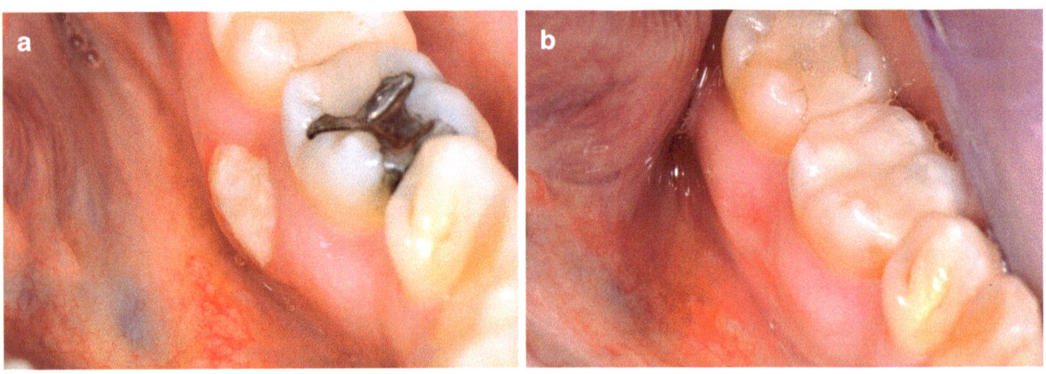

Fig. 7.83 (a) "Lingual sequestrum," probably of traumatic origin. (b) Spontaneous healing within 3 weeks

Etiology

Most cases of osteomyelitis of the jaw bones are the result of an odontogenic infection, e.g., extension from a periapical granuloma. Non-odontogenic causes include secondary inflammation after a fracture or orthognathic surgery of the mandible. Specific infections of the jaw bones, such as tuberculosis, are exceedingly rare. Osteomyelitis may also occur in abnormal bone as is, for instance, the case in osteopetrosis.

Tooth extraction in previous irradiated bone may lead to a severe type of osteomyelitis, referred to as osteoradionecrosis (ORN). When a diagnosis of ORN is suspected, one should always consider the possibility of recurrent cancer, usually a squamous cell carcinoma.

Prolonged oral or intravenously administered bisphosphonates may result in necrosis of the bone, referred to as chemonecrosis (bisphosphonate-related osteonecrosis of the jaws; BONJ). Because also some drugs other than bisphosphonates may cause osteonecrosis, the term "medication-related osteonecrosis of the jaws" (MONJ) seems more appropriate. In the majority of cases of MONJ, there has been an odontogenic cause, e.g., a previous tooth extraction. A classification of osteomyelitis and allied inflammatory lesions and disorders of the jaws is depicted in Table 7.2.

Table 7.2 Classification of osteomyelitis of the jaws

Acute primary osteomyelitis; rare type of osteomyelitis, probably caused by hematogenous spread of microorganisms, e.g., after a sore throat
Chronic osteomyelitis, *purulent* or *sequestrating* type, producing fragments of non-vital bone, so-called sequesters
Chronic osteomyelitis, *sclerosing* type (osteomyelitis sicca; no formation of sequesters), being subdivided in a focal and a diffuse type; the focal type is probably identical to the so-called enostosis (idiopathic focal osteopetrosis, dense bone island)
Chronic osteomyelitis with proliferative periostitis ("periostitis ossificans"), particularly occurring in children in the mandible ("juvenile chronic mandibular osteomyelitis")
Chronic periostitis in denture wearers ("pulse granuloma")
Osteoradionecrosis
Medication-related osteomyelitis, including bisphosphonate-related osteonecrosis

Clinical Aspects

Osteomyelitis of the jaws almost exclusively affects the mandible, probably due to its somewhat limited vascularization compared to the maxilla.

The acute type may cause severe pain and may be accompanied by fever; there is often increased mobility of the teeth in the affected part of the jaw.

In chronic purulent or sequestrating osteomyelitis, bone exposure and intraoral or extraoral fistulas may develop (Fig. 7.84a–c). This type of osteomyelitis is usually painful.

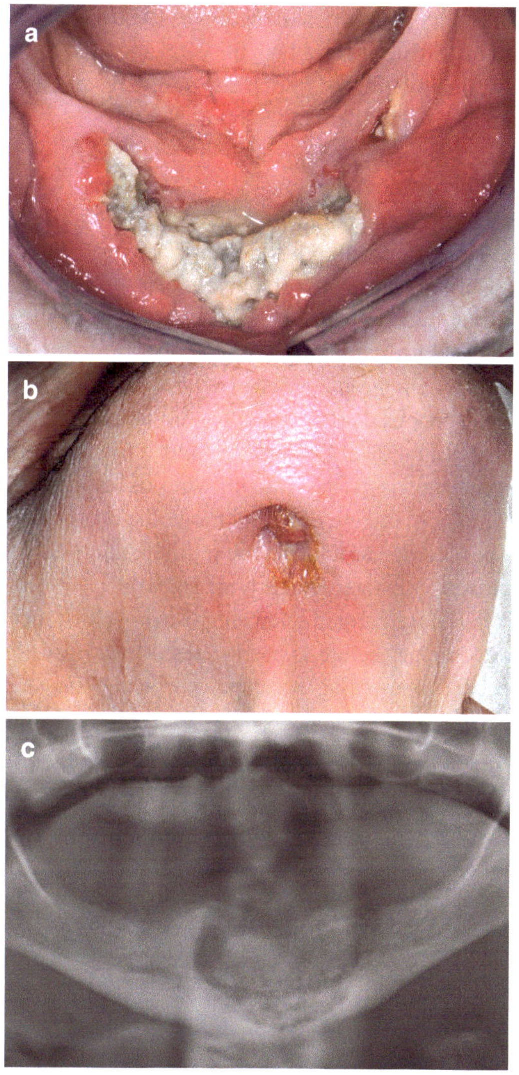

Fig. 7.84 (**a**) Purulent, sequestrating osteomyelitis in the anterior part of the mandible. (**b**) Cutaneous fistula in the submental region. (**c**) The radiographic features are compatible with sequestrating osteomyelitis

Focal chronic sclerosing osteomyelitis is usually asymptomatic, being detected as an incidental finding on a radiograph. Diffuse chronic sclerosing osteomyelitis may be painful and may be accompanied by recurrent swelling of the mandible and also trismus.

In case of chronic periostitis in denture wearers, the alveolar mucosa may become swollen and painful.

The clinical presentation of ORN and MONJ may be somewhat similar as in chronic osteomyelitis with or without bone exposure; both conditions can be very painful. On the specialist level, there are several staging systems both for ORN and MONJ.

Osteomyelitis of the jaws rarely results in infections elsewhere in the body.

Radiographic Aspects

In the early stage of acute primary osteomyelitis, the radiograph will not show any changes.

Chronic purulent osteomyelitis is characterized by mixed opaque and lucent changes of the bony and formation of sequesters.

In focal chronic sclerosing osteomyelitis, a homogeneous dense opaque pattern is seen at the apex of a tooth, not being surrounded by a radiolucent rim as is the case in osseous dysplasia (Fig. 7.85). In case of a vital tooth, the opacity is to be regarded as a focal type of idiopathic osteopetrosis (enostosis, dense bone island).

In diffuse chronic sclerosing osteomyelitis, the radiographic picture is characterized by a diffuse opacity, often being accompanied by a periostal reaction in the form of parallel opaque pericortical lines ("onion skin appearance") (Fig. 7.86).

In case of chronic periostitis in denture wearers, often a cup-shaped radiolucent defect of the alveolar ridge can be observed (Fig. 7.87).

In ORN and MONJ, a mixture of opaque and radiolucent changes can be observed, with or without signs of sequestration (Figs. 7.88a, b and 7.89). CT scans provide much more detailed information about the extent and the severity of the necrosis.

Scintigraphic examination will in most cases of osteomyelitis show an increased uptake of the radioisotope.

Microbiology

Culturing of infected bone or discharge from the infected bone will rarely show the presence of pathogenic microorganisms; in rare cases actinomycetes or *M. tuberculosis* may be cultured.

Blood Examination

Only in acute osteomyelitis, an increased erythrocytic sedimentation rate or reactive C-protein level may be seen.

Histopathology

Histopathologically, signs of acute or chronic inflammation may be observed. In chronic sclerosing osteomyelitis, dense bone without obvious signs of inflammation is encountered.

Rarely, specific microorganisms such as *M. tuberculosis* can be demonstrated. The possible presence of actinomycetes is in general

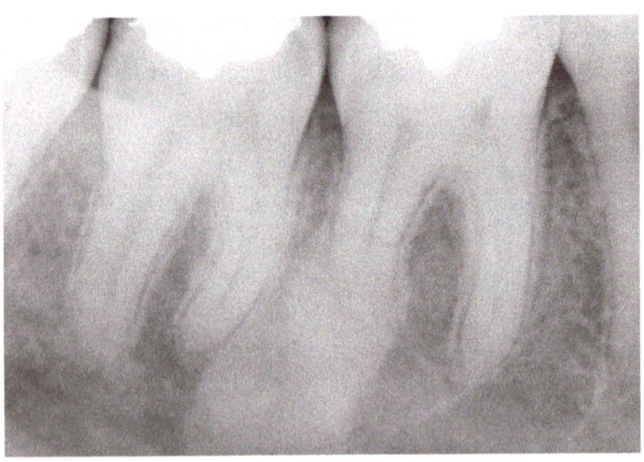

Fig. 7.85 Focal sclerosering osteomyelitis (or dense bone island?) at 46; incidental finding

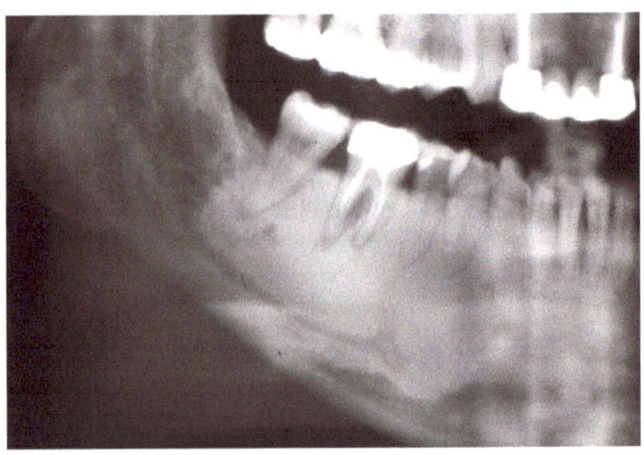

Fig. 7.86 Diffuse sclerosering osteomyelitis of the mandible

considered to represent a secondary finding, not being the cause of the osteomyelitis (Fig. 7.90).

The presence of squamous cell epithelium around possible sequesters can misleadingly mimic a squamous cell carcinoma. In case of chronic periostitis in denture wearers, the so-called pulse granulomas can be encountered around remnants of vegetables that have been forced through the oral mucosa into the periosteum (Fig. 7.91).

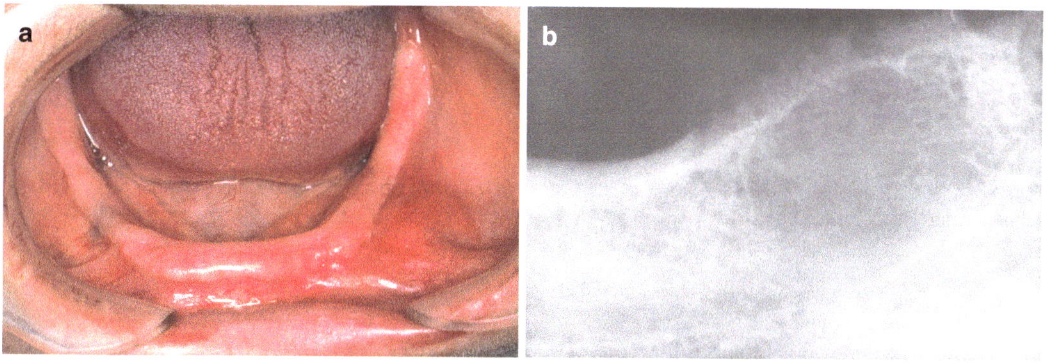

Fig. 7.87 (**a**) Periostitis of the lower left bicuspid region in a denture wearer. (**b**) Somewhat circumscribed radiolucency compatible with a diagnosis of periostitis

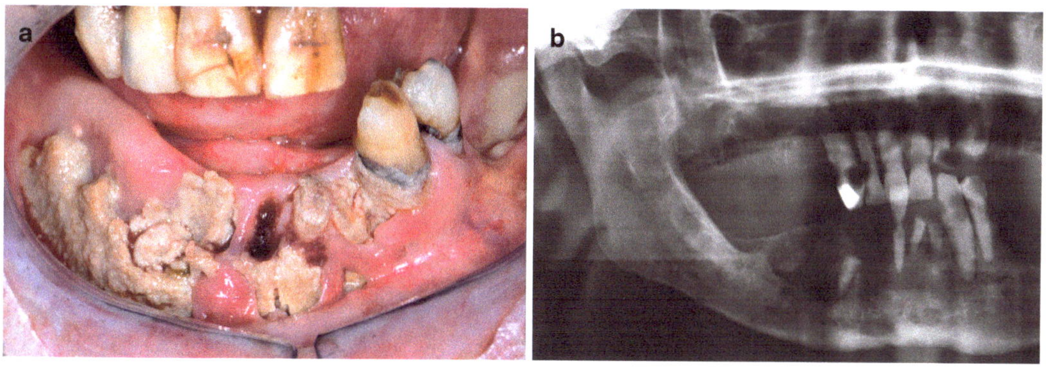

Fig. 7.88 (**a**) Osteoradionecrosis of the mandible. (**b**) On the panoramic view rather limited bone destruction is observed

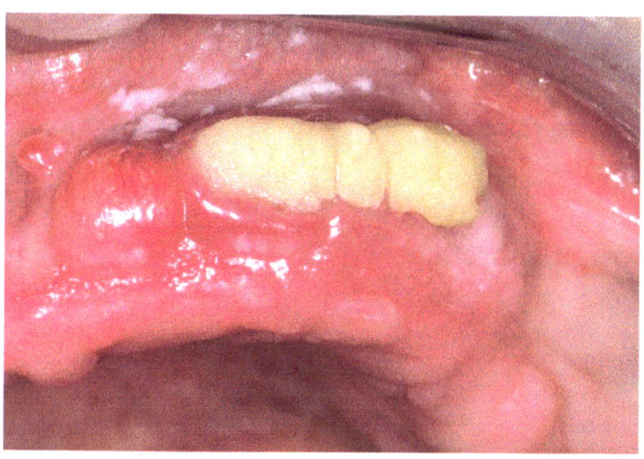

Fig. 7.89 Bisphosphonate-related osteonecrosis of the anterior maxilla

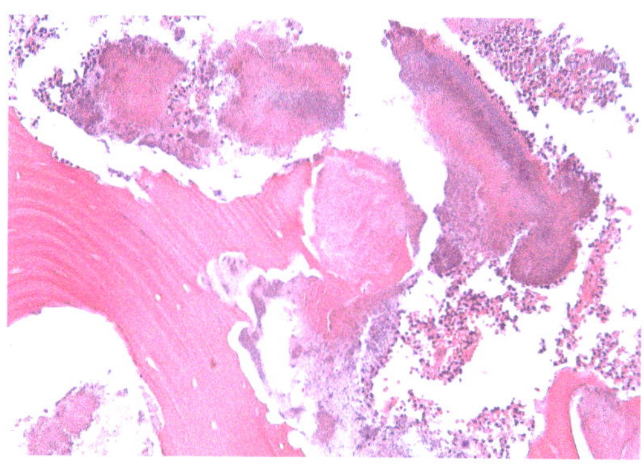

Fig. 7.90 Sequester of the necrotic bone surrounded by clusters of microorganisms

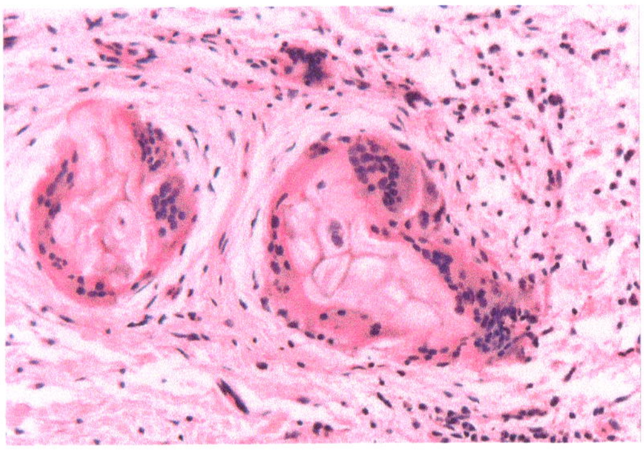

Fig. 7.91 "Pulse granuloma" showing multinucleated foreign body cells around food particles

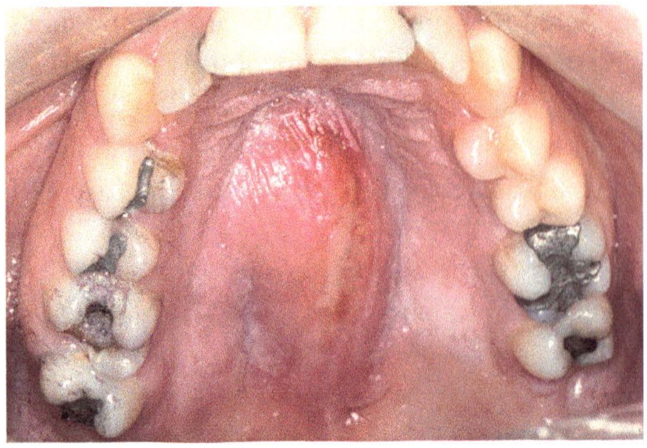

Fig. 7.92 Palatal abscess caused by a periapical inflammation of non-vital 12

Treatment

Elimination of the causative factor, if identified, is obviously of importance in all types of osteomyelitis and inflammatory diseases of the jaws. In primary acute osteomyelitis, the (intravenously) administration of antibiotics is indicated.

In chronic purulent osteomyelitis, the removal of sequesters is recommended. The use of antibiotics in this type of osteomyelitis is questionable. In otherwise asymptomatic focal chronic osteomyelitis (dense bone island?), there is no need for treatment.

The treatment of diffuse chronic osteomyelitis is cumbersome. Some recommend surgical decortication of the involved part of the mandible in order to remove the necrotic or inflamed bone and at the same time improve the vascularization of the bone. The use of antibiotics in this condition is at least questionable. This also applies to the use of hyperbaric oxygen. Some authors have reported favorable results by the use of night guards and physiotherapy directed at the jaw muscles based on the concept of tendoperiostitis.

In chronic periostitis in denture wearers, thorough excochleation of the defect is advised and, of course, adjustment of the denture.

In ORN one may consider to remove the necrotic bone with or without additional antibiotic treatment. The value of hyperbaric oxygen in the treatment or prevention of ORN has never been proven scientifically. To some extent this also applies to the prophylactic use of antibiotics in case of extraction of teeth in previously irradiated bone. Even the pre-irradiation dental screening procedure is perhaps less effective in preventing ORN than generally thought of, except for the importance of optimal oral hygiene during and after radiotherapy.

In MONJ cessation of the drug ("drug holiday") does not seem to be effective. Much attention should be paid at the possible prevention of this type of necrosis by dental screening before the commencement of intravenously administered bisphosphonates and other medications that may induce necrosis of the jaws.

7.13.4 Periapical Granuloma

Definition

Inflammatory reaction at the apex of a tooth.

Etiology

Necrosis of the pulpa, most often due to progression of caries but sometimes due to traumatic injury to the tooth, results in a periapical inflammation, usually of a chronic nature.

Clinical Aspects

A periapical granuloma is often asymptomatic but may occasionally flare up and may cause abscess formation with or without producing a fistula into the oral cavity or through the skin (Figs. 7.92, 7.93, and 7.94a, b). It is actually unknown why some periapical granulomas transform into a cyst (radicular cyst) or give rise to osteomyelitis, while others remain unchanged. The tooth with a periapical granuloma may become painful at percussion. A non-vital tooth usually becomes darkly colored.

Radiographic Aspects

On the radiograph a periapical radiolucency will be observed, being somewhat circumscribed but not being "corticated" as is seen in a radicular cyst. There are, however, no reliable radiographic aspects to differentiate a periapical granuloma from a radicular cyst. In case of a vital tooth, a periapical radiolucency may be based on osseous dysplasia, as being discussed elsewhere in this chapter.

Histopathology

In case of periapical curettage, the tissue should always be forwarded to the pathologist for confirmation of the diagnosis. The histopathologic features consist of an inflammatory infiltrate, acute or chronic, without true granuloma formation; in fact, the term periapical granuloma is a misnomer. Cholesterol clefts, being the result of degradation of erythrocytes, are a common finding, as are macrophages with often a foamy appearance ("foam cells"). There may be proliferation of odontogenic epithelium without the formation of a cyst as is the case in a radicular cyst.

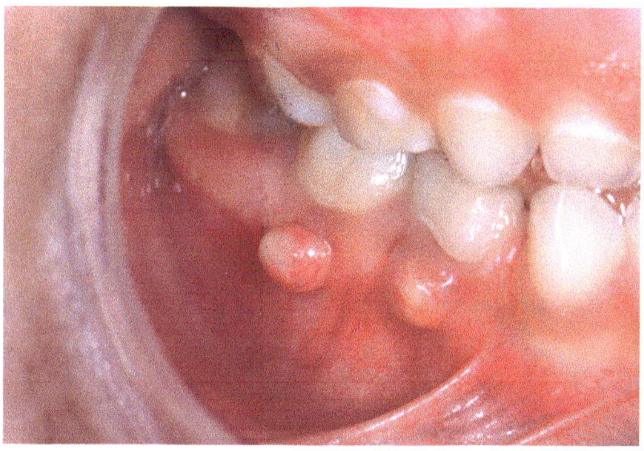

Fig. 7.93 Multiple odontogenic fistulas in the deciduous dentition; otherwise asymptomatic

Treatment

In case of a non-vital tooth, a root canal treatment is indicated. Additional periapical curettage or apicoectomy is rarely needed. Badly decayed teeth may be extracted.

7.14 Sarcomas of the Bone

7.14.1 Chondrosarcoma

Definition

Malignant neoplasm of cartilaginous tissue. Interestingly, benign neoplasms of cartilaginous tissue (chondromas) rarely occur in the jaw bones with the exception of the condylar region of the mandible.

Clinical Aspects

Slowly enlarging, non-characteristic swelling of the jaw with or without other signs or symptoms.

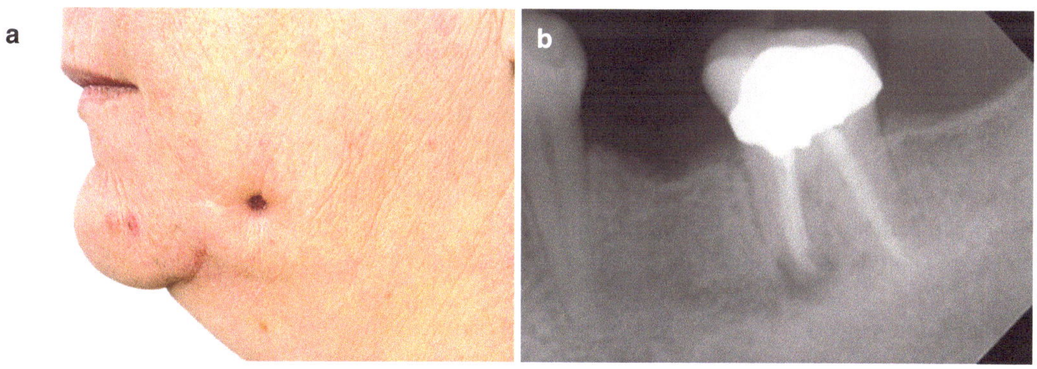

Fig. 7.94 (a) Cutaneous fistula of odontogenic origin (37), being asymptomatic otherwise. (b) Periapical radiolucency at the mesial apex of 37

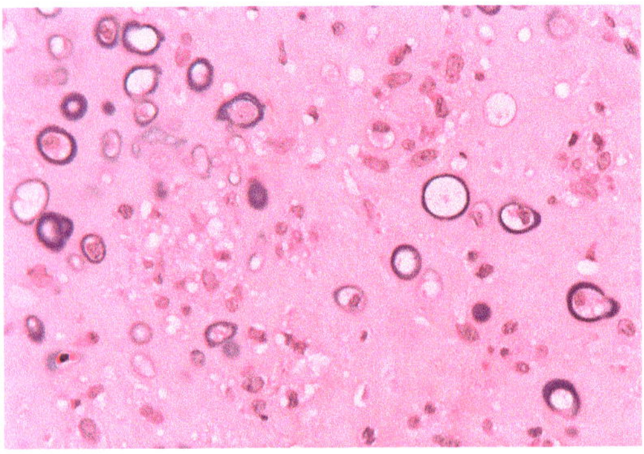

Fig. 7.95 High-power view of well-differentiated chondrosarcoma

Radiographic Aspects
Ill-defined radiolucent, radiopaque, or mixed aspect, non-characteristic.

Histopathology
Proliferation of atypical chondroblasts (Fig. 7.95). May occasionally be difficult to distinguish from chondroblastic osteosarcoma.

Treatment
Aggressive surgical removal with or without (neo)adjuvant chemotherapy.

7.14.2 Ewing's Sarcoma

Definition
Malignant neoplasm of immature blastic round cells of unknown origin.

Epidemiology
Rare neoplasm; may occur already at an early age in children and adolescents.

Clinical Aspects
Fast-growing tumor, painful, and initially presenting as a soft tissue swelling (Fig. 7.96a–c).

Radiographic Aspects
Ill-defined radiolucency; the crypts around the apices of non-erupted teeth may disappear.

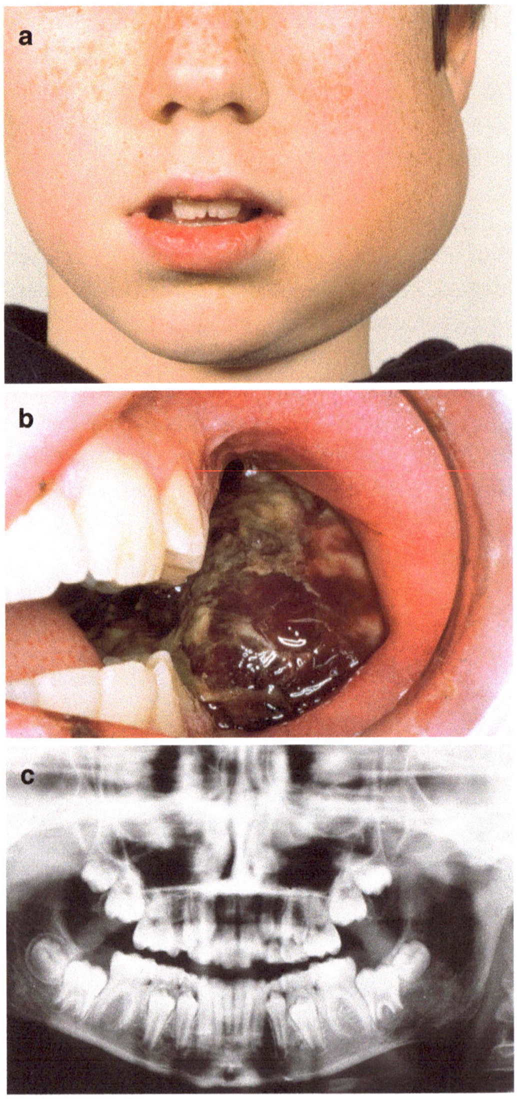

Fig. 7.96 (**a**) Rapidly growing swelling of the cheek due to Ewing's sarcoma. (**b**) Intraoral view shows the extent of the lesion. (**c**) Diffuse radiolucency of the left angle of the mandible; notice the loss of cortication around 37 and 38

Histopathology
Proliferation of round cells ("round cell sarcoma"); immunohistochemical stains are usually needed to arrive at the final diagnosis.

Treatment
Treatment consists of a combination of surgery, radiotherapy, and chemotherapy. Poor prognosis.

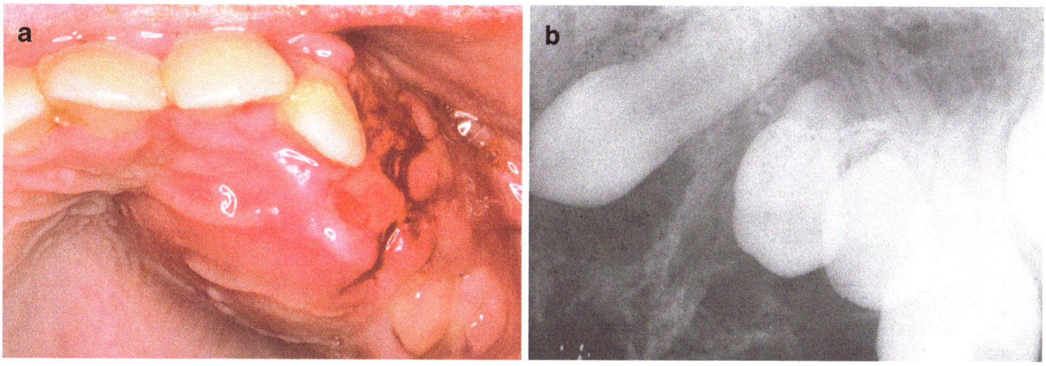

Fig. 7.97 (**a**) Osteosarcoma in a 12-year-old girl. (**b**) Loss of cortication around the non-erupted teeth, highly suspicious of malignancy

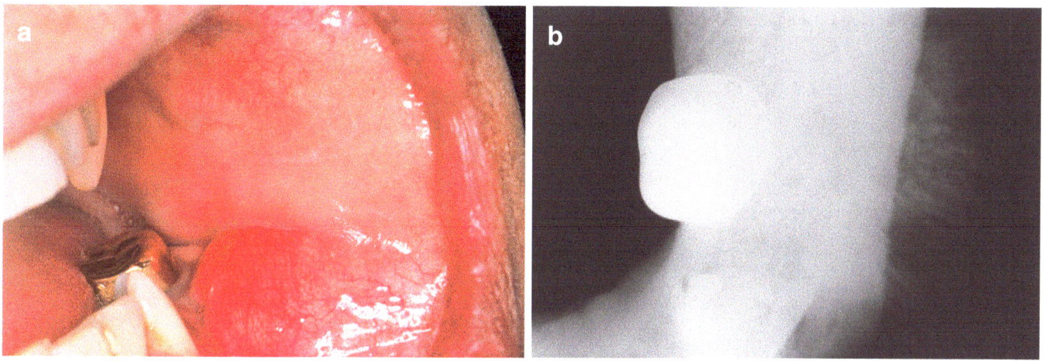

Fig. 7.98 (**a**) Osteosarcoma of the mandible causing one-sided anesthesia of the lower lip. (**b**) The "sunray" aspect as shown on the occlusal view is almost diagnostic of osteosarcoma

7.14.3 Osteosarcoma

Definition

Malignant neoplasm of bone.

Epidemiology

Osteosarcomas are the most common sarcomas that may occur in the jaw bones. Some 5 % of all osteosarcomas that arise in the body arise in the jaws. The estimated incidence of osteosarcoma of the jaws is one per million population per year. May occur already in children and adolescents.

Clinical Aspects

May occur in the mandible or the maxilla. The clinical presentation consists of an often slowly enlarging tumor with or without associated symptoms such as increased mobility of teeth, pain, or anesthesia of the lower lip in case of a mandibular osteosarcoma (Figs. 7.97a, b, 7.98a, b, and 7.99a, b). Occasionally, hematogenous metastases are present already at the time of the initial presentation.

Radiographic Aspects

Radiolucent or radiopaque ill-defined changes of the bone, occasionally showing a radiation aspect of the periosteum ("sunray appearance"). In dentate parts of the jaws, an important sign of malignancy consists of an irregularly widening of the periodontal ligament. Tooth follicles of unerupted teeth may lose their cortication.

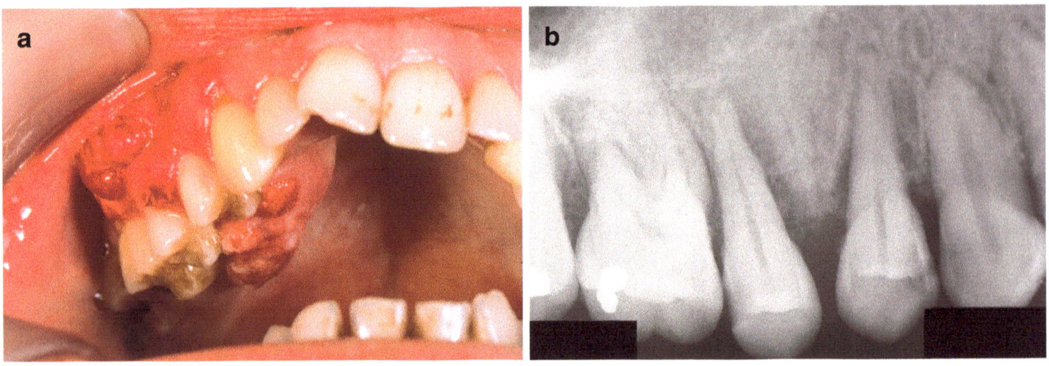

Fig. 7.99 (**a**) Osteosarcoma of the maxilla. (**b**) The widening of the periodontal ligaments is almost diagnostic of osteosarcoma

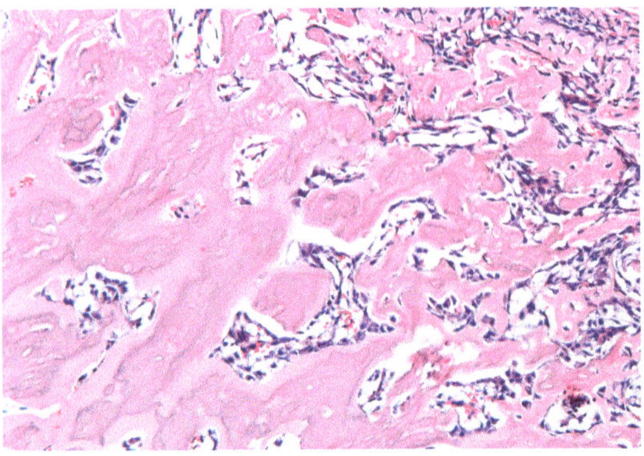

Fig. 7.100 Newly formed bone in osteosarcoma surrounded by numerous osteoblasts

Histopathology

Formation of osteoid and abnormal bone surrounded by large osteoblasts (Fig. 7.100); sometimes presence of chondroid structures. Cementum-like osseous tissue may be present with or without multinucleated giant cells in the surrounding stromal tissue. The differential diagnosis may include the extremely rare osteoblastoma, an osteoma, a cementoblastoma, a central giant cell lesion, a fibrosarcoma, and a metastasis.

Histopathologically, osteosarcomas are graded in low-grade, intermediate-grade, and high-grade malignancies.

Treatment

Treatment consists of aggressive surgical treatment with or without (neo)adjuvant chemotherapy and postoperative radiotherapy. If local radicality is obtained, the prognosis is rather favorable.

7.15 Some Uncommon Generalized Bone Diseases and Syndromes Involving the Jaw Bones

7.15.1 Cherubism

Some Characteristics

Genetic disorder resulting in activation of the osteoclasts and disturbed jaw formation sometimes, but not always, resulting in a facial appearance that resembles little angels ("cherubs"). Cherubism is a rare disorder that develops during early childhood.

The clinical presentation consists of painless, bilateral swellings of the posterior mandible (Fig. 7.101a–c); occasionally, also the maxilla is involved. There may be displacement of teeth and delayed eruption. Although the clinicoradiographic features are almost diagnostic, a biopsy is recommended for confirmation of the diagnosis.

Radiographically, bilateral multilobulated radiolucencies are observed. Histopathologically, the lesions strongly resemble (central) giant cell lesions and brown tumors as expression of hyperparathyroidism.

In the majority of patients, remission occurs before puberty.

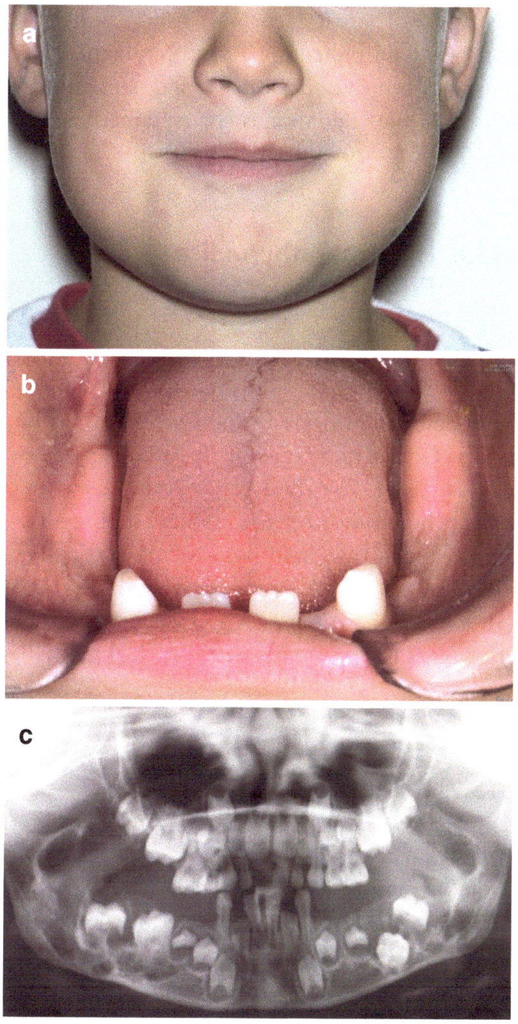

Fig. 7.101 (**a**) A 7-year-old boy suffering from cherubism. (**b**) Intraoral view shows oligodontia. (**c**) Bilateral radiolucencies in the ascending ramus of the mandible, almost diagnostic of cherubism

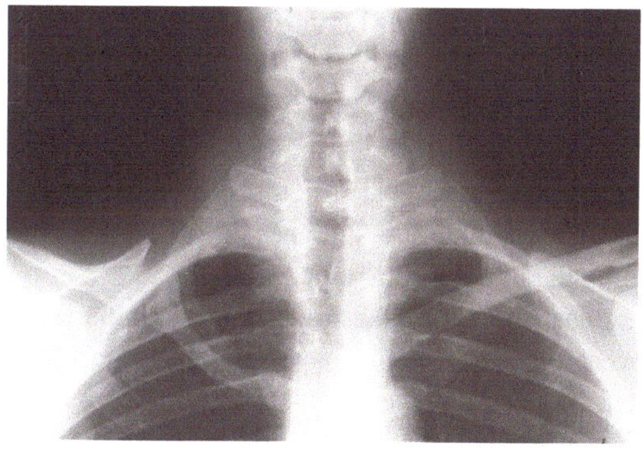

Fig. 7.102 Underdeveloped right clavicle in a patient with cleidocranial dysplasia

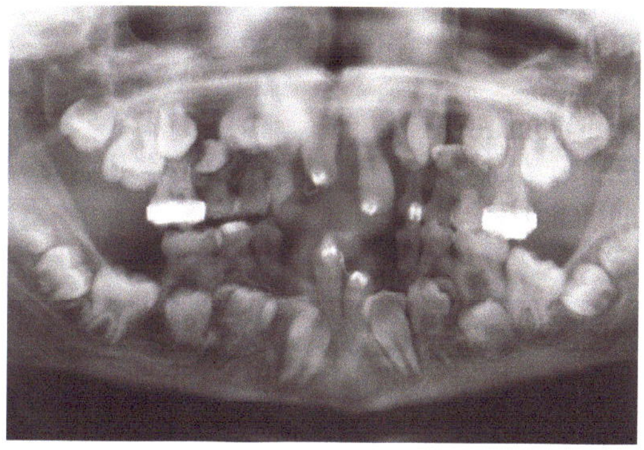

Fig. 7.103 Multiple retained teeth in the mandible and maxilla in cleidocranial dysplasia in a 12-year-old boy

7.15.2 Cleidocranial Dysplasia

Some Characteristics

Often inherited disorder in which osteoblastic differentiation and bone formation are disturbed. Mainly affects the skull and the clavicles. The latter may be hyperplastic or absent (Fig. 7.102), enabling the patient to approximate the shoulders. Oral abnormalities include a high palatal arch, sometimes a cleft palate, and the presence of numerous unerupted permanent and supernumerary teeth (Fig. 7.103). There is no effective treatment for this disorder.

7.15.3 Cortical Hyperostosis (Van Buchem's Disease)

Some Characteristics

Extremely rare inherited disorder characterized by thickening of the calvarium, the jaws, the clavicles, and the ribs as a result of excessive endosteal and subperiosteal deposition of bone. In most cases there are no physical abnormalities, but there may be hearing loss and loss of vision due to narrowing of the foramina in the skull base. Radiographically, the lower border of the mandible may show sclerotic changes (Fig. 7.104). There is no treatment available.

7.15.4 Ectodermal Dysplasia

Some Characteristics

Rare, inherited disorder in which two or more ectodermal anatomical structures fail to develop. There are numerous subtypes, the best known being the hypohidrotic type.

Because of the lack of sufficient numbers of sweat glands, patients have an intolerance for heat. Often presence of thin hairs and atrophic nails. The dental abnormal findings include oligodontia or hypodontia; the teeth may be cone shaped (Fig. 7.105).

7.15.5 Gardner's Syndrome

Some Characteristics

Gardner's syndrome is a hereditary disorder characterized by multiple intestinal polyps (having a strong tendency to become malignant, being an indication for prophylactic colectomy), multiple osteomas, and sometimes also multiple odontomas or retained teeth (Fig. 7.106).

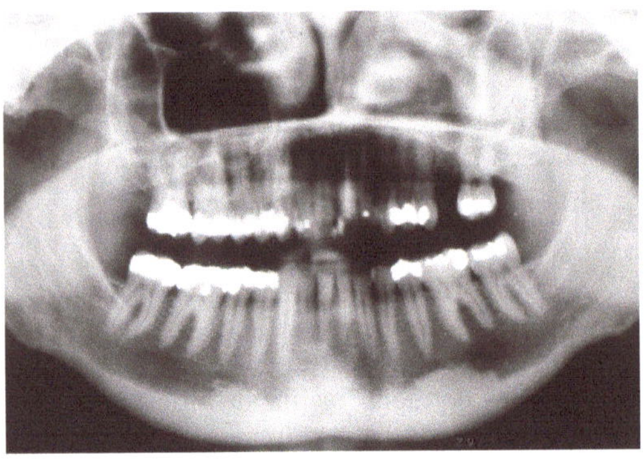

Fig. 7.104 Diffuse sclerosing changes of the inferior border of the mandible in a patient suffering from generalized cortical hyperostosis

7.15.6 Hyperparathyroidism, Primary

Some Characteristics

Primary hyperparathyroidism is usually caused by an adenoma of one of the four parathyroid glands. One of the signs of this disease is the occurrence of so-called brown tumors in the bones, including the jaw bones. Clinically, radiographically, and histopathologically, these lesions may strongly resemble giant cell lesions of the bone (Fig. 7.107a, b). After removal of the adenoma, the bone lesions will regress.

7.15.7 Osteopetrosis

Some Characteristics

Often hereditary disorder characterized by increased density of the bone due to a defect in the normal osteoclast function; as a result the thickness of the cortical bone increases, while the cancellous bone becomes sclerotic. Tooth extraction in involved bone may result in a fracture or may give rise to osteomyelitis (Fig. 7.108a, b). Treatment can only be symptomatic.

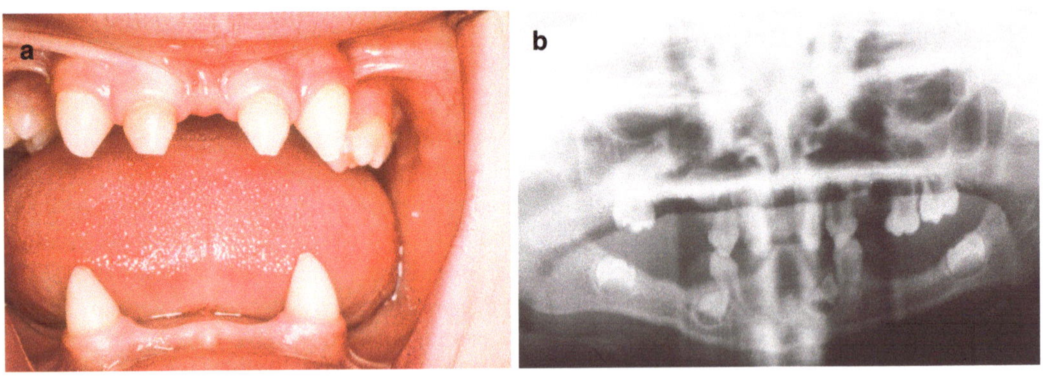

Fig. 7.105 (**a**) Oligodontia in a patient suffering from ectodermal dysplasia. (**b**) The panoramic view confirms the lack of many teeth in the mandible and maxilla

7.15.8 Paget's Disease

Some Characteristics

Idiopathic disorder of bone characterized by abnormal deposition and resorption of bone. May be monostotic or polyostotic. The affected bones become thickened and enlarged. The maxilla is more often involved than the mandible. There may be hypercementosis of the teeth (Fig. 7.109).

The serum value of alkaline phosphatase is increased, while the levels of calcium and phosphor may be normal. A biopsy will show increased osteoblastic and osteoclastic activity resulting in a mosaic pattern (Fig. 7.110). Treatment may consist of administration of bisphosphonates. In a few percent of patients, an osteosarcoma may arise, but rarely do so in the jaws.

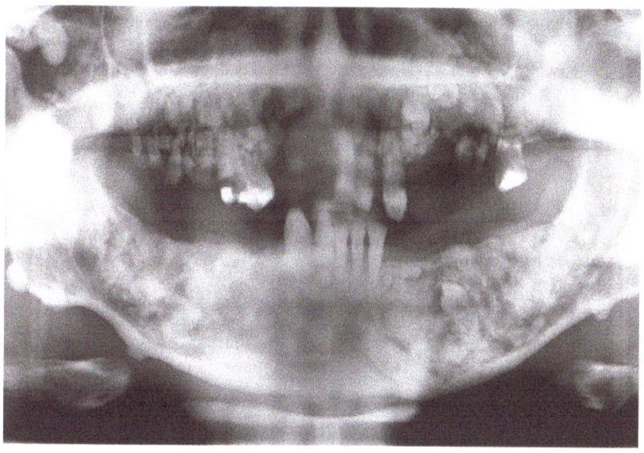

Fig. 7.106 Multiple osteomas and multiple retained teeth in a patient suffering from Gardner's syndrome

7.15.9 Pseudohypoparathyroidism

Some Characteristics

Disorder in the biochemical chain of the parathyroid hormone.

Apart from osteomas of the skin, osteomas of the oral mucosa may occur (Fig. 7.111a, b). Oligodontia, delayed eruption, enamel

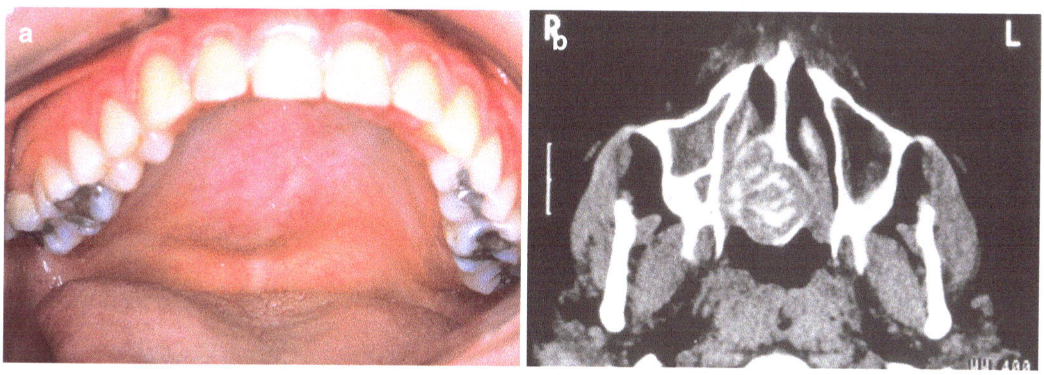

Fig. 7.107 (**a**) Palatal swelling in a 14-year-old girl suffering from hyperparathyroidism. (**b**) CT scan shows the extent of the giant cell containing lesion ("brown tumor")

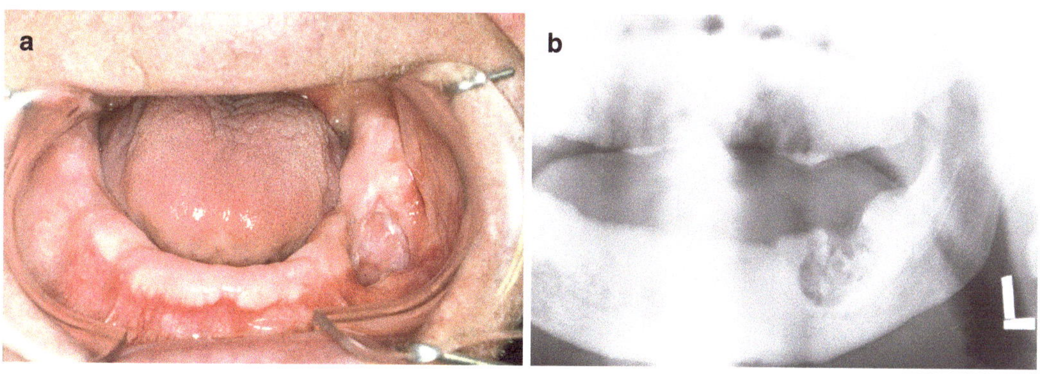

Fig. 7.108 (**a**) Broadening of the mandible due to osteopetrosis; notice defect in the region of 36. (**b**) Secondary osteomyelitis in a patient suffering from osteopetrosis; notice sclerotic bone of the maxilla and the mandible

hypoplasia, and widened pulp chambers are common features in these patients. Treatment consists of administration of calcium and vitamin D.

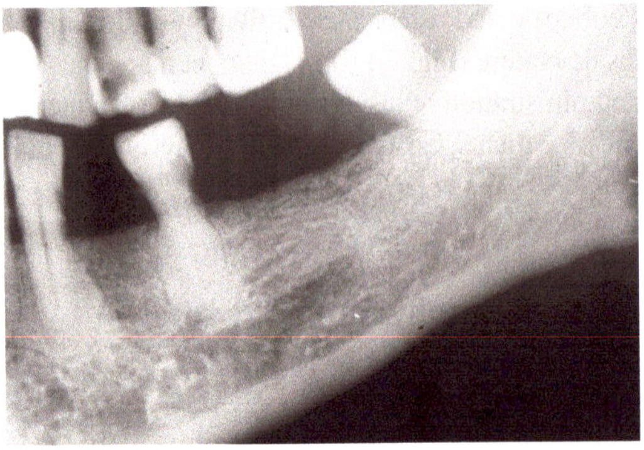

Fig. 7.109 Hypercementosis in a patient suffering from Paget's disease

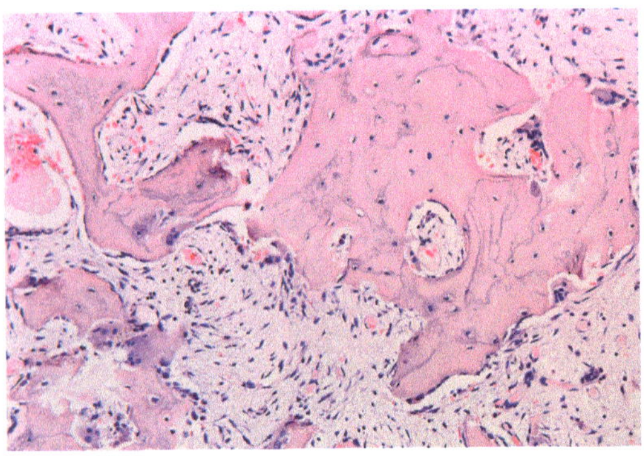

Fig. 7.110 Low-power view of osseous changes ("mosaic pattern") in Paget's disease

7.15.10 Pycnodysostosis

Some Characteristics

Rare autosomal recessive form of osteosclerosis in which there is a malfunction of the osteoclasts. Pyknodysostosis is a form of short-limbed dwarfism. The eruption of teeth may be delayed. Simple tooth extraction may lead to a jaw fracture. The radiographs show a generalized increase in bone density (Fig. 7.112). The mandibular angles are flattened. There is no treatment available.

7.15.11 Thalassemia

Some Characteristics

Inherited disorder of hemoglobin synthesis initially mainly reported from Mediterranean

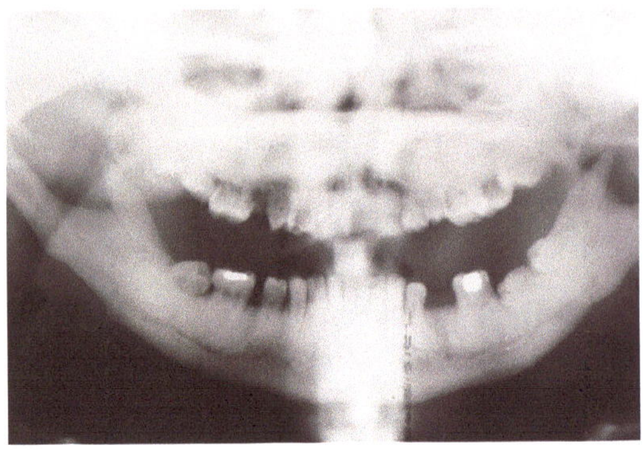

Fig. 7.112 Characteristic aspects of the radiograph in a patient suffering from pycnodysostosis

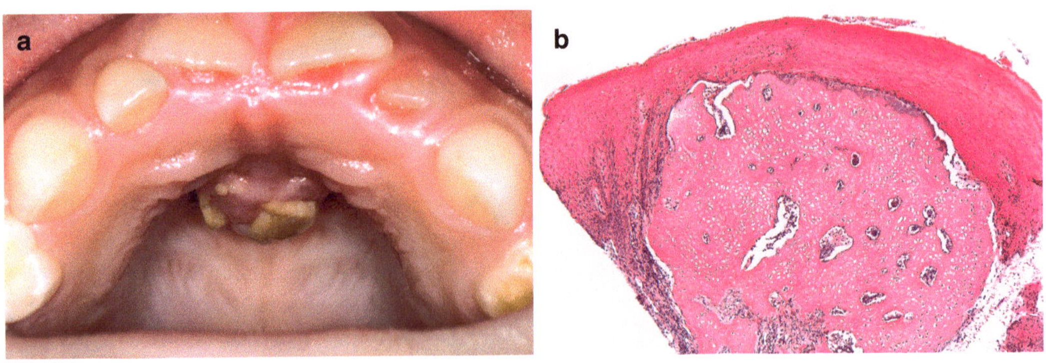

Fig. 7.111 (a) Osteoma in the palatal mucosa in a patient suffering from pseudohypoparathyroidism. (b) Low-power view of palatal osteoma in pseudohypoparathyroidism

populations. There are several subtypes. The resulting bone marrow hyperplasia may affect the jaws, resulting in enlargement of the mandible and maxilla; also frontal bossing may occur (Fig. 7.113a–c). Radiographically, a delicate trabecular pattern is a rather characteristic feature. There is no treatment available.

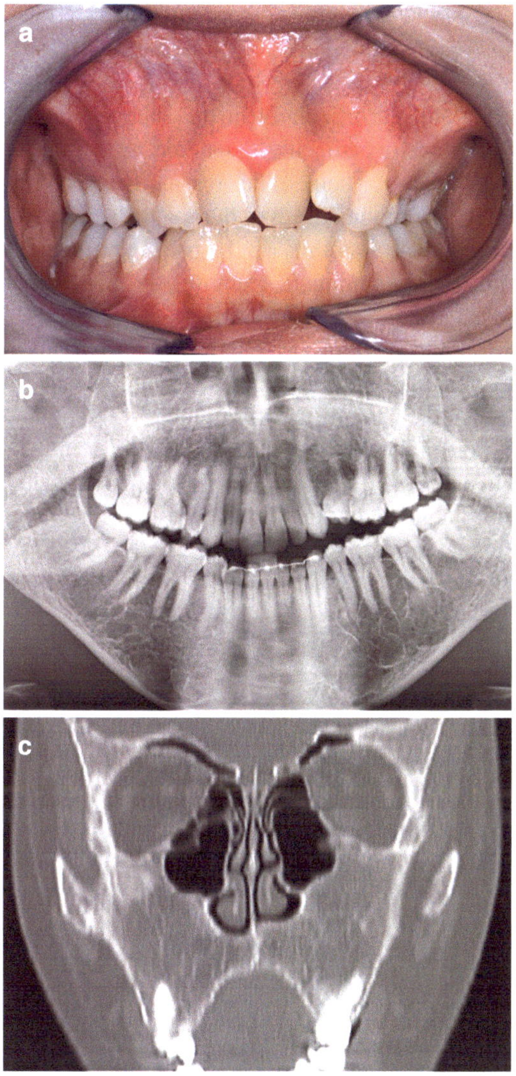

Fig. 7.113 (**a**) Some broadening of the jaw bones in a patient suffering from thalassemia. (**b**) Panoramic view; notice the delicate trabecular pattern in the mandible. (**c**) The CT scan shows almost complete replacement of the maxillary sinuses as a result of compensatory bone marrow formation

7.16 Overprojection of Opaque Structures in the Jaw Bones or the Oral and Perioral Soft Tissues

7.16.1 Calcifications of the Carotid Artery

In elderly people calcifications of the carotid artery in the neck, often bilaterally, are rather common incidental findings on a routine panoramic view (Fig. 7.114). There is an ongoing debate as whether such calcifications need further attention and possibly surgical removal or should be left alone with or without the prescription of antithrombotics. Anyhow, the observation of the calcification should be communicated with the patient, and the further management policy should be discussed.

7.16.2 Other Opacities Projected on a Radiograph

In a venous malformation, thrombi may become calcified already at an early age resulting in so-called phleboliths. These phleboliths are painless and do not need to be removed (Fig. 7.115).

Occasionally, calcified lymph nodes in the neck are seen on a radiograph; at times, it may be difficult to know whether the calcifications are located in lymph nodes, indeed. Occasionally, the medical history reveals a previously treated tuberculosis (Fig. 7.116).

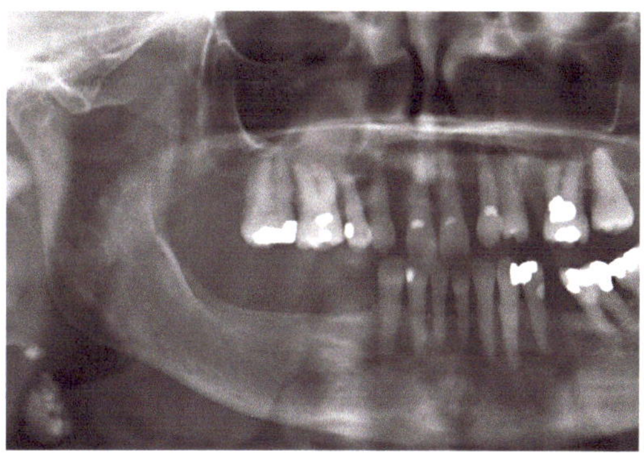

Fig. 7.114 Calcification of the carotid as an incidental finding on a panoramic view

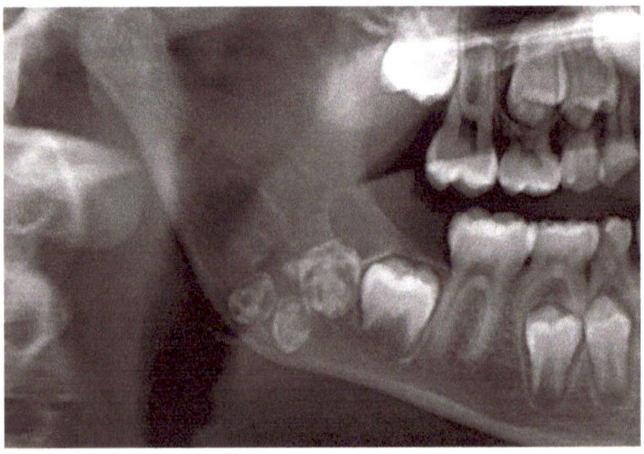

Fig. 7.115 Phleboliths in a vascular malformation projected on the angle of the mandible

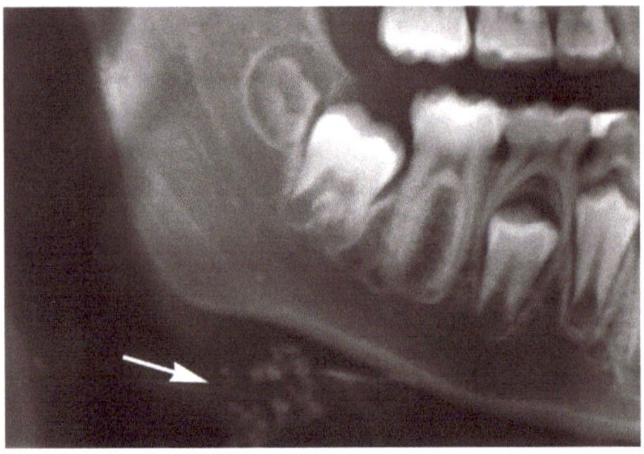

Fig. 7.116 Calcifications in the right submandibular region due to tuberculous involvement of the lymph nodes

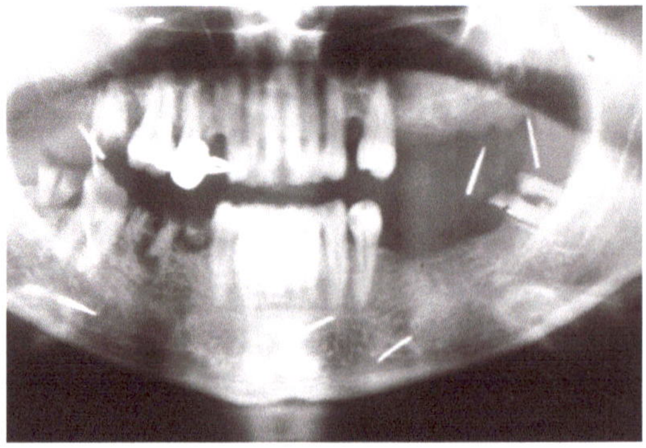

Fig. 7.117 "Charm needles" inserted in the perioral soft tissues being partly projected on the mandible

Sialoliths, particularly in the submandibular region, are occasionally diagnosed on a radiograph taken for some other reason, being completely asymptomatic, even during mails. If large enough, such sialoliths can be palpated bimanually. If asymptomatic, removal is not truly indicated.

Calcifications in the skin, such as in pilomatrixoma, may be projected on a dental film.

In some parts of the world, there is the tradition of implanting gold or platina needles in the skin of the shoulders or the cheeks, being thought to promote health and beauty; these needles are often referred to as "charm needles" (Fig. 7.117).

Index

I. van der Waal, *Atlas of Oral Diseases: A Guide for Daily Practice*,
DOI 10.1007/978-3-662-48122-6

MIX
Papier aus verantwortungsvollen Quellen
Paper from responsible sources
FSC® C105338

If you have any concerns about our products,
you can contact us on
ProductSafety@springernature.com

In case Publisher is established outside the EU,
the EU authorized representative is:
Springer Nature Customer Service Center GmbH
Europaplatz 3, 69115 Heidelberg, Germany

Printed by Libri Plureos GmbH
in Hamburg, Germany